STRESS AND PERFORMANCE IN SPORT

Wiley Series
Human Performance and Cognition

Acquisition and Performance of Cognitive Skills
*Edited by Ann M. Colley
and John R. Beech*

Stress and Performance in Sport
Edited by J. Graham Jones and Lew Hardy

Further titles in preparation

STRESS AND PERFORMANCE IN SPORT

Edited by

J. Graham Jones
Loughborough University

AND

Lew Hardy
University of Wales, Bangor

JOHN WILEY & SONS

Chichester · New York · Brisbane · Toronto · Singapore

Copyright ©1990 by John Wiley & Sons Ltd.
            Baffins Lane, Chichester
            West Sussex PO19 1UD, England

Other Wiley Editorial Offices
John Wiley & Sons, Inc., 605 Third Avenue, New York, NY 10158–0012, USA
Jacaranda Wiley Ltd, G.P.O. Box 859, Brisbane, Queensland 4001, Australia
John Wiley & Sons (Canada) Ltd, 22 Worcester Road, Rexdale, Ontario M9W 1L1, Canada
John Wiley & Sons (SEA) Pte Ltd, 37 Jalan Pemimpin 05–04, Block B, Union Industrial
Building, Singapore 2057

Library of Congress Cataloging-in-Publication Data:
Stress and performance in sport   /   edited by J. Graham Jones and Lew
   Hardy.
        p.   cm.—(Wiley series in human performance and cognition)
   Includes bibliographical references.
   ISBN 0471–920843
   1. Sports—Psychological aspects.   2. Stress management.
   3. Performance.   4. Stress (Psychology)   5. Stress (Physiology)
   I. Series.
   GV706. 4. S745   1990
   796′. 01—dc20   90–34579
                                                              CIP

British Library Cataloguing in Publication Data:
Stress and performance in sport.—(Human performance and
   cognition).
   1. Sportsmen. Stress
   I. Jones, J. Graham   II. Hardy, Lew   III. Series
   796.01

ISBN 0 471 92084 3

Typeset by Associated Publishing Services, Salisbury, Wiltshire
Printed and bound in Great Britain by Biddles Ltd., Guildford, Surrey.

Contents

3.   STRESS IN SPORT: FUTURE RESEARCH DIRECTIONS

Series Preface

Books in the original Series on Human Performance were designed to provide clear explanations of the main issues affecting human performance, based on a broad range of experimental research. The earlier volumes dealt with such topics as the analysis of human skills, the effects of sleep and biological rhythms, the sustainment of attention during vigilance performance, the effects of noise on human efficiency, the changes resulting from aging, and the consequences of sex differences in human performance. In each of these volumes it became evident that it was necessary to take account of the cognitive processes that underlie the overt expression of human performance variables. It was clearly desirable to devote more attention to those cognitive processes, and to the relevant research findings. These considerations were evidenced in the publication of the most recent volume, on the acquisition and performance of cognitive skills, which began the Series in Human Performance and Cognition.

The extended series now has a broader scope. One advantage of the change in title is to give explicit recognition to what was hitherto implicit, acknowledging that human performance is governed by cognitive processes. However, the change in title is not merely an improvement in nomenclature. Rather, it provides an opportunity to offer books dealing with a much wider range of topics, ranging from cognitive science to cognitive ergonomics. It is intended for the new series to include volumes concerning issues such as human–computer interaction, risk-taking and error, and cognitive skills under stress. At the same time the series will preserve the distinguishing features, such as clarity of exposition, that account for its present measure of success.

As before, many of the books in the series take the form of edited volumes. However, the end products of the editing process are not haphazard collections of papers, but systematically organized texts that utilize the advantages of multiple authorship. Although writing a monograph is often regarded as the more difficult assignment, producing an edited volume presents a considerable challenge. On one hand, it provides an opportunity to bring to bear on the subject matter a concentration of expertise that would otherwise be unavailable; on the other hand, the need for a multiplicity of contributors carries with it the risk that the overall result might lack coherence. In the present series, every effort has been made to counter the potential disadvantages of the edited format while preserving the positive advantages that stem from the opportunity to draw on specialized knowledge. The individual chapters have been commissioned in accordance with an integrated plan for each volume. Information about chapter content has been circulated among the contributors to ensure cohesiveness, and editorial control has been extended to the level of difficulty as well as to the format of each text. The books have thus been designed to combine readability with high standards of scholarship.

The present volume continues this tradition. It succeeds in satisfying two related objectives in the context of sport psychology and stress. First, it conveys an understanding of the ways in which anxiety, or excitement, affect performance in competitive sports, and describes the cognitive mechanisms underlying these effects. To this end, the book goes well beyond the traditional explanations based on arousal theory, acknowledging that more complex explanations are required and providing coverage for modern contributions such as catastrophe theory and reversal theory. The second objective that the book accomplishes is to evaluate methods for dealing with the stresses surrounding sports performance. It considers the effects of goal setting on achievement and the effectiveness of combined, multimodal techniques for managing stress effects. It evaluates the methods of cognitive behavioral therapy in the context of sports anxiety, and deals with the sometimes odd but effective routines that athletes tend to develop in preparation for perform-ance. Finally, interviews with selected medallists help to confirm the basic soundness of the concepts selected to explain performance under stress.

One of the strengths of the volume is that it draws on a great deal of research based directly on activities such as javelin throwing, hockey and basketball. However, although the book should be prescribed reading for all sport psychologists, it makes a sufficient theoretical contribution to interest a much wider audience. The effects of anxiety on performance are also felt by musicians, by actors and by politicians. In fact, there have also been studies of anxiety in connection with writing skills, military skills, interpersonal skills, test-taking skills, and laboratory motor skills. It seems reasonable to claim that the present book has something to offer to persons concerned with all of these topics, since many of its conclusions have broad generality. Despite the breadth of the contribution, the editors have maintained a high level of expository skill throughout the volume. Hence, the book is a valuable addition to the Series in Human Performance and Cognition, extending the tradition created by its predecessors.

Dennis Holding
University of Louisville

Preface

This book is directed at sport psychologists, psychologists with a particular interest in (sport) performance, researchers in human performance and students of sport psychology. The fact that a whole text is devoted to such a specific and specialized topic as 'stress in sport' reflects the amount of research interest in this area in recent years. However, this book does not owe its existence to an urge to review the large amount of literature in the area so much as to signal the editors' concerns over the relatively slow theoretical advancement pertaining to the stress–performance relationship in sport. Consequently, a major part of the book, Section 1, is devoted to a direct examination of the competitive stress–performance relationship. The section is entitled 'Stress in Sport: Conceptual Considerations and Effects on Performance' and comprises five chapters. Chapter 1, by Jones and Hardy, identifies three general areas which have attracted research interest and presents a brief overview of major research directions in those areas. Chapter 2, by Jones, argues that the inverted-U hypothesis is an outdated and inappropriate description of the stress–performance relationship and goes on to discuss more recent and detailed models which have been developed in experimental psychology and which have potential for application in sport psychology. The separation of the anxiety response into cognitive and somatic components forms the basis of Chapter 3, by Parfitt, Jones and Hardy. This chapter focuses on the differential effects of the multidimensional anxiety components on global, as well as subcomponents of, sports performance. Hardy's application of catastrophe theory to anxiety in sport is described in Chapter 4, together with a discussion of some supporting evidence. Finally, Chapter 5, by Kerr, discusses the application of reversal theory to stress in sport.

The second section again comprises five chapters and is entitled 'Stress Management and Self-regulation in Sport.' The first chapter, by Beggs, focuses on goal setting, not only as a method of enhancing motivation and self-confidence, but also as a technique which may be used as a form of stress management. Chapter 7, by Burton, discusses a multidimensional approach to stress management which is based on the proposal that anxiety reduction techniques should be matched to the anxiety symptoms. Mace's chapter examines the possible mediating role of cognitions in sports performance and reviews research examining the effects of cognitive behavioural interventions in sport. This chapter also considers the planning of mental training programmes for coping with stress in sport. Chapter 9, by Boutcher, reviews research examining the use of performance routines in sport and considers several possible explanations for their success, including attentional control, warm-up decrement and automatic functioning. The final chapter in this section is by Jones and Hardy and is based on a series of structured interviews with elite performers. The aim of this chapter is to examine the practical application of the theoretical issues discussed in the previous chapters.

The final section, 'Stress in Sport: Future Research Directions', comprises only one chapter, by Hardy and Jones, which attempts to draw together the major findings of the previous chapters in the form of a series of consensus statements and questions for future research.

In summary, this book represents an attempt to integrate the work of several authors towards an understanding of stress in sport. As editors, we were concerned that most edited volumes are characterized by a series of discrete contributions which do not always tie together very well. Consequently, each author was requested to relate their material as much as possible to other topics and approaches represented in the book. We thank the authors for their efforts to help achieve this aim and trust that it has led to an integrated and cohesive perspective on stress in sport. We would also like to thank the performers, Steve Backley, Sue Challis, Alan Edge, David Hemery, James May and Mary Nevill, who so willingly gave up their time for our interviews, without which the book really would have been incomplete. The insight which we gained from these interviews was far greater than could ever be expressed in a single chapter of a book. As always, it seems that our theoretical understanding may lag some way behind the practice of really skilled performers.

Finally, we would like to express our warmest appreciation to our families and loved ones for their help, support and patience during the preparation of this book. Unfortunately, we no longer have an excuse for being grumpy.

Graham Jones
Lew Hardy

List of Contributers

W. D. Alan Beggs

Blind Mobility Research Unit, Department of Psychology, Nottingham University, Nottingham, NG7 2RD, UK

Stephen H. Boutcher

Department of Health and Physical Education, 205 Memorial Gymnasium, University of Virginia, Charlottesville, Virginia 22903, USA

Damon Burton

107 Physical Education Building, Division of Health, Physical Education, Recreation and Dance, University of Idaho, Moscow, Idaho 83843, USA

Lew Hardy

Sport, Health and Physical Education, University of Wales, Bangor, Gwynedd, LL57 2DG, UK

J. Graham Jones

Department of Physical Education and Sports Science, Loughborough University, Loughborough, Leicestershire, LE11 3TU, UK

John H. Kerr

Department of Physical Education, Nijenrode, Netherlands School of Business, Straatweg 25, 3621 BG Breukelen, The Netherlands

Roger Mace

Newman College, Genners Lane, Bartley Green, Birmingham, B32 3NT, UK

C. Gaynor Parfitt

Sport, Health and Physical Education, University of Wales, Bangor, Gwynedd, LL57 2DG, UK

Chapter 1

The academic study of stress in sport

J. Graham Jones and Lew Hardy

Loughborough University and University of Wales, Bangor

I was practically paralytic with fear—John too—although somehow we were able to crack bad jokes in our attempt to relieve the tension, wishing we were anywhere but there at the time. John Cooper and Denis sat at the end of the beds smoking furiously, and looking, perhaps, even more overwrought than Sherwood and myself. My fingers and feet were damp and freezing cold. I felt weak, my breath was short and I felt a slight constriction in my throat. The back of my neck ached a bit and my prevailing thoughts were of impending unpleasantness. Sherwood and I just wanted to get the whole thing over and done with. The waiting was agony but my mind, conditioned through long training and experience, warned 'wait to warm up! Wait! Wait'. . . . (Hemery, 1976, pp. 1–2)

These were the thoughts of David Hemery, one of Britain's greatest ever athletes, waiting for the start of his Olympic gold medal winning 400 metre hurdles race in 1968.

The study of stress in sport lies within the realms of the relatively new academic discipline of sport psychology. The recent growth in the popularity of sport psychology, particularly in Western Europe, has reflected the realization that sports performance is not simply the product of physiological (e.g. strength, fitness) and biomechanical (e.g. technique) factors, but that psychological factors also play a crucial role in determining performance. Indeed, in a study of the factors influencing the Olympic performances of 235 Canadian Olympians, Orlick and Partington (1988) concluded that:

Stress and Performance in Sport. Edited by J. Graham Jones and Lew Hardy.
©1990 John Wiley & Sons Ltd.

Of the three major readiness factors rated by the athletes—mental, physical, technical—mental readiness provided the only statistically significant link with final Olympic ranking. (p. 129)

Orlick and Partington also suggested that a large proportion of the athletes failed to perform to potential because they were unable to maintain their concentration in the face of distractions. This is clearly not just a problem for Olympic athletes; it is a problem for all serious sports performers, no matter what their ability level. Consider, for example, golf, a sport which the legendary Arnold Palmer has suggested is at least 90 per cent psychological (Hemery, 1986, p. 104). Patmore (1986) calculated that in a professional tournament a golfer takes at least 16 hours to complete the 72 holes. However, Patmore also calculated that the total time spent by the golfer actually swinging and striking the ball during those 72 holes is approximately seven minutes and 30 seconds, leaving 15 hours, 52 minutes and 30 seconds (99.2 per cent) of 'thinking time'. Clearly, this is ample time for even the most skilled performers to distract themselves.

One of the major concerns of many sports performers striving for peak performance is to reach a psychological state which will facilitate that level of performance. There are, of course, many factors which can influence the performer's psychological state and so alter it from the optimum required for a particular type of performance; these forces will be referred to as 'stressors' (Jones and Hardy, 1989). Sport, by its very nature, is highly visible and competitive, and the rewards for success are often great. The sport environment provides, therefore, many of the ingredients which invariably create stress in those who participate (Cratty, 1984; King, Stanley and Burrows, 1987). Returning briefly to the example of golf, Jack Nicklaus once said of putting, '. . . it doesn't take much technique to roll a 1.68 inch ball along a smooth, level surface into, or in the immediate vicinity of, a 4.5 inch hole. With no pressure on you, you can do it one-handed most of the time. But there is always pressure on the shorter putts'. Nicklaus further stated that '. . . 90 per cent of the rounds I play in major championships, I play with a bit of a shake' (quoted in Patmore, 1986, p. 75). Another indication of the extent of stress in sport is provided by Gould, Horn and Spreeman (1983), who reported findings that elite wrestlers between the ages of 15 and 19 were anxious or worried in 66 per cent of their matches.

Situational stressors like competition may be thought of as imposing a mental load or cognitive demand on the individual which has to be met in order to produce effective performance (Fisher, 1984). Of course, many sports performers would argue that meeting these cognitive demands is the very essence of competitive sport. Indeed, Patmore (1986) has described sport at the highest levels as an 'experiment' in which the central factor determining the quality of performance is the individual's ability to cope with stress:

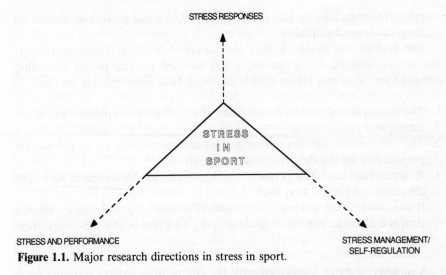

Figure 1.1. Major research directions in stress in sport.

The technical skills of the contestants, if the experiment has been set up correctly, cancel each other out. The sport experiment is not concerned with the particular technical skills the subject has brought with him to the contest. His [technical] skill is not really at issue—although he fervently believes it is—since his fellow contestants also have it; they have been screened and selected very carefully indeed to ensure that their [technical] skill compares with his. The deciding factor is not his [technical] skill, but his ability to perform it under stress. (Patmore, 1986, p. 13)

MAJOR RESEARCH DIRECTIONS IN STRESS IN SPORT

Stress in sport has proved a popular and widely studied research area in sport psychology. This research may be categorized into three broad areas, as depicted in Figure 1.1. The following sections provide a brief overview of issues addressed within these three areas.

Stress responses

Recent research in this area has been characterized by the adoption of a cognitive-based interactional model in which stress occurs as a result of cognitive appraisals that one's coping resources will be taxed or even inadequate to meet the demands imposed by a particular situation. This move away from the traditional behavioural-based analysis of stress in sport psychology has meant that competition is no longer regarded as a uniformly stressful event;

competitive stress may be interpreted negatively by one performer, but as an exciting challenge by another.

The majority of research into the competitive stress response (almost universally referred to as 'anxiety') has focused on the period preceding competition. Silva and Hardy (1984) identified four main reasons for this:

1. The assumption that the athlete's mental set prior to competition can affect subsequent performance;
2. The assumption that the athlete has some control over his or her mental preparation during the pre-competition period;
3. At a practical level, this period is much more accessible to researchers than the period of competition itself;
4. If pre-competition anxiety is a (negative) source of performance variance then the clinician can assist in developing an appropriate pre-competition state.

A number of issues concerned with the competitive anxiety response have been addressed in this research area, including the concept of anxiety, measurement, antecedents, temporal patterning and individual differences. These issues are discussed in detail in later chapters and are referred to only briefly here.

The concept of anxiety

Recent research has addressed the issue of multidimensionality in competitive anxiety from two perspectives. First, the notion of traits and states is now widely accepted, a fact that is reflected in the wide use of state–trait anxiety inventories in sport psychology research (see Spielberger, 1989). Secondly, competitive state anxiety is now viewed as a multidimensional construct which can be separated into at least two components, popularly known as cognitive and somatic anxiety (Gould, Petlichkoff and Weinberg, 1984; Jones and Hardy, 1989; Martens et al., 1990). Cognitive anxiety is characterized by negative expectations, lack of concentration and images of failure, while somatic anxiety refers to the perception of physiological symptoms such as sweaty hands or tension. These conceptual advancements have considerable potential for aiding the development of our understanding of the anxiety–performance relationship.

Measurement

State anxiety can broadly be measured via three types of indicator: cognitive, physiological and behavioural. The measurement of anxiety at the cognitive level has mainly relied upon self-report questionnaires. Several sport-specific questionnaires have been developed for the purpose of measuring sport-

1

STRESS IN SPORT: CONCEPTUAL CONSIDERATIONS AND EFFECTS UPON PERFORMANCE

---

specific trait anxiety (Sport Competition Anxiety Test; Martens, 1977), state anxiety (Competitive State Anxiety Inventory; Martens *et al.*, 1980) and, more recently, multidimensional competitive state anxiety (Competitive State Anxiety Inventory-2; Martens *et al.*, 1990). Hackfort and Schwenkmezger (1989) classified physiological indicators of anxiety into:

1. Respiratory and cardiovascular indicators, such as pulse rate, blood pressure and respiration rate;
2. Biochemical indicators, including adrenaline and noradrenaline;
3. Electrophysiological indicators, such as EEG and skin resistance.

Behavioural indicators of anxiety present obvious problems in sport-related research as it is extremely difficult to distinguish between anxious behaviour and coping behaviour. Consequently, Hackfort and Schwenkmezger (1989) have stated that '. . . observation methods become useful only in conjunction with procedural data, and observational data only in conjunction with self statements' (p. 62).

The notion of a multilevel approach to the measurement of anxiety is attractive and has led to what could be termed 'sport psychophysiology' (e.g. Landers *et al.* 1980; Stern, 1976). The major problem with this approach is the low covariation reported in the majority of empirical research between psychological and physiological indices. Nevertheless, the approach does provide a more detailed perspective on anxiety and other affective responses.

Antecedents

The search for effective methods of achieving optimal performance states means that the identification of precursors of anxiety is likely to prove valuable. However, to date, relatively little systematic and structured research has been carried out which examines the antecedents of competitive state anxiety. Of this scant amount, the majority has focused upon identification of the antecedents of the different anxiety components (e.g. Gould, Petlichkoff and Weinberg, 1984; Jones, Swain and Cale, in press; McAuley, 1985).

Temporal patterning

The temporal patterning of anxiety in the period leading up to and during competition has attracted notable research interest. Early researchers (e.g. Fenz and Epstein, 1967; Highlen and Bennett, 1979; Mahoney and Avener, 1977) examined the potential of the temporal patterning of competitive anxiety as a means of distinguishing between successful and less successful athletes. Utilizing the multidimensional approach, later investigators have examined the pre-competitive temporal patterning of anxiety components in a variety of sports (e.g. Gould, Petlichkoff and Weinberg, 1984; Gould *et al.*, 1987; Jones and Cale, 1989a, Martens *et al*, 1990; Parfitt and Hardy, 1987; Ussher and Hardy, 1986).

Individual differences

Another area which has stimulated research interest is the role of individual differences in the stress response. The most popular individual difference variables which have so far been investigated include competitive trait anxiety (e.g. Martens, 1977; Martens and Gill, 1976), sex (e.g. Jones and Cale, 1989a; Jones, Swain and Cale, in press; Martens *et al*, 1990), gender role (e.g. Wark and Wittig, 1979; Wittig, 1984), skill level (e.g. Martens *et al.*, 1990) and type of sport (e.g. Krane and Williams, 1987; Martens *et al.* 1990).

Stress and performance

Precise identification of the relationship between stress and performance has proved elusive. This elusiveness has been at least partly due to a general lack of precision in defining and distinguishing between key concepts such as arousal and anxiety. There has been relatively little in the way of theory development pertaining to the relationship between stress and performance within sport psychology. Many researchers have debated the relative merits of drive theory (Hull, 1943; Spence and Spence, 1966) and the inverted-U hypothesis, both of which depend upon the assumption that the stress–performance relationship can be explained as a function of changes in a very general arousal system (e.g. Martens *et al.*, 1980; Oxendine, 1970; Sonstroem and Bernardo, 1982). In particular, a considerable amount of research effort has been expended on the investigation of the inverted-U hypothesis (e.g. Klavora, 1978; Martens and Landers, 1970). The findings from this research have been equivocal but, more importantly, a situation has been created in which terms such as stress, arousal and anxiety have been used interchangeably in many cases.

Multidimensional anxiety and performance

Recent empirical work has adopted more precise definitions and terminology, and has attempted to directly examine the relationship between anxiety and performance. This approach is based on the assumption that anxiety is multidimensional and has examined the effects on performance of specific components of the anxiety response (e.g. Burton, 1988; Gould, Petlichkoff and Weinberg, 1984; Gould *et al.*, 1987; Jones and Cale, 1989b; Parfitt and Hardy, 1987). The findings from this research have been used as the basis for an interesting theoretical conceptualization of the stress–performance relationship: catastrophe theory (Hardy and Fazey, 1987). This represents a behavioural application of Thom's (1975) mathematical theory of catastrophes (see Chapter 4 in this book) and is currently stimulating research interest in both Britain and the United States.

Reversal theory

Although not principally concerned with performance, Kerr's (1987, 1989) application of reversal theory (Apter, 1982) to sport is another interesting approach which has attracted research activity (e.g. Kerr and Cox, 1988; see Chapter 5 in this book).

Subcomponents of performance

Finally, a further development in this area relates to the performance measure under investigation. Some studies have examined global sports performance such as swimming (Burton, 1988), wrestling (Gould, Petlichkoff and Weinberg, 1984) and pistol shooting (Gould et al, 1987) as the dependent variable. However, more recent work has examined performance in terms of those subcomponents which are thought to be important in sports performance: for example, reaction time (Jones, Cale and Kerwin, 1988; Parfitt, 1988), working memory and perceptual speed (Idzikowski and Baddeley, 1987; Jones and Cale, 1989b; Parfitt, 1988; Parfitt and Hardy, 1987). What is becoming increasingly clear from this type of research is that competitive stress does not necessarily impair performance and can, in some circumstances, enhance it.

Stress management and self-regulation

If stress is such an important factor in sports performance (Patmore, 1986), then the ability to cope with it is clearly crucial. However, it is important to recognize that according to the interactional approach stress does not always have negative connotations. Rather, the stress of competition may cause (negative) anxiety in one performer but (positive) excitement in another. Furthermore, of those who do experience anxiety, some may use it to facilitate performance, while others may find that it debilitates their performance. The implication, therefore, is that stress management techniques should be individually tailored to cater for these individual differences.

There are several forms of stress management. In recent years, self-regulation training has become recognized as an important aspect of coping with stress and enhancing the likelihood of peak performance (Hardy and Nelson, 1988). As mentioned earlier in the discussion, there are many stressors in the competitive environment which may prevent peak performance (Czikszentmihalyi, 1975; Privette and Landsman, 1983). However, Hardy (1989) has identified a growing body of knowledge which suggests that '. . . at least four metacognitive skills can be identified which the experimental literature suggests are important determinants of peak performance. These are goal setting, imagery, anxiety and activation control, and attention control skills' (p. 224). This appears to be consistent with Mahoney and associates' finding that elite performers are characterized by greater motivation and self-confidence, more highly developed attention control strategies and lower levels of anxiety than lesser performers (Mahoney and Avener, 1977; Mahoney, Gabriel and Perkins, 1987).

Goal setting

Goal setting is viewed as an important technique for the enhancement of both motivation (Deci and Ryan, 1985; Latham and Locke, 1975; Roberts, 1986) and self-confidence in sport (Bandura, 1977; Locke et al., 1984). Based largely on empirical findings from organizational psychology, Locke and Latham (1985) have made a number of proposals concerning goal setting in sport, including: specific, challenging goals lead to better performance than moderate or easy goals; short-term goals or subgoals are important in the attainment of long-term goals; feedback is crucial to the goal setting process; the acceptance of goals is important if goal setting is to be effective; and, competition may improve performance through the setting of higher goals. A small number of studies have also begun to address the potentially very interesting relationship between goal setting and competitive anxiety. Hardy, Maiden and Sherry (1986), for example, found that goal acceptance was lowered under conditions of high competitive anxiety. Examining the relationship from another perspective, Cale and Jones (1989) reported that levels of cognitive anxiety and self-confidence were also a function of goal difficulty level. Furthermore, Jones, Swain and Cale (1990) have reported that cognitive anxiety in a sample of elite intercollegiate middle-distance runners was predicted by goal difficulty level and the runners' perceptions of whether or not they could achieve their goals. The relationship between goal setting and anxiety appears, therefore, to be a fruitful and important area for future research.

Imagery

Imagery has been shown to be a powerful skill in both learning and performing physical skills. More specifically, imagery can be used to enhance learning (Feltz and Landers, 1983), reduce warm-up decrement (Ainscoe and Hardy, 1987; Hardy and Wyatt, 1986), to reduce anxiety (Suinn, 1983) and to increase self-confidence (Bandura, 1977). However, Hardy and Nelson (1988) concluded that despite considerable evidence in favour of imagery as a valuable skill in sport, the precise mechanisms by which it exerts its influence are still poorly understood.

Anxiety and activation control

The most popular and widely researched method of anxiety control in sport is through relaxation. A large number of different relaxation strategies exist, but it is possible to broadly categorize them into somatic (e.g. progressive muscular relaxation) and cognitive (e.g. meditation) relaxation strategies (Davidson and Schwartz, 1976). This distinction is important following the adoption within sport psychology of a multidimensional conceptualization of the competitive anxiety response. Furthermore, the general consensus of the available literature is that anxiety reduction may be more effective when relaxation strategies are matched to the precise modes of the anxiety response (Davidson, 1978; Lehrer *et al.*, 1980; Schwartz, Davidson and Goleman, 1978).

As Hardy and Nelson (1988) have pointed out, techniques for controlling activation are less fully researched. Studies which have examined whether performance can be enhanced by increasing general activation levels, or 'psyching up', seem to indicate that 'psyching up' enhances performance in sports which require gross strength, speed or power, but inhibits performance in skills which require fine control.

Attention control

Empirical studies of attention control skills in sport psychology are few. This is perhaps surprising considering the evidence which suggests that cognitive anxiety can impair performance by disrupting attention (Wine, 1971, 1980) and causing warm-up decrement (Jones and Hardy, 1988). Hardy (1989) has suggested the following areas as worthy of research effort: the identification of attentional processes (e.g. perceptual attention, working memory) required for different sports; the identification of process availability and disruption under high-performance anxiety; and the development of techniques to enhance attention control. One strategy that has been proposed as a means of enhancing concentration is the systematic routinization of actions and thoughts prior to performance (Boutcher and Rotella, 1987), and this use of performance routines is examined in some detail in Chapter 9 in this book.

In conclusion, Hardy and Nelson (1988) have identified two distinct forms of self-regulation training for the skills outlined above: 'one-to-one' teaching by clinicians and sport psychologists; and programmed learning using mental training packages which are currently available in the form of books (e.g. Syer and Connolly, 1984; Weinberg, 1988) or cassette tapes and workbook packages (e.g. Unestahl, 1983; Gauron, 1984; Hardy and Fazey, 1990). Athough relatively little empirical work has been published which systematically evaluates these approaches, that which has been performed is generally supportive of their use (Seabourne *et al.*, 1985; Straub, 1986).

SUMMARY AND OUTLINE OF THE BOOK

It is evident from the preceding discussion that stress in sport has developed into a popular and specialized area for academic enquiry. A significant factor in this development is that the sport environment provides a natural laboratory in which to study behaviour in general, and stress-related behaviour in particular. The issues which have been identified in this chapter have already attracted considerable research attention and seem likely to continue to do so for some time in the foreseeable future.

These issues will be addressed in more detail in the remaining chapters in this section and the two sections which follow. The remainder of this section comprises four chapters, the first two of which examine the multidimensionality of the anxiety response, its nature, its antecedents and its effects upon performance. The other two chapters examine two recent developments in the anxiety–performance literature: catastrophe theory and reversal theory. Interestingly, although these two models come from rather different theoretical backgrounds, it will be seen that they could have more than a little in common.

The second section of the book is largely concerned with the management and self-regulation of stress. Many of the implications of the first section for intervention are discussed in five chapters which focus upon goal setting, stress management skills, cognitive behavioural interventions such as imagery and stress inoculation, and the use of performance routines to enhance concentration. This section concludes with a chapter which is based on a series of structured interviews conducted with elite performers. This chapter attempts to bring the experiences of these performers to bear on the issues which have been raised in the more theoretical preceding chapters.

The final section comprises one chapter which attempts to draw together the major findings of the previous chapters in a series of consensus statements and questions for future research.

REFERENCES

Ainscoe, M. W. and Hardy, L. (1987). Cognitive warm up in a cyclical gymnastics skill, *International Journal of Sport Psychology*, **18**, 269–275.
Apter, M. J. (1982). *The Experience of Motivation: The Theory of Psychological Reversals*. London: Academic Press.

Bandura, A. (1977). Self-efficacy: toward a unifying theory of behavioural change, *Psychological Review*, **84**, 191–215.

Boutcher, S. H. and Rotella, R. J. (1987). A psychological skills educational program for closed-skill performance enhancement, *The Sport Psychologist*, **1**, 127–137.

Burton, D. (1988). Do anxious swimmers swim slower? Reexamining the elusive anxiety–performance relationship, *Journal of Sport and Exercise Psychology*, **10**, 45–61.

Cale, A. and Jones, J. G. (1989). Relationships between expectations of success, multidimensional anxiety and perceptuo-motor performance. Paper presented at the Annual Conference of the North American Society for the Psychology of Sport and Physical Activity, Kent State University, Ohio, USA.

Cratty, B. J. (1984). *Psychological Preparation and Athletic Excellence*. Ithaca, New York: Mouvement Publications.

Czikszentmihalyi, M. (1975). Play and intrinsic rewards, *Journal of Humanistic Psychology*, **15**, 41–63.

Davidson, R. J. (1978). Specificity and patterning in biobehavioural systems: implications for behaviour change, *American Psychologist*, **33**, 430–436.

Davidson, R. J. and Schwartz, G. E. (1976). The psychobiology of relaxation and related states: a multiprocess theory, in D. Mostofsky (ed.). *Behavioural Control and Modification of Physiological Activity*. Englewood Cliffs, New Jersey: Prentice-Hall.

Deci, E. L. and Ryan, R. M. (1985). *Intrinsic Motivation and Self-Determination in Human Behaviour*. New York: Plenum Press.

Feltz, D. L. and Landers, D. M. (1983). The effects of mental practice on motor skill learning and performance: a meta-analysis, *Journal of Sport Psychology*, **5**, 25–57.

Fenz, W. D. and Epstein, S. (1967). Changes in gradients of skin conductance, heart rate and respiration rate as a function of experience, *Psychosomatic Medicine*, **29**, 33–51.

Fisher, S. (1984). *Stress and the Perception of Control*. Hillsdale, New Jersey: Lawrence Erlbaum.

Gauron, E. F. (1984). *Mental Training for Peak Performance*. Lansing, New Jersey: Sports Science International.

Gould, D., Horn, T. and Spreeman, J. (1983). Sources of stress in junior elite wrestlers, *Journal of Sport Psychology*, **5**, 159–171.

Gould, D., Petlichkoff, L. and Weinberg, R. S. (1984). Antecedents of, temporal changes in, and relationships between CSAI-2 subcomponents, *Journal of Sport Psychology*, **6**, 289–304.

Gould, D., Petlichkoff, L., Simons, J. and Vevera, M. (1987). Relationship between Competitive State Anxiety Inventory-2 subscale scores and pistol shooting performance, *Journal of Sport Psychology*, **9**, 33–42.

Hackfort, D. and Schwenkmezger, P. (1989). Measuring anxiety in sports: perspectives and problems, in D. Hackfort and C. D. Spielberger (eds). *Anxiety in Sports*. New York: Hemisphere.

Hardy, L. (1989). Sport psychology, in A. M. Colman and J. G. Beaumont (eds). *Psychology Survey 7*. London: British Psychological Society and Routledge.

Hardy, L. and Fazey, J. A. (1987). The inverted-U hypothesis—a catastrophe for sport psychology and a statement of a new hypothesis. Paper presented at the Annual Conference of the North American Society for the Psychology of Sport and Physical Activity, Vancouver, Canada, June.

Hardy, L. and Fazey, J. A. (1990). *Mental Training*. Leeds: National Coaching Foundation.

Hardy, L., Maiden, D. S. and Sherry, K. (1986). Goal setting and performance: the effects of performance anxiety, *Journal of Sports Sciences*, **4**, 233–234.

Hardy, L. and Nelson, D. (1988). Self-regulation training in sport and work, *Ergonomics*, **31**, 1573–1583.

Hardy, L. and Wyatt, S. (1986). Immediate effects of imagery upon skilful motor performance, in D. G. Russell and D. Marks (eds). *Imagery 2*. New Zealand: Human Performance Associates.

Hemery, D. (1976). *Another Hurdle*. London: Heinemann.

Hemery, D. (1986). *The Pursuit of Sporting Excellence*. London: Collins.

Highlen, P. S. and Bennett, B. B. (1979). Psychological characteristics of successful and nonsuccessful elite wrestlers, *Journal of Sport Psychology*, **1**, 123–137.

Hull, C. L. (1943). *Principles of Behavior*. New York: Appleton-Century.

Idzikowski, C. and Baddeley, A. (1987). Fear and performance in novice parachutists, *Ergonomics*, **30**, 1463–1474.

Jones, J. G. and Cale, A. (1989a). Precompetition temporal patterning of anxiety and self-confidence in males and females, *Journal of Sport Behavior*, **12**, 183–195.

Jones, J. G. and Cale, A. (1989b). Relationships between multidimensional competitive state anxiety and cognitive and motor subcomponents of performance, *Journal of Sports Sciences*, **7**, 229–240.

Jones, J. G., Cale, A. and Kerwin, D. G. (1988). Multidimensional competitive state anxiety and psychomotor performance, *Australian Journal of Science and Medicine in Sport*, **20**, 3–7.

Jones, J. G. and Hardy L. (1988). The effects of anxiety upon psychomotor performance, *Journal of Sports Sciences*, **6**, 59–67.

Jones, J. G. and Hardy, L. (1989). Stress and cognitive functioning in sport, *Journal of Sports Sciences*, **7**, 41–63.

Jones, J. G., Swain, A. and Cale, A. (1990). Antecedents of multidimensional competitive state anxiety and self-confidence in elite intercollegiate middle-distance runners, *The Sport Psychologist*, **4**, 107–118.

Jones, J. G., Swain, A. and Cale, A. (in press). Gender differences in precompetition temporal patterning and antecedents of anxiety and self-confidence. *Journal of Sport and Exercise Psychology*.

Kerr, J. H. (1987). Structural phenomenology, arousal and performance, *Journal of Human Movement Studies*, **13**, 211–229.

Kerr, J. H. (1989). Anxiety, arousal and sports performance: an application of Reversal Theory, in D. Hackfort and C. D. Spielberger (eds). *Anxiety in Sports*. New York: Hemisphere.

Kerr, J. H. and Cox, T. (1988). Effects of telic dominance and metamotivational state on squash task performance, *Perceptual and Motor Skills*, **67**, 171–174.

King, M., Stanley, G. and Burrows, G. (1987). *Stress: Theory and Practice*. London: Grune and Stratton.

Klavora, P. (1978). An attempt to derive inverted-U curves based on the relationship between anxiety and athletic performance, in D. M. Landers and R. W. Christina (eds). *Psychology of Motor Behaviour and Sport*. Champaign, Illinois: Human Kinetics.

Krane, V. and Williams, J. M. (1987). Performance and somatic anxiety, cognitive anxiety and confidence changes prior to competition, *Journal of Sport Behavior*, **10**, 47–56.

Landers, D. M., Christina, R., Hatfield, B. D., Daniels, F. S. and Doyle, L. A. (1980). Moving competitive shooting into the scientist's lab, *American Rifleman*, **128**, 36–37 and 76–77.

Latham, G. P. and Locke, E. A. (1975). Increasing productivity with decreasing time limits: a field replication of Parkinson's law, *Journal of Applied Psychology*, **60**, 524–526.

Lehrer, P. M., Schoicket, S., Carrington P. and Woolfolk, R. L. (1980). Psychophysiological and cognitive response to stressful stimuli in subjects practising progressive relaxation and clinically standardized meditation, *Behavioral Research and Therapy*, **18**, 293–303.

Locke, E. A., Frederick, E., Lee, C. and Bobko, P. (1984). Effect of self-efficacy, goals, and task strategies on task performance, *Journal of Applied Psychology*, **69**, 241–251.

Locke, E. A. and Latham. G. P. (1985). The application of goal setting to sports, *Journal of Sport Psychology*, **7**, 205–222.

Mahoney, M. J. and Avener, M. (1977). Psychology of the elite athlete: an exploratory study, *Cognitive Therapy and Research*, **1**, 135–141.

Mahoney, M. J., Gabriel, T. J. and Perkins, T. S. (1987). Psychological skills and exceptional athletic performance, *The Sport Psychologist*, **1**, 181–199.

Mahoney, M. J. and Meyers, A. W. (1989). Anxiety and athletic performance: traditional and cognitive-developmental perspectives, in D. Hackfort and C. D. Spielberger (eds). *Anxiety in Sports*. New York: Hemisphere.

Martens, R. (1977). *Sport Competition Anxiety Test*. Champaign, Illinois: Human Kinetics.

Martens, R., Burton, D., Rivkin, F. and Simon, J. (1980). Reliability and validity of the Competitive State Anxiety Inventory (CSAI), in C. H. Nadeau, W. R. Halliwell, K. M. Newell and G. C. Roberts (eds). *Psychology of Motor Behavior and Sport*. Champaign, Illinois: Human Kinetics.

Martens, R., Burton, D., Vealey, R. S., Bump, L. A. and Smith, D. E. (1990). The Competitive State Anxiety Inventory-2, in R. Martens, R. S. Vealey and D. Burton (eds). *Competitive Anxiety in Sport*. Champaign, Illinois: Human Kinetics.

Martens, R. and Gill, D. L. (1976). State anxiety among successful competitors who differ in competitive trait anxiety, *Research Quarterly*, **47**, 698–708.

Martens, R. and Landers, D. M. (1970). Motor performance under stress: a test of the inverted-U hypothesis, *Journal of Personality and Social Psychology*, **16**, 29–37.

McAuley, E. (1985). State anxiety: antecedent or result of sport performance, *Journal of Sport Behavior*, **8**, 71–77.

Orlick, T. and Partington, J. (1988). Mental links to excellence, *The Sport Psychologist*, **2**, 105–130.

Oxendine, J. B. (1970). Emotional arousal and motor performance, *Quest*, **13**, 23–32.

Parfitt, C. G. (1988). Interactions between models of stress and models of motor control. Unpublished doctoral thesis, University College of Wales, Bangor.

Parfitt, C. G. and Hardy, L. (1987). Further evidence for the differential effects of competitive anxiety upon a number of cognitive and motor sub-systems, *Journal of Sports Sciences*, **5**, 62–63.

Patmore, A. (1986). *Sportsmen Under Stress*. London: Stanley Paul.

Privette, G. and Landsman, T. (1983). Factor analysis of peak performance: the full use of potential, *Journal of Personality and Social Psychology*, **44**, 195–200.

Roberts, G. C. (1986). The growing child and the perception of competitive stress in sport, in G. Gleeson (ed.). *The Growing Child in Competitive Sport*. London: Hodder and Stoughton.

Schwartz, G. E., Davidson, R. J. and Goleman, D. (1978). Patterning of cognitive and somatic processes in the self-regulation of anxiety: effects of meditation versus exercise, *Psychosomatic Medicine*, **40**, 321–328.

Seabourne, T. G., Weinberg, R. S., Jackson, A. and Suinn, R. M. (1985). Effect of individualized, non-individualized and package intervention strategies on karate performance, *Journal of Sport Psychology*, **7**, 40–50.

Silva, J. M. and Hardy, C. J. (1984). Precompetitive affect and athletic performance, in W. F. Straub and J. M. Williams (eds). *Cognitive Sport Psychology*. Lansing, New York: Sport Science Associates.

Sonstroem, R. J. and Bernardo, P. (1982). Intraindividual pregame state anxiety and basketball performance: a re-examination of the inverted-U curve, *Journal of Sport Psychology*, **4**, 235–245.

Spence, J. T. and Spence, K. W. (1966). The motivational components of manifest anxiety: drive and drive stimuli, in C. D. Spielberger (ed.). *Anxiety and Behavior*. New York: Academic Press.

Spielberger, C. D. (1989). Stress and anxiety in sports, in D. Hackfort and C. D. Spielberger (eds). *Anxiety in Sports*. New York: Hemisphere.

Stern, R. M. (1976). Reaction time and heart rate between the GET SET and GO of stimulated races, *Psychophysiology*, **13**, 149–154.

Straub, W. F. (1986). The effect of three different methods of mental training on motor performance, in J. H. Salmela, B. Petiot and T. B. Hoshizaki (eds). *Psychological Nurturing and Guidance of Gymnastic Talent*. Montreal: Sport Psyche Editions.

Suinn, R. M. (1983). Imagery and sports, in A. A. Sheikh (ed.). *Imagery: Current Theory, Research and Application*. New York: Wiley.

Suinn, R. M. (1989). Behavioral interventions for stress management in sports, in D. Hackfort and C. D. Spielberger (eds). *Anxiety in Sports*. New York: Hemisphere.

Syer, J. and Connolly, C. (1984). *Sporting Body, Sporting Mind: An Athlete's Guide to Mental Training*. Cambridge: Cambridge University Press.

Thom, R. (1975). *Structural Stability and Morphogenesis*, translated by D. H. Fowler. New York: Benjamin–Addison Wesley.

Unestahl, L. E. (ed.) (1983). *The Mental Aspects of Gymnastics*. Orebro, Sweden: Veje.

Ussher, M. H. and Hardy, L. (1986). The effects of competitive anxiety on a number of cognitive and motor sub-systems, *Journal of Sports Sciences*, **4**, 232–233.

Wark, K. A. and Wittig, A. F. (1979). Sex role and sport competition anxiety, *Journal of Sport Psychology*, **1**, 248–250.

Weinberg, R. S. (1988). *The Mental Advantage: Developing Your Psychological Skills in Tennis*. Champaign, Illinois: Human Kinetics.

Wine, J. D. (1971). Test anxiety and direction of attention *Psychological Bulletin*, **76**, 92–104.

Wine, J. D. (1980). Cognitive-attentional theory of test anxiety, in I. G. Sarason (ed.). *Test Anxiety: Theory Research and Applications*. Hillsale, New Jersey: Lawrence Erlbaum.

Wittig, A. F. (1984). Sport competition anxiety and sex role, *Sex Roles*, **10**, 469–473.

Chapter 2

A cognitive perspective on the processes underlying the relationship between stress and performance in sport

J. Graham Jones
Loughborough University

Precise identification of the relationship between stress and performance has proved elusive for many years but still continues to intrigue researchers. Despite rather slow progress, advancement of knowledge concerning this relationship has occurred within a general, cognitive psychological framework, although this knowledge has largely failed, or at least been very slow, to filter through to the discipline of sport psychology. This may, of course, be due to problems of ecological validity. Sport psychology research is becoming increasingly applied in nature, with limited concern being devoted to the measurement of precise parameters in controlled environments. Martens (1979) was a leading protagonist of the move towards ecologically valid field settings and away from laboratories. This drive towards achieving the identity and autonomy of sport psychology as a credible academic discipline in its own right, rather than subsumed under general or 'mainstream' psychology, is to be applauded but it has also had some drawbacks. While there is clearly dissatisfaction among some sport psychologists over the lack of sport-specific psychological theories, there remains much to be learned from applying recent cognitive psychological theories to the sport environment. This is nowhere more evident than in the investigation of the relationship between stress and performance in sport.

Slow advancement of knowledge in this area within sport psychology is mainly due to sport psychologists' reluctance to question the merits of traditional optimal arousal theory. This is evident in virtually all sport psychology textbooks under headings or labels which make little or no distinction between concepts such as arousal, activation, anxiety and stress in

Stress and Performance in Sport. Edited by J. Graham Jones and Lew Hardy.
©1990 John Wiley & Sons Ltd.

formulating an inverted-U relationship with performance. The inverted-U hypothesis is firmly embedded in the history of psychology and the basis of its attraction to sport psychologists probably lies in its relative simplicity and intuitive appeal. The continued acceptance of the inverted-U has, however, resulted in what amounts to a disregard of advances in cognitive psychology which suggest that the relationship between stress and performance is much more complex than the inverted-U hypothesis could ever allow for.

This chapter discusses the validity of the inverted-U hypothesis, particularly in the context of the relatively recent move towards 'cognitive sport psychology', in which the concern is not necessarily directed towards global performance effectiveness, but rather towards specific aspects of information processing or cognitive efficiency. The move towards a cognitive approach to sport psychology is well documented in Straub and Williams (1984), who emphasized that this approach is not concerned only with information processing, but that:

> general cognitive sport psychology might be defined as the specific study of the mental processes and memory structures of athletes in order to enhance their individual and collective behaviours. According to this perspective, athletes are seen as organisms who search, filter, selectively act on, reorganise and create information. (p. 7)

The current preoccupation with field-based research in sport psychology is providing rich and valuable data. It is argued here, however, that it may be more appropriate to strive for a better balance between field and laboratory-based research. There remains much to be learned in the laboratory and this is particularly evident in the context of the stress–performance relationship. It is also argued that a better understanding of this complex relationship within a sport psychological framework is unlikely without a careful consideration of findings and models from the realms of experimental and cognitive psychology which have largely superseded the inverted-U hypothesis.

The emphasis of this chapter is centred around the premise that athletes are processors of information and that the stress of competition has potential, and possibly differential, effects on specific aspects of the information-processing system. Conceptual models of information processing may be classified under two major frameworks: resource allocation and linear stage models. Resource allocation models are primarily concerned with the strategical allocation of attentional resources to various mental functions. Linear stage models, on the other hand, emphasize cognitive computational processing mechanisms in an attempt to describe the flow of information through the organism as a sequence of processing stages mediating the transformation from signals into responses (Sanders, 1983). These two approaches have largely been viewed as competing analyses of performance, particularly when considered in the context of the relationship between stress and information processing (Rabbit, 1979). Hockey, Coles and Gaillard (1986) suggested that experimental psychologists have increasingly adopted models of human behaviour based on the operation of the digital computer so that they are concerned with structural relationships between computational systems. These approaches were described by these authors as 'dry' models due to their assumptions of 100 per cent reliability and zero variability in their information-processing characteristics. Consequently, they do not allow for variability arising under different environmental or internal states. Hockey *et al.* (1986) proposed that the emphasis should be on developing 'wet' models which take into account factors such as: variability resulting from changes in state (such as changes in behaviour under stress); relationships between information processing and the typical underlying pattern of biological activity; and individual differences. Hockey *et al.* used the term 'energetics' to refer to the intensive aspects of behaviour which are likely to affect information processing.

An important feature of this approach is the much more precise definitions required of 'energetic' concepts such as stress, arousal and activation. Arousal and activation will be addressed as separate, but interacting, concepts later in this discussion, but it is important that the definition of stress be confronted at this point. One of the major problems in examining the stress–performance relationship has been a lack of consensus over a precise definition of stress. Stress has been treated as both a dependent and an independent variable (Cox, 1978; Meister, 1981). The independent variable approach treats stress mainly in terms of the stimulus characteristics of a disturbing environment. The second approach, which treats stress as a dependent or response-based variable, describes it in terms of the person's response to disturbing environments (Cox, 1978). Selye (1956) defined stress as the non-specific response of the body to any demand. Since a person is always experiencing demands of some kind (e.g. air, food and water), a person is, according to Selye, always under stress. Jick and Payne (1980) argued that such a definition means that the result or response is not always negative or 'stressful' in nature. Cherry (1978) similarly proposed that stress is a combination of external factors or 'stressors' which are potentially, but not necessarily, disturbing to the individual. Thus, it is the response to the stressor which is crucial. Cherry (1978) and Jick and Payne (1980) referred to 'strain' as the potentially stressful response. As Selye's conceptualization of stress implies, individuals are not necessarily strained by a stressor: some sports performers, for example, will cope perfectly well with the 'stress' of competition. What is important, therefore, is the interaction between the stressor and the individual. Consequently, the individual experiences strain only if he or she perceives him or herself as being unable to meet the demands imposed by a particular stressor (Cherry, 1978; Jick and Payne, 1980; Lazarus, 1966; McGrath, 1970). If an individual does not exhibit strain symptoms then, of course, he or she is coping with the stressor.

This recognition of the crucial role of cognition in the stress response, and in behaviour in general, has had important implications for sport psychology. Gone are the days when 'behaviourism beheaded . . . athletes' (Straub and Williams, 1984, p. 3). These are the days of cognitive sport psychology in which athletes are active processors of information, requiring exceptional powers of perception, decision-making and response execution. The problem for athletes, of course, is that all of these performance subcomponents are open to all sorts of influences, both in the competitive environment and within the athlete him or herself. How, for example, do energetical factors such as arousal, activation and effort affect particular subcomponents of performance, and how are individual differences likely to mediate these relationships? The remainder of this chapter will consider various models and discuss their usefulness in addressing such questions within the context of sports performance.

THE INVERTED-U HYPOTHESIS: A CONCEPTUAL IMPEDIMENT

The most simple and common interpretations of the relationship between stress and performance are based on the notion that performance changes under stress are the result of changes in a single underlying dimension of arousal. Arousal, as used in this context, was defined as '. . . the extent of release of potential energy, stored in the tissues of the organism, as this is shown in activity or response' (Duffy, 1962, p. 179). The relationship between unidimensional arousal and performance has been most popularly conceptualized as taking the form of an inverted-U, the origins of which are credited to the early work of Yerkes and Dodson in 1908. The major assumptions of optimal arousal theorists are that for every type of behaviour there exists an optimum level of arousal, usually of moderate intensity, that produces maximum performance and that this optimum level decreases as performance complexity increases. Levels of arousal above or below this optimum amount are seen to produce inferior performance. Thus, the hypothesis simply states that increases in arousal are accompanied by increases in performance up to a certain point but further increases cause a deterioration in performance.

This theoretical framework formed the basis of Oxendine's (1970, 1984) proposed relationship between arousal and sports performance as a function of task characteristics. His ideas were based upon three assumptions: (1) a slightly above average level of arousal is preferable to a normal or subnormal arousal state for all motor tasks; (2) a high level of arousal is essential for optimum performance in gross motor activities involving strength, endurance and speed; and (3) a high level of arousal interferes with performance involving complex skills, fine muscle movements, coordination, steadiness and general concentration. Oxendine attempted to classify sports skills on the basis of the optimum arousal level required for maximum performance. His classification comprised five levels of arousal ranging from 'slight arousal' at one extreme (i.e. level 1) to 'extremely excited' at the other (i.e. level 5). Sports skills requiring extreme arousal, according to Oxendine, include blocking in American football, sprinting and weightlifting, while skills requiring only slight arousal include field goal kicking, archery and golf putting.

There is no doubt that this attempt to match different types of sports performance with different levels of arousal is appealing at an intuitive level. However, several criticisms can be levelled at Oxendine's hypotheses. First, the scant amount of empirical research carried out to examine his proposals generally supports the third prediction (e.g. Weinberg and Genuchi, 1980) but not the other two (Landers, 1977). Secondly, his classification is oversimplified in that it assumes one particular arousal level to be appropriate for all skills within a particular sport. He classified basketball skills, for example, as requiring an intermediate level of arousal (i.e. level 3) for optimum performance. However, there are instances within a basketball game when a player may need a high level of arousal, perhaps when rebounding for example, and other instances when the player may need a relatively low level of arousal, perhaps in the case of a free throw. Thus, no consideration is given to situational factors. Consider, for example, the field goal kicker attempting a kick from 15 metres as compared to an attempt from 50 metres. In the first instance, a 'slight' arousal level may well be appropriate, as Oxendine suggested, but the kicker may need an 'extreme' level of arousal if he is to generate the power necessary to be successful from 50 metres. Thus, Oxendine's classification fails to take into account the need for sports performers to shift arousal levels to suit the specific requirements of individual skills within a sporting performance. Finally, Oxendine did not seriously consider the cognitive requirements of different sports skills. For example, consider the distinction made between football blocking as a gross, 'low in complexity' skill requiring strength, speed and endurance, and the finer, more 'complex' skill of golf putting requiring fine-muscle movements, coordination and steadiness. This is essentially a distinction between 'simple' and 'complex' sports skills based primarily upon bodily movements and energy requirements. However, careful consideration of the cognitive requirements of these skills reveals some problems with the criteria underlying this type of task analysis. In the case of golf putting, both the object to be struck (i.e. the ball) and the target (i.e. the hole) are stationary and the environment is constant. Golfers can take all the time they need to process the necessary information and then perform the skill when they are satisfied that they are sufficiently prepared. Football blockers, on the other hand, have to contend with a constantly changing environment and a moving target. They are not able to predetermine their rate of information processing. They must process information as quickly as possible and have little chance of recovery should their opponent deceive them. Weinberg (1989) similarly proposed that this whole approach is too simplistic in that it takes little account of factors such as perceptual require-ments of the task, decision-making components and skill level. Landers and Boutcher (1986) have recently proposed a system for estimating the complexity of sports performance which goes some way towards addressing those issues raised above. This system is centred on the analysis of three major dimensions of skilled performance: decision characteristics of the skill, comprising number of decisions necessary, number of alternatives per decision, speed and sequence of decisions; perceptual characteristics of the skill, comprising number of stimuli needed, number of stimuli present, duration and intensity of stimuli and clarity of the correct stimulus among competing stimuli; and motor act characteristics of the skill, comprising number of muscle actions to execute the skill, amount of coordination of actions, precision steadiness and fine motor skill required. This approach may prove useful in the basic analysis of the criteria for establishing the complexity of different sport skills and accompanying energetical states required for effective performance.

Levi (1972) effectively extended the inverted-U hypothesis by proposing a relationship between arousal and stress. He argued that both high and low levels of arousal are experienced as stressful, with stress increasing as arousal deviates further from the optimum level. Combining these functions produces a linear relationship between stress and performance, with performance efficiency decreasing as stress increases (Cox, 1978). A problem with Levi's (1972) approach concerns the rather mechanistic nature of the stress–arousal relationship: underarousal or overarousal is associated with increased stress. This approach does not, of course, sit well with the more recent and now prevalent interactionist approach to stress discussed earlier in which the active role of the individual is taken into account and stress is viewed as one's perception of being unable to meet the demands imposed by a particular situation. Thus, it is the individual's perception or cognitive appraisal of the situation which is the crucial factor (Cox, 1978; Lazarus, 1966; Sanders, 1983; Welford, 1973). For example, a low level of arousal may not be stressful to a person who wishes to go to sleep. Neiss (1988) similarly argued that the inverted-U is incapable of distinguishing between different states, and is consequently '. . . an impediment to the understanding of individual differ-ences' (p. 535). For example, is the athlete who is experiencing a high level of arousal anxious (negative) or 'psyched-up' (positive)? The assumption of the inverted-U hypothesis is that very high levels of arousal are negative and debilitative to performance. This may be the case for many individuals, but other individuals may perceive the same arousal state as being positive and label it as facilitative to performance (see, for example, Hollandsworth et al., 1979). Only an interactionist approach would permit such an analysis. Further-more, Selye's (1974) notion of 'eustress', together with recent research findings (e.g. Jones and Cale, 1989a; Parfitt and Hardy, 1987), suggests that Levi's proposal that stress impairs performance may not always be accurate.

A further problem is that this approach is purely descriptive and does not explain why performance is impaired at levels of arousal above or below the optimum (Eysenck, 1982, 1984; King, Stanley and Burrows, 1987). Weinberg (1989) argued that perhaps the best explanation of the inverted-U hypothesis is Easterbook's (1959) hypothesis that the observed effects on performance are due to the effects of arousal upon attentional selectivity. The basic assumption here is that heightened arousal, emotionality and anxiety all have comparable effects upon cue utilization. The hypothesis simply states that an individual's breadth of perceptual attention narrows as his or her level of arousal increases. Thus, increases in arousal from a low to a moderate level are accompanied by an increase in perceptual selectivity whereby irrelevant task cues are eliminated and performance improves. As arousal level continues to increase beyond the optimum, breadth of attention continues to decrease, causing a 'tunnelling' effect, so that relevant cues are also eliminated, resulting in a deterioration in performance. In this context, therefore, arousal progressively reduces the range of environmental events considered by the cognitive system, producing a monotonic increase in the selectivity of attention. Eysenck (1984) questioned the assumed automaticity of attentional narrowing accompanying increasing arousal and suggested that any such narrowing might well be an active coping response. In other words, when the information processing demands are too great for the available processing capacity, then individuals may adopt a coping response by restricting attention to only a small amount of the information available.

It is rather simplistic, however, to assume that breadth of perceptual attention is the only change associated with increased arousal. Hockey and Hamilton (1983) argued that research should also focus on how other components of performance, such as speeded throughput of information and short-term memory, also change as a function of arousal. The basic premise of this approach, which is discussed in greater detail in the following section, is that arousal states have specific effects upon different subcomponents of performance, rather than general effects upon global performance. It is argued, therefore, that the inverted-U hypothesis merely relates to global performance effectiveness rather than specific processing efficiency (Eysenck, 1984) and is incapable of describing and explaining the much more complex relationship which almost certainly exists. Hardy and Fazey (1987) and Hardy (see Chapter 4 in this book) have even criticized the face validity of the shape of the inverted-U curve in proposing a relationship between stress and performance which is based on catastrophe theory (Zeeman, 1976). They argued that it is unrealistic to assume that once performers become overaroused and performance drops off then a reduction in arousal to previous levels will regain optimum performance (see Chapter 4 in this book).

What of the empirical evidence for the inverted-U hypothesis? Hockey, Coles and Gaillard (1986) argued that no clear supporting evidence has emerged from the vast amount of literature. Naatanen (1973) similarly proposed that the inverted-U lacks adequate empirical support and provided evidence of his own to suggest that changes in performance at higher levels of arousal are an artefact of divided attention. Certainly, laboratory-based findings do not generally favour an inverted-U relationship. Supporting evidence has tended to emerge from field studies of arousal and motor behaviour (e.g. Klavora, 1978; Martens and Landers, 1970), although these too are character-ized by inconsistent results. Neiss (1988) strongly condemned the inverted-U as not having received clear support from a single study:

> . . . the inverted-U hypothesis is effectively immune to falsification. An exami-nation of the empirical evidence relating arousal to motor performance will reveal that current support for the inverted-U hypothesis is psychologically trivial. (p. 353)

A problem of even more serious proportions which is associated with the whole inverted-U approach lies in the lack of clarity over the definition and operationalization of the arousal concept. This problem essentially concerns the unidimensional conceptualization of arousal, which owes much to Moruzzi and Magoun's (1949) identification of the brainstem reticular formation as the neurophysiological structure which mediated generalized drive. The retic-ular activating system was assumed to serve as a generalized arousal mechanism which responded to sensory input of all kinds, energized behaviour and produced both electroencephalograph (EEG) and sympathetic nervous system activation (Fowles, 1980). Arousal was regarded, therefore, as a unidimen-sional activation response which prepared the organism for action (Duffy, 1962) and lying on a continuum of neural excitation ranging from comatose states of deep sleep to extreme excitement (Malmo, 1959). Consequently, arousal or activation conceptualized in this way was viewed as a unitary concept in which increases in arousal were accompanied by increases in behavioural, physiological and cognitive indices.

Recent approaches to the arousal–performance relationship are character-ized by a general dissatisfaction with the use of arousal as a unitary concept (Hockey, Coles and Gaillard, 1986) due to its incapacity to account for the highly differentiated pattern of arousal accompanying the primary emotions (Posner and Rothbart, 1986). The notion of unidimensional arousal responses was challenged as long ago as 1967 by Lacey, who argued that it is possible to distinguish between three forms of arousal: electrocortical (i.e. cognitive), referring to the degree of electrical activity in the cortex and measured by the EEG; autonomic (i.e. somatic), referring to the degree of physiological activity primarily under the control of the automatic nervous system and measured by such indices as palmar sweating, skin conductance, respiration, heart rate, blood pressure, etc.; and behavioural arousal, referring to the overt activity of the organism. Lacey's argument was based on demonstrations of increases in the activity of one system occurring simultaneously with decreases in the activity of another (e.g. Dureman and Edstrom, 1964; Mirksy and Cardon, 1962). It was also based on evidence from studies which showed that measures within each of these three arousal systems sometimes vary in opposite directions (i.e. directional fractionation) and thus elicit different patterns of response (i.e. situational stereotypy) (e.g. Davis, 1957; Schachter, 1957). Lacey's arguments and supporting evidence for directional fractionation and situational stereotypy presented insurmountable problems for unidimensional arousal theory. Consequently, it is impossible for the inverted-U, while still based on an undifferentiated, global arousal concept, to accommodate the complexity of these proposals.

The arguments against the inverted-U hypothesis appear, therefore, to be overwhelming. King, Stanley and Burrows (1987) even referred to it it as 'a terrible myth' (p. 11), while Hardy and Fazey (1987) described its continued adoption and acceptance as a 'catastrophe for sport psychology'. Gould and Krane (in press) have similarly recognized the problems with this approach in an interesting review of some much more recent approaches to this area. In spite of these objections, the inverted-U has maintained a high degree of recognition (Oxendine, 1984), almost to the extent that its validity is taken for granted, particularly among sport pyschologists and coaches. It is argued, however, that this hypothesized relationship is too vague and simplistic, so that it is incapable, in its present form, of explaining the complex relationship between stress and performance. The following sections will discuss some alternative approaches to examining this relationship.

MULTIDIMENSIONAL AROUSAL SYSTEMS

Unidimensional arousal theory assumes that behaviour and performance is influenced directly by the level of undifferentiated arousal. This rather mechanistic notion of the arousal–performance relationship ignores the fact that individuals actively attempt to cope with and ameliorate any potentially harmful effects arising from factors within the environment, such as competition. Broadbent (1971) proposed a hierarchical, two-dimensional arousal system which attempted to accommodate this active coping response. He first described a relatively passive lower arousal mechanism, the state of which is induced by the demands of the task in question as well as by extraneous determinants. Broadbent's second mechanism, the upper arousal mechanism, was conceived of as an active cognitive control system responsible for monitoring the first mechanism and making an effortful, compensatory response in the case of unsatisfactory arousal levels in an attempt to maintain performance. The assumption here, of course, is that inefficiency in the lower mechanism will not impair performance as long as the upper mechanism is able to function effectively. Performance impairment only occurs, therefore, when the upper mechanism is unable to meet the compensatory demands placed upon it.

Eysenck (1982) also proposed a two-dimensional arousal system, much along the lines of Broadbent's ideas. The first system is a passive, undifferentiated physiological arousal state which influences performance according to its suitability for the processing demands of a particular task. The second system, which is akin to Broadbent's upper mechanism, is the control system which attempts to rectify any adverse effects of the first arousal system on performance. Consequently, high levels of performance can be obtained by two different methods: by near-optimal arousal in the first system and minimal involvement of the second system, or by sufficient compensatory activity in the second system (Eysenck, 1984). According to this approach, therefore, performance is not always impaired at sub- or supra-optimal physiological arousal levels, since it should be possible to maintain performance through the efficient action of a higher-order cognitive control system. Using this approach, Eysenck (1984) made an important conceptual distinction between 'processing efficiency' and 'performance effectiveness':

> Effectiveness is a measure of the quality of performance, whereas efficiency refers to the relationship between the quality of performance and the effort invested in it. More specifically, the relationship between processing efficiency and performance effectiveness can be expressed in the following formula: processing efficiency = performance effectiveness/effort. Compensatory activity in the second arousal system tends to reduce the effects of arousal on performance effectiveness, and so arousal will often affect processing efficiency more than performance effectiveness. (p. 339)

The notion that arousal influences processing efficiency rather than general performance effectiveness forms the basis of Hockey and Hamilton's (1983) proposals for the form of the stress–performance relationship. They argued that different stressors, such as noise, incentives, etc., create qualitatively different cognitive activation states which then influence performance *via* different cognitive processes. This approach focuses on the differences between the performance patterns which emerge under different environmental conditions. The underlying premise is that different stressors affect performance in different ways. Hockey and Hamilton (1983) attempted to map out detailed patterns of performance for individual stressors imposed in laboratory-based studies using indicator variables such as speed, accuracy, alertness, selectivity and capacity of short-term memory. While there are clearly more dimensions to cognitive performance (Mulder, 1986), the concept of multidimensional activation states itself provides an interesting basis for future research into the effects of stress on sports performance.

The majority of recent research in this area in the North American sport psychology literature has tended to focus on global sports performance (or what in Eysenck's (1984) terms would be referred to as 'performance effectiveness') and has, on occasions, even been as gross as to merely distinguish between a win or a loss as the performance measure. While this line of research has provided some valuable and ecologically valid data and findings, this type of performance measure appears to be too imprecise to facilitate a more comprehensive understanding of the relationship between stress and sports performance. The adoption of the type of approach employed by Hockey and Hamilton (1983) would allow a much more detailed analysis of how conditions within the competitive sport environment relate to the perceptuo-motor processes ('processing efficiency') underlying performance (Jones, 1988). This research strategy is characterized, then, by the investigation of a single stressor, perhaps competitive state anxiety, upon a variety of subcomponents of performance (Jones and Hardy, 1989). While this approach is discussed in much more detail within the realms of multidimensional competitive state anxiety by Parfitt, Jones and Hardy (Chapter 3 in this book), it is worth noting that several studies have already examined the relationship between competitive state anxiety and the cognitive and motor processes underlying sports performance, including: simple and discrimination reaction time in cricket players (Jones, Cale and Kerwin, 1988); perceptuo-motor speed and working memory in hockey players (Jones and Cale, 1989a); logical reasoning, verbal fluency and learned handgrip in rowers (Ussher and Hardy, 1986); and spatial relations, time estimation and agility in basketball players (Parfitt and Hardy, 1987). Future research in this area may benefit from the use of Landers and Boutcher's (1986) proposals for identifying important perceptual, decision and response components involved in specific sports skills, particularly in the context of maximizing the ecological validity of findings from this line of research. This approach also goes some way towards satisfying Hockey, Coles and Gaillard's (1986) criteria for developing 'wet' models of performance, but within the specific context of sports performance and with competitive state anxiety as the energetical factor.

The approach outlined above appears to have important implications for intervention strategies in sport. The specific implication is that interventions could focus upon developing information-processing strategies which stressed performers can use, rather than emotional control strategies to reduce the amount of stress which they experience. For example, to counter deficits in working memory, one could train performers using dual-task paradigms in which they have to make relevant decisions while under sport-related stress, such as physical fatigue and competition. Indeed, recent research by Guttman (1987) and Kuhn (1987) has shown that such paradigms do differentiate between elite and club level performers. Alternatively, distraction training and attention control strategies could be employed (Hardy and Nelson, 1988; Schmid and Peper, 1983) to reduce the hyperdistractability which might be associated with increased selectivity of attention in highly anxious performers. For example, relevant 'distractions' such as other performers, bad refereeing decisions, etc., could be gradually introduced to desensitize performers to them.

The extension of the ideas of Hockey and Hamilton to performance in sport is accompanied by the implicit assumption that the relationship between stress and sports performance is a very complex one. However, the gradual 'mapping' of the effects of different stressors present within sports environments on subcomponents of performance is likely to lead to a much more accurate and detailed knowledge. An important implication for sport psychologists who pursue this line of research concerns its ecological validity, as much of it is likely to be carried out in a laboratory or in an environment which will almost certainly incorporate some degree of artificiality. Jones, Cale and Kerwin (1988) did make strenuous efforts to examine reaction time performance in cricket players in the players' dressing room just prior to batting. However, although the setting for this data collection may have increased the ecological validity of the experiment, it was certainly artificial for batsmen to perform reaction time tasks before going out to bat. However, like Eysenck (1984), this author is not in favour of what Eysenck referred to as '. . . a wholesale abandonment of experimental rigour in favour of a totally naturalistic approach' (p. 364). The large number of variables influencing behaviour in sport, particularly within the context of the stress–performance relationship, means that without the facility to manipulate them in a systematic manner, it is extremely difficult to assess the relative importance of each variable in determining behaviour. A satisfactory combination of experimental rigour and ecological validity is very difficult to achieve, but the type of approach adopted by Jones et al. (1988) may provide a step forwards. The problems of ecological validity are further considered within the context of multidimensional competitive state anxiety and performance subcomponents in the chapter by Parfitt, Jones and Hardy (see Chapter 3 in this book).

THE ROLE OF AROUSAL, ACTIVATION AND EFFORT IN THE RELATIONSHIP BETWEEN STRESS AND PERFORMANCE

This section discusses a (wet) model of stress and performance which was developed by Sanders (1983) and which is based on more clearly defined concepts than many previous approaches. While this model provides a more definitive structure to the stress–performane relationship, it is necessarily very specific and limited in its application. The model adopts an interactional approach to stress and is interesting in that it attempts to integrate two approaches to information processing which have previously been viewed as competing: resourse allocation and linear stage models. The underlying proposition is that the effects of stress are the result of transactions between resource or energetical states and cognitive processes. Different stressors are viewed as affecting specific energetical supply mechanisms which, in turn, affect specific cognitive processes. The processes identified in the model are those arising from linear stage additive factor analyses (Sternberg, 1969) of choice reactions and essentially comprise perception, decision-making and response preparation. Consideration of the ecological validity of such an approach to sports performance is important since Sanders (1986) emphasized that '. . . it is clear that the additive factor approach is at best limited to a strict subset of behavioural variables subsumed in choice reaction processes' (p. 146). While this model is clearly not appropriate for considering subcomponents of performance such as problem-solving, reasoning, etc., it does provide an approach which is applicable to specific situations in sport which require rapid responses. A tennis player receiving a serve, for example, has to first of all identify the characteristics of the ball as it approaches him or her in terms of velocity, amount of spin, etc. (i.e. perception). He or she then has to make a rapid decision about an appropriate shot to intercept and return the serve. Finally, he or she must 'programme' this decision into a response before transmitting this response to the appropriate muscles (see Note 1).

As mentioned earlier, much of the confusion in the stress–performance area stems from the lack of precise definitions of key concepts: arousal and activation, for example, are commonly used interchangeably. However, the work of Pribram and McGuinness (1975), McGuinness and Pribram (1980) and Tucker and Williamson (1984) suggests that there are strong arguments for distinguishing between arousal and activation as different physiological states in terms of the primary central nervous system function (Hockey, Coles and Gaillard, 1986). Pribram and McGuinness' (1975) proposals also included the existence of a third separate, but interacting, system—effort. The resource framework adopted by Sanders (1983) is based upon Pribram and McGuiness' proposals. The assumption of Sanders' model is that the efficiency of each of the processing stages in the linear stage framework is influenced by the different energetical resource states of arousal, activation and effort. Arousal is viewed as a response to input which affects or 'energizes' perceptual processes. The activation system is viewed as being responsible for the organism's readiness to respond so that it affects motor preparation. Finally, the effort or coordination system is responsible for the coordination of the arousal and activation systems in establishing the more difficult relationships between perception and action, for example decision-making. This coordination is viewed as demanding effort on the part of the organism. Effort is, therefore, a coordinating mechanism in the sense that it attempts to correct any imbalances in the basal arousal and activation mechanisms in order to produce maximal performance. This whole process is dependent upon the efficient functioning of an evaluation mechanism which receives feedback about the state of the system so that effort can attempt to restore any perceived imbalance in state levels. The idea is that stress will arise whenever the effort mechanism is either seriously overloaded or fails to accomplish the necessary energetical adjustments. Thus, stress may arise because effort fails in correcting too low or too high a level of arousal, too low or too high a level of activation, or because there is a failure to supply sufficient energetical resources to decision-making due to the 'cost' of performing its coordinating function. This notion of energetical mechanisms under the control of a more powerful mechanism is akin to the proposals of Broadbent (1971) and Eysenck (1984) discussed earlier.

This model is, of course, far removed from predictions about general arousal levels affecting general performance. The emphasis, like Hockey and Hamilton's (1983) approach, is on specific states and how they affect different components of performance. In the case of the earlier example of a tennis player receiving a serve, Sanders' model predicts that effective perception of the ball in flight is affected by the player's arousal state (which is influenced by the intensity of the stimuli in the performing environment), that effective decision-making in the form of choosing an appropriate shot is influenced by effort, and that the cognitive preparation of the shot is affected by the state of activation (see Figure 2.1). It is also possible for decision-making to be bypassed in the case of a very high level of arousal resulting in an 'overflow' to the activation system. This is likely to cause faster responses, which will be beneficial in high stimulus–response compatibility situations or when the skill is well learned, but it also carries the danger of causing errors or inappropriate responses.

Research carried out to test the predictions of the model using depressant drugs, stimulant drugs and sleep loss to manipulate arousal and activation states (Frowein, 1981; Frowein, Reitsma and Aquarius, 1981; Sanders, Wijnen and Van Arkel, 1982) suggests that increased arousal and activation states are associated with more rapid execution of perceptual and response preparation processes respectively, although they do not necessarily predict the quality of

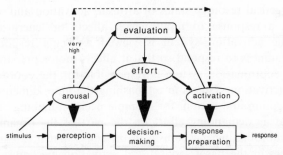

Figure 2.1. A simplified and modified version of Sanders' (1983) model of stress and human performance (reproduced by permission of Chapman & Hall from Jones and Hardy, 1989).

their operation. The relationship between effort and decision-making is potentially complex, depending on the complexity of the task being performed and on the suitability of arousal and activation states for effective performance. A task which is relatively complex will place high cognitive demands upon effort so that its ability to effectively coordinate the arousal and activation mechanisms is reduced, thus increasing the likelihood of stress. Where decision-making is relatively simple, the cognitive demands upon effort are relatively low so that it has more resources available to devote to the energetical state of the system, thus reducing the probability of stress occurring.

Sanders' model represents another approach which emphasizes the complexity of the stress–performance relationship. It also provides a very definitive and specific framework within which to examine the relationship between stress and sports performance in particular. This line of research would, of course, be limited to examining those skills which require rapid reactions and would need to be preceded by an accurate and detailed analysis of the underlying processes involved in that skill. Abernethy and associates (Abernethy and Russell, 1984; Howarth *et al.*, 1984) have provided a lead in this area. Abernethy and Russell (1984), for example, examined and identified the specific processing components preceding response initiation (together with their durations) involved in the batting performance of skilled cricket players. These were essentially stimulus detection, response selection and response organization. It would be interesting to examine how the durations, and quality of the operation, of these processes are influenced under varying states of arousal, effort and activation respectively.

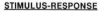

STIMULUS-RESPONSE

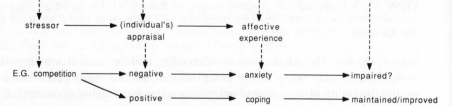

INTERACTIONIST

Figure 2.2. Comparison between stimulus–response and interactional approaches to the relationship between stress and performance.

INDIVIDUAL DIFFERENCES, STRESS AND PERFORMANCE

It is clear from the discussion thus far that the relationship between stress and performance is a complex one. The adoption of an interactionist approach to stress has meant that it is impossible to ignore the additional complexity arising from consideration of individual differences. This is depicted in Figure 2.2, which also incorporates speculative predictions about performance. As discussed earlier in this chapter, the stimulus–response conceptualization of stress essentially assumes that stress impairs performance. However, in the context of the interactionist approach, distinctions are often drawn between stress(or) and strain. Strain is the response to an individual's negative cognitive appraisal of his or her adaptation to the demands of a particular environment (i.e. the stressor) (Lazarus, 1966), which may result in avoidance motivation and possible decrements in performance. Another individual's perception of the same environment may be positive, resulting in approach motivation and possibly improved, or at least maintained, performance levels.

One individual difference variable which has received considerable attention, particularly within the context of competitive anxiety, is that of gender. It has consistently been demonstrated that females report higher levels of sport-specific trait anxiety (Martens, 1977) than males. Females have also been shown to report higher levels of competitive state anxiety than males (Jones and Cale, 1989b). Andersen and Williams (1987) suggested that this is because traditional socialization of the sexes has favoured males in terms of preparation for athletic competition in that they are exposed to and taught a competitive orientation to life more than females. Gender differences in expectations of success may also be an important factor in determining competitive state anxiety. Gill *et al.* (1984) suggested that competitive situations actually exaggerate gender differences in achievement cognitions, with females generally reporting less confidence and lower expectations of success than males (Benton, 1973; House, 1974; Lenney, 1977). Lenney (1977) emphasized, however, that these differences vary according to the task and the situation, with gender differences being particularly evident in tasks which are perceived to be masculine.

There may be an alternative explanation relating to gender differences in reporting anxiety symptoms. It has generally been found that females have a greater willingness to report more feelings, particularly of an unpleasant nature, than males (Briscoe, 1985; Verbrugge, 1985). Several authors have drawn attention to the possible effects of the greater social acceptability of the reporting of anxiety symptoms by females than males (Durkin, 1987). Certainly, there is no strong evidence to suggest that females who report greater anxiety than males produce inferior performance.

Another intriguing area concerns the relationship between personality, stress and performance. Humphreys and Revelle (1984) proposed a model which attempted to predict the combined effects of selected personality dimensions (i.e. achievement motivation, trait anxiety and impulsivity (see Note 2)), situational moderators (i.e. stressors) and motivational states upon information processing. A simplified version of their model is presented in Figure 2.3. The model incorporates two systems: arousal and on-task effort. Contrary to evidence discussed thus far, Humphreys and Revelle adopted the unidimensional notion of arousal as '. . . a conceptual dimension defined as that factor common to various indicants of alertness' (p. 158). (This is clearly a conceptual drawback with the model but it is discussed here because it has some interesting implications for sports performance.) The authors' conceptualization of 'on-task effort' is more specific than the general feeling of trying hard in that it refers to the allocation of available resources to the task at hand. In discussing this model, Mulder (1986) viewed arousal as the current state of the system and on-task effort as a compensatory control system, so that this approach is similar to those proposed by Broadbent (1971), Eysenck (1982, 1984) and Sanders (1983). Humphreys and Revelle also distinguished between the effects of cognitive and biological (physiological) stressors upon the two systems. They suggested that physiological stressors (e.g. time of day, sleep loss) affect arousal while cognitive stressors (such as incentives and importance) affect on-task effort.

The model attempts to predict performance on two types of task (skill): sustained information transfer (SIT) and short-term memory (STM) tasks. SIT tasks involve rapid throughput but no appreciable retention of informa-

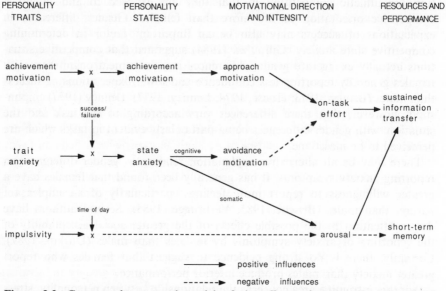

PERSONALITY   PERSONALITY   MOTIVATIONAL DIRECTION   RESOURCES AND
TRAITS   STATES   AND INTENSITY   PERFORMANCE

Figure 2.3. Conceptual structural model of the effects of personality, situational moderators and motivational states on information processing and cognitive performance (modified from Humphreys and Revelle, 1984) (reproduced by permission of Chapman & Hall from Jones and Hardy, 1989).

tion. They are similar to those which form the basis of Sanders' model, requiring individuals to process a stimulus, associate a response to that stimulus and execute the response. STM skills differ from SIT skills in that they require either information to be maintained in an available state or information to be retrieved that has not been attended to for a short period of time.

A major premise of the model is that these skills are differentially affected by arousal and on-task effort. Increases in both on-task effort and arousal are hypothesized to produce an increase in the number of resources used to sustain SIT skills. Humphreys and Revelle further proposed that performance on SIT tasks is a monotonically increasing function of the number of resources applied and concluded that increases in both arousal and on-task effort should improve SIT performance. Empirical evidence suggests, however, that high levels of arousal cause performance decrements on STM tasks. In summary, performance of SIT skills is enhanced by increases in both (cognitive) on-task effort and (physiological) arousal while STM skills are likely to show deficits associated with high levels of (physiological) arousal. Thus, high arousal is a good state for speeded throughput but a poor one for the retention, recall or manipulation of information.

Finally, the model incorporates predictions concerning interactions between the three personality dimensions, the on-task effort and arousal systems, and specific task requirements. Humphreys and Revelle proposed that impulsivity is related to physiological manipulations, such as time of day, and is therefore related to arousal. In the morning, low impulsives are more aroused than high impulsives so that increases in arousal are more likely to enhance SIT performance in high impulsives than low impulsives. In the evening, low impulsives are less aroused than high impulsives so that increased arousal should benefit SIT performance in low impulsives more than high impulsives. However, low impulsives should be more likely to experience deficits on tasks with a STM load than high impulsives in the morning, and *vice versa* in the evening. According to Humphreys and Revelle, achievement motivation is affected by cognitive manipulations, such as success and failure feedback, so that this dimension is positively related to on-task effort. The model predicts that high achievers are likely to demonstrate larger increases in on-task effort and hence better performance on SIT tasks than low achievers.

The authors adopted a two-component model of anxiety (Davidson and Schwartz, 1976; Liebert and Morris, 1967) so that some anxiety inductions are viewed as affecting primarily cognitive anxiety and hence (cognitive) on-task effort, and others as affecting somatic anxiety and/or (physiological) arousal. Consequently, the situation regarding trait anxiety is complex since it is possible for performance to be affected in two different ways: first, increased somatic anxiety may lead to increased arousal, thus improving performance upon SIT tasks; conversely, cognitive anxiety may be associated with avoidance motivation and reduced on-task effort, normally producing decrements in SIT performance. However, the findings from Parfitt and Hardy's (1987) study of basketball players contradict the latter proposal. Their findings suggest that cognitive anxiety is not necessarily associated with avoidance motivation. Parfitt and Hardy provided their subjects with an 'instructional set' which emphasized the relevance of the experimental task to subsequent basketball performance, hence inducing approach motivation and enhanced task performance under elevated cognitive anxiety (this argument is addressed in greater detail in Chapter 3 in this book). The situation regarding STM performance is more straightforward in that higher levels of somatic anxiety in high trait anxiety individuals will cause inferior STM performance compared to low trait anxiety individuals.

Humphreys and Revelle's model is both a general model of the effects of motivation upon performance and also a much more specific model of the ways in which certain personality traits relate to motivation and subsequent performance. It is not clear, however, as to the amount of performance variance which each of these personality dimensions accounts for. As Eysenck (1986) emphasized, it is perhaps too early, given the limited empirical base, to attempt such an analysis: '. . . theorizing about individual differences has not yet reached the point where it is routinely possible to account for substantial amounts of performance variance in terms of judiciously selected dimensions of individual differences' (p. 255). While Humphreys and Revelle's model is not specifically related to sports performance, it has important implications for sport both at a research and at a practical level. At a research level, it reflects once again the importance of the detailed investigation of different stressors on specific components of performance rather than on global performance. At a practical level, it has implications for the sport psychologist and the coach, the general message being that the same mental preparation techniques are unlikely to be appropriate for all individuals, in terms of both their responses to specific situations and their performances on particular types of skill.

CONCLUSIONS

It is the author's firm opinion that the development of research into, and the understanding of, the relationship between stress and performance has been hindered by sport psychologists' continued acceptance of unidimensional descriptions of the relationship between stress and performance and the inverted-U hypothesis in particular. The inverted-U relationship is too simple and is incapable of reflecting the extremely complex relationship which actually exists. It is argued that alternative methods of conceptualizing stress and performance which have been developed outside the sports context offer more appropriate, informative and testable approaches. The emphasis of these approaches is placed firmly upon cognitive considerations and is far removed from Oxendine's (1970, 1984) analysis of bodily movements and energy requirements.

The models discussed have important implications both for future research into stress and sports performance and for the development of methods of improving sports performance in stressful conditions. First, at a theoretical level, it is clear that the effects of stress on performance cannot be explained within the confines of one general arousal system. Unfortunately, it is still not evident as to the exact number of stress states or 'energetical' resource systems which actually exist, but the general agreement among the various approaches discussed (Broadbent, 1971; Eysenck, 1982, 1984; Hockey and Hamilton, 1983; Humphreys and Revelle, 1984; Sanders, 1983) is that there is more than one. At a practical level, these approaches do not always present obvious simple implications for improving performance under stress. At a theoretical level, however, they do provide the basis on which to construct a much more detailed analysis of the stress–performance relationship.

Secondly, the various models discussed strongly suggest that stress effects are situation-specific, and, more specifically, that they are dependent upon the nature of the stressor. This suggests, therefore, that competitive anxiety, fatigue, fear, etc., may all have different effects upon different components of sports performance. The implications for sports performers are that they should train in conditions that simulate those aspects of the competitive environment which most trouble them. Another conclusion which may be drawn from consideration of the various approaches discussed is that stress effects are task-specific. In other words, stress effects are dependent upon the cognitive (information-processing) requirements of the task, so that different task components can be affected in different ways by the same stressor. Consequently, 'vulnerable' task components should be identified and practices designed to help performers learn how to maintain performance on these components under conditions of competitive stress.

Finally, the model developed by Humphreys and Revelle (1984) proposes that stress effects are individual- and individual-by-situation- specific: individuals differing in personality type may react differently in response to an interaction between the stressor and the specific demands of the task they are performing. This implies that, in addition to simulating competition conditions and practising specific skills under those conditions, training programmes and pre-competition preparation should also cater for individual differences. For example, general 'psyching-up' routines which are frequently used in the precompetition period in many team sports may be inappropriate for many individuals in their particular team roles.

In summary, the relationship between stress and sports performance is clearly an extremely complex one, involving an interaction between the nature of the stressor, the cognitive and motor demands of the task to be performed and the psychological characteristics of the individual performing it. Future research carried out by sport psychologists in this area needs to be very vigorous in order to clarify some of the details of this interaction. Hopefully, this can be achieved *via* a balanced combination of laboratory and field-based research.

NOTES

1. A potential problem in applying this model to sports, or any, performance requiring rapid responses concerns the validity of the assumptions of Sternberg's (1969) additive factor method (AFM) which underlies the linear stage framework. Can a sports skill, such as receiving and returning a tennis serve, be broken down into distinct, independent processing stages? Do sports performers process information in a strict serial manner, so that a stage becomes passive once it has processed information and passed it on to the next stage? Many theorists believe that the notion of additive, exclusive, serial processes is too simple (e.g. Grice, Nullmeyer and Spiker,

1982; Vaughan and Ritter, 1973), arguing instead in favour of parallel processing. Even as long ago as 1938, Woodworth suggested that '. . . there is nothing to prevent two cerebral processes from occurring simultaneously' (p. 305). Sanders (1980) agreed that the information flow is almost certainly multidimensional but did not view this as a basis for rejecting the AFM, countering with '. . . the one-dimensional scheme can be used as a frame of reference for interpreting when and how a second dimension operates' (p. 335).

2. Although Humphreys and Revelle reviewed the extraversion literature, they actually developed their model in terms of the lower-order factor of impulsivity as studies have suggested that many of the arousal-based effects associated with extraversion are actually impulsivity effects (Amelang and Breit, 1983; Campbell, 1983; Eysenck and Folkard, 1980).

REFERENCES

Abernethy, B. and Russell, D. G. (1984). Advance cue utilisation by skilled cricket batsmen, *Australian Journal of Science and Medicine in Sport*, **16**, 2–10.

Amelang, M. and Breit, C. (1983). Extraversion and rapid tapping: reactive inhibition or general cortical activation as determinants of performance differences, *Personality and Individual Differences*, **4**, 103–105.

Andersen, M. B. and Williams, J. M. (1987). Gender and sport competition anxiety: a reexamination, *Research Quarterly for Exercise and Sport*, **58**, 52–56.

Benton, A. A. (1973). Reactions to demands to win from an opposite-sex opponent, *Journal of Personality*, **41**, 430–442.

Briscoe, M. (1985). Sex differences in psychological well-being, *Psychological Medicine*, Monograph Suppl. 1, 1–46.

Broadbent, D. E. (1971). *Decision and Stress*. London: Academic Press.

Campbell, J. B. (1983). Differential relationships of extraversion, impulsivity and sociability to study habits, *Journal of Research in Personality*, **17**, 308–314.

Cherry, N. (1978). Stress, anxiety and work: a longitudinal study, *Journal of Occupational Psychology*, **51**, 259–270.

Cox, T. (1978). *Stress*. London: MacMillan.

Davidson, R. J. and Schwartz, G. E. (1976). The psychobiology of relaxation and related states: a multiprocess theory, in D. Mostofsky (ed). *Behavioural Control and Modification of Physiological Activity*. Englewood Cliffs, New Jersey: Prentice-Hall.

Davis, R. C. (1957). Response patterns, *Transactions of the Academy of Science*, **19**, 731–739.

Duffy, E. (1962). *Activation and Behaviour*. New York: Wiley.

Dureman, I. and Edstrom, R. (1964). EEG and time perception. 22nd Report from the Department of Psychology, University of Uppsala, Sweden.

Durkin, K. (1987). Social cognition and social context in the construction of sex differences, in M. A. Baker (ed). *Sex Differences in Human Performance*. Chichester: Wiley.

Easterbrook, J. A. (1959). The effect of emotion on the utilisation and the organisation of behaviour, *Psychological Review*, **66**, 183–201.

Eysenck, M. W. (1982). *Attention and Arousal: Cognition and Performance*. New York: Springer-Verlag.

Eysenck, M. W. (1984). *A Handbook of Cognitive Psychology*. London: Lawerence Erlbaum.

Eysenck, M. W. (1986). Individual differences in anxiety, cognition and coping, in G. R. J. Hockey, A. W. K. Gaillard and M. G. H. Coles (eds). *Energetics and Human Information Processing*. Dordrecht, The Netherlands: Martinus Nijhoff.

Eysenck, M. W. and Folkard, S. (1980). Personality, time of day and caffeine: some theoretical and conceptual problems in Revelle *et al.*, *Journal of Experimental Psychology: General*, **109**, 32–41.

Fowles, D. C. (1980). The three arousal model: implications of Gray's two-factor learning theory for heart rate, electrodermal activity, and psychopathy, *Psychopysiology*, **17**, 87–104.

Frowein, H. W. (1981). Selective effects of barbiturate and amphetamine on information processing and response execution, *Acta Psychologica*, **47**, 105–115.

Frowein, H. W., Reitsma, D. and Aquarius, C. (1981). Effects of two counteracting stresses on the reaction process, in A. D. Baddeley and J. L. Long (eds). *Attention and Performance IX*. Hillsdale, New Jersey: Lawrence Erlbaum.

Gill, D. L., Gross, J. B., Huddleston, S. and Shifflett, B. (1984). Sex differences in achievement cognitions and performance in competition, *Research Quarterly for Exercise and Sport*, **55**, 340–346.

Gould, D. and Krane, V. (in press). The arousal–athletic performance relationship: current status and future directions, in T. Horn (ed). *Advances in Sport Psychology*. Champaign, Illinois: Human Kinetics.

Grice, G. R., Nullmeyer, R. and Spiker, V. A. (1982). Human reaction time: toward a general theory, *Journal of Experimental Psychology: General*, **111**, 135–153.

Guttman, G. (1987). Emotions and their correlations with cognition and performance. Paper presented at the 7th European Congress on Sport Psychology, Bad Blankenburg, DDR, September.

Hardy, L. and Fazey, J. A. (1987). The inverted-U hypothesis—a catastrophe for sport psychology and a statement of a new hypothesis. Paper presented at the Annual Conference of the North American Society for the Psychology of Sport and Physical Activity, Vancouver, Canada, June.

Hardy, L. and Nelson, D. (1988). Self-regulation training in sport and work, *Ergonomics*, **31**, 1573–1583.

Hockey, G. R. J., Coles, M. G. H. and Gaillard, A. W. K. (1986). Energetical issues in research on human information processing, in G. R. J. Hockey, A. W. K. Gaillard and M. G. H. Coles (eds). *Energetics and Human Information Processing*. Dordrecht, The Netherlands: Martinus Nijhoff.

Hockey, G. R. J. and Hamilton, P. (1983). The cognitive patterning of stress states, in G. R. J. Hockey (ed). *Stress and Fatigue in Human Performance*. Chichester: Wiley.

Hollandsworth, J. G., Glazeski, R. C., Kirkland, K., Jones, G. E. and Van Norman, L. R. (1979). An analysis of the nature and effects of test anxiety: cognitive, behavioural and physiological components, *Cognitive Therapy and Research*, **3**, 165–180.

House, W. C. (1974). Actual and perceived differences in male and female expectancies and minimal goal levels as a function of competition, *Journal of Personality*, **42**, 493–509.

Howarth, C., Walsh, W. D., Abernethy, B. and Snyder, C. W. (1984). A field examination of anticipation in squash: some preliminary data, *Australian Journal of Science and Medicine in Sport*, **16**, 7–11.

Humphreys, M. S. and Revelle, W. (1984). Personality, motivation, and performance: a theory of the relationship between individual differences and information processing, *Psychological Review*, **91**, 153–184.

Jick, T. and Payne, R. L. (1980). Stress at work, *Exchange: The Organisational Behaviour Teaching Journal*, **5**, 50–53.

Jones, J. G. (1988). Pre-competition multidimensional anxiety, self-confidence and performance. Paper presented at the Annual Conference of the British Psychological Society, University of Leeds, UK, April.

Jones, J. G. and Cale, A. (1989a). Relationships between multidimensional competitive state anxiety and cognitive and motor subcomponents of performance, *Journal of Sports Sciences*, **7**, 129–140.

Jones, J. G. and Cale, A. (1989b). Precompetition temporal patterning of anxiety and self-confidence in males and females, *Journal of Sport Behavior*, **12**, 183–195.

Jones, J. G., Cale, A. and Kerwin, D. G. (1988). Multidimensional competitive state anxiety and psychomotor performance, *Australian Journal of Science and Medicine in Sport*, **20**, 3–7.

Jones, J. G. and Hardy, L. (1989). Stress and cognitive functioning in sport, *Journal of Sports Sciences*, **7**, 41–63.

King, M., Stanley, G. and Burrows, G. (1987). *Stress: Theory and Practice*. London: Grune and Stratton.

Klavora, P. (1978). An attempt to derive inverted-U curves based on the relationship between anxiety and athletic performance, in D. M. Landers and R. W. Christina (eds). *Psychology of Motor Behaviour and Sport*. Champaign, Illinois: Human Kinetics.

Kuhn, W. (1987). The dual task paradigm to diagnose tactical abilities in soccer. Paper presented at the International Conference on Sport, Leisure and Ergonomics, Burton Manor, Cheshire, UK, November.

Lacey, J. I. (1967). Somatic response patterning and stress: some revisions of activation theory, in M. H. Appley and R. Trumbell (eds). *Psychological Stress: Issues in Research*. New York: Appleton-Century-Crofts.

Landers, D. M. (1977). Motivation and performance: the role of arousal and attentional factors, in L. Geduilas and M. E. Kneer (eds). *Proceedings of the NCPESM/ NAPECW National Conference*. Chicago: University of Chicago Circle, Office of Publication.

Landers, D. M. and Boutcher, S. H. (1986). Arousal–performance relationships, in J. M. Williams (ed.). *Applied Sport Psychology*. Palo Alto, California: Mayfield.

Lazarus, R. S. (1966). *Psychological Stress and the Coping Process*. New York: McGraw-Hill.

Lenney, E. (1977). Women's self-confidence in achievement settings, *Psychological-Bulletin*, **84**, 1–13.

Levi, L. (1972). Stress and distress in response to psychosocial stimuli, *Acta Medico-logica Scandinavia*, Suppl. 528.

Liebert, R. M. and Morris, L. W. (1967). Cognitive and emotional components of test anxiety: a distinction and some initial data, *Psychological Reports*, **20**, 975–978.

Malmo, R. B. (1959). Activation: a neuropsychological dimension, *Psychological Review*, **66**, 367–386.

Martens, R. (1977). *Sport Competition Anxiety Test*. Champaign, Illinois: Human Kinetics.

Martens, R. (1979). About smocks and jocks, *Journal of Sport Psychology*, **1**, 94–99.
Martens, R. and Landers, D. M. (1970). Motor performance under stress: a test of the inverted-U hypothesis, *Journal of Personality and Social Psychology*, **16**, 29–37.
McGrath, J. E. (1970). *Social and Psychological Factors in Stress*. New York: Holt, Rinehart and Winston.
McGuinness, D. and Pribram, K. H. (1980). The neuropsychology of attention: emotional and motivational controls, in M. C. Wittrock (ed). *The Brain and Psychology*. Los Angeles: University of California Press.
Meister, D. (1981). The problem of stress definition, in G. Salvendy and M. J. Smith (eds). *Machine Pacing and Occupational Stress*. London: Taylor and Francis.
Mirsky, A. F. and Cardon, P. V. (1962). A comparison of the behavioural and physiological changes accompanying sleep deprivation and chlorpromazine administration in Man, *Electroencephalography and Clinical Neurophysiology*, **14**, 1–10.
Moruzzi, G. and Magoun, H. W. (1949). Brainstem reticular formation and activation in the EEG, *Electroencephalography and Clinical Neurophysiology*, **1**, 455–473.
Mulder, G. (1986). The concept and measurement of mental effort, in G. R. J. Hockey, A. W. K. Gaillard and M. G. H. Coles (eds). *Energetics and Human Information Processing*. Dordrecht, The Netherlands: Martinus Nijhoff.
Naatanen, R. (1973). The inverted-U relationship between activation and performance: a critical review, in S. Kornblum (ed.). *Attention and Performance IV*. New York: Academic Press.
Neiss, R. (1988). Reconceptualizing arousal: psychobiological states in motor performance, *Psychological Bulletin*, **103**, 345–366.
Oxendine, J. B. (1970). Emotional arousal and motor performance, *Quest*, **13**, 23–32.
Oxendine, J. B. (1984). *Psychology of Motor Learning*. Englewood Cliffs, New Jersey: Prentice-Hall.
Parfitt, C. G. and Hardy, L. (1987). Further evidence for the differential effects of competitive anxiety upon a number of cognitive and motor sub-systems, *Journal of Sports Sciences*, **5**, 62–63.
Pribram, K. H. and McGuinness, D. (1975). Arousal, activation and effort in the control of attention, *Psychological Review*, **82**, 116–149.
Posner, M. I. and Rothbart, M. K. (1986). The concept of energy in psychological theory, in G. R. J. Hockey, A. W. K. Gaillard and M. G. H. Coles (eds). *Energetics and Human Information Processing*. Dordrecht. The Netherlands: Martinus Nijhoff.
Rabbit, P. M. A. (1979). Current paradigms and models in human information processing, in V. Hamilton and D. M. Warburton (eds). *Human Stress and Cognition: An Information Processing Approach*. Chichester: Wiley.
Sanders, A. F. (1980). Stage analysis of reaction processes, in G. Stelmach and J. Requin (eds). *Tutorials on Motor Behaviour*. Amsterdam: North-Holland.
Sanders, A. F. (1983). Towards a model of stress and human performance, *Acta Psychologica*, **53**, 64–97.
Sanders, A. F. (1986). Energetical states underlying task performance, in G. R. J. Hockey, A. W. K. Gaillard and M. G. H. Coles (eds). *Energetics and Human Information Processing*. Dordrecht, The Netherlands: Martinus Nijhoff.
Sanders, A. F., Wijnen, J. L. C. and Van Arkel, A. E. (1982). An additive factor analysis of the effects of sleep loss on reaction processes, *Acta Psychologica*, **51**, 41–59.
Schachter, J. (1957). Pain, fear and anger in hypertensives and normotensives, *Psychosomatic Medicine*, **19**, 17–29.
Schmid, A. B. and Peper, E. (1983). Do your thing when it counts, in L. E. Unestahl (ed.). *The Mental Aspects of Gymnastics*. Orebro, Sweden: Veje Publications.

Selye, H. (1956). *The Stress of Life*. New York: McGraw-Hill.
Selye, H. (1974). *Stress Without Distress*. Philadelphia: Lippincott.
Sternberg, S. (1969). On the discovery of processing stages: some extensions of Donders' method, *Acta Psychologica, 30*, 276–315.
Straub, W. F. and Williams, J. M. (1984). Cognitive sport psychology: historical, contemporary and future issues, in W. F. Straub and J. M. Williams, (eds). *Cognitive Sport Psychology*. Lansing, New York: Sport Science Associates.
Tucker, D. M. and Williamson, P. A. (1984). Asymmetric neural control in human self-regulation, *Psychological Review, 91*, 185–215.
Ussher, M. H. and Hardy, L. (1986). The effects of competitive anxiety on a number of cognitive and motor sub-systems, *Journal of Sports Sciences, 4*, 232–233.
Vaughan, H. G. and Ritter, W. (1973). Physiologic approaches to the analysis of attention and performance, in S. Kornblum (ed.). *Attention and Performance IV*. New York: Academic Press.
Verbrugge, L. (1985). Gender and health: an update on hypotheses and evidence, *Journal of Health and Social Behaviour, 26*, 156–182.
Weinberg, R. S. (1989). Anxiety, arousal and motor performance: theory, research and applications, in D. Hackfort and C. D. Spielberger (eds). *Anxiety in Sports: An International Perspective*. New York: Hemisphere.
Weinberg, R. S. and Genuchi, M. (1980). Relationship between competitive trait anxiety, state anxiety and golf performance: a field study, *Journal of Sport psychology, 2*, 148–154.
Welford, A. T. (1973). Stress and performance, *Ergonomics, 16*, 567–580.
Woodworth, R. S. (1938). *Experimental Psychology*. New York: Holt.
Yerkes, R. M. and Dodson, J. D. (1908). The relation of strength of stimulus to rapidity of habit formation, *Journal of Comparative and Neurological Psychology, 18*, 459–482.
Zeeman, E. C. (1976). Catastrophe theory. *Scientific American, 234*, 65–83.

Chapter 3

Multidimensional anxiety and performance

C. Gaynor Parfitt,[1] J. Graham Jones[2] and Lew Hardy[1]
[1]*University of Wales, Bangor*
[2]*Loughborough University*

This chapter discusses the anxiety–performance relationship from a multi-dimensional perspective. The appropriateness of considering anxiety, stress or arousal as multidimensional is well documented elsewhere in the literature. For example, Jones (Chapter 2 in this book) and Jones and Hardy (1989) have critically discussed the unidimensional approach to the stress/anxiety/arousal–performance relationship and concluded that the complex relationship which actually exists cannot be reflected in such a simple approach. Further-more, Hardy (Chapter 4 in this book) and Hardy and Fazey (1987) have proposed an alternative (multidimensional) model to describe the anxiety–performance relationship. Consequently, rather than considering the appro-priateness or otherwise of a multidimensional conceptualization of anxiety, this chapter will trace the development, consider the existing evidence, and discuss the future direction of multidimensional anxiety and performance research.

THE COMPONENTS OF ANXIETY

The identification of components of anxiety

One of the earliest distinctions between different aspects of the anxiety response came from the test anxiety literature. Liebert and Morris (1967) discussed the identification of two factors present in Mandler and Sarason's Test Anxiety Questionnaire (TAQ; Mandler and Sarason, 1952; Sassenrath, 1964; Sassenrath, Kight and Kaiser, 1965). These factors were labelled 'worry' and 'emotionality', and were defined as cognitive or intellectual concerns

Stress and Performance in Sport. Edited by J. Graham Jones and Lew Hardy.
©1990 John Wiley & Sons Ltd.

about one's performance, and autonomic reactions to the stress of the situation, respectively. Similar components had also been identified in other research areas. For example, Hamilton (1959) and Buss (1962) obtained factor analytic results which also suggested that there were two main components of anxiety reflecting the symptoms of psychiatric disorder. These components were labelled psychic and somatic anxiety. Later, again in clinical psychology, Davidson and Schwartz (1976) proposed a multidimensional model of anxiety which also hypothesized the existence of at least two components to the anxiety response. These factors were labelled cognitive and somatic anxiety. Davidson and Schwartz discussed the possibility of specific interference patterns for cognitive anxiety and somatic anxiety, based upon the principle of psychophysiological specificity. More precisely, the work of Segal and Fusella (1970) had indicated that auditory and visual imagery inhibited the perception of stimuli in the same mode more than in the other mode. Davidson and Schwartz (1976) linked these and other results to the notion of finite capacity and limited channel information processing to hypothesize that anxiety represented a recycling of negative information in a particular channel, thereby reducing available processing space (Wine, 1971). They further argued that relaxation strategies worked by replacing this negative information with positive or neutral information. Consequently, Davidson and Schwartz proposed that relaxation strategies should exert specific effects upon cognitive and somatic anxiety in accordance with the channel which they occupy.

Another clinical model developed by Borkovec (1976) proposed three components of the anxiety response: physiological arousal, cognition and overt behaviour. Borkovec's physiological arousal response can clearly be linked to Davidson and Schwartz's (1976) somatic anxiety (that is to say, somatic anxiety is the perception of physiological responses), and Borkovec's cognition can be linked to Davidson and Schwartz's cognitive anxiety. However, overt behaviour is not independently accommodated in Davidson and Schwartz's model. Thus, although the terminology and precise nature and number of components varied, there was a general consensus of opinion that different components of anxiety should be taken into account when attempting to control it.

Further consideration of the components identified in the test anxiety literature, and those just discussed, confirmed that some of these components were in fact similar. For example, Morris, Davis and Hutchings (1981) indicated that the cognitive–somatic distinction was essentially the same as the worry–emotionality distinction made by Liebert and Morris (1967). Morris, Davis and Hutchings consolidated this opinion by describing worry as:

the cognitive elements of anxiety, such as negative expectations and cognitive concerns about oneself, the situation at hand, and potential consequences

and emotionality as:

one's perception of the physiological–affective elements of the anxiety experience, that is, indications of autonomic arousal and unpleasant feeling states such as nervousness and tension. (p. 541)

While these components have been shown to covary in a number of studies (for example Holroyd *et al.*, 1978; Smith and Morris, 1977), they have also been shown to vary independently in others (for example Deffenbacher, 1978; Morris and Liebert, 1973; Schwartz, Davidson and Goleman, 1978; Spiegler, Morris and Liebert, 1968). With respect to the covariation of cognitive and somatic responses, Borkovec (1976) suggested that each component might serve a conditional or discriminative function for the other. More precisely, he argued that:

changes in one response component due to direct manipulation of its conditions may ultimately affect subsequent changes in the response of one or both of the remaining components. (p. 267)

For example, a sudden increase in physiological arousal (somatic anxiety) can be a source of worry, while conversely, worrying about a threatening event may cause an increase in physiological arousal.

The independent manipulation of the anxiety components

The cognitive and somatic components of anxiety have been manipulated in two different ways: by the introduction of specific stressors and by observing the temporal patterning of each component. Morris and Liebert (1973) independently manipulated worry and emotionality, as measured by the TAQ, using two different treatment conditions: threat of electric shock and threat of failure. The threat of electric shock resulted in an increase in emotionality only, while the threat of failure (negative) feedback resulted in an increase in worry only. Other support for the independence of worry and emotionality includes work which considers ego-threat situations (Deffenbacher, 1978) and social evaluation (Morris, Harris and Rovins, 1981). In both of these studies worry was increased independently of emotionality. Finally, Hardy and Whitehead (1984) conducted a study which also independently manipulated the components. Furthermore, they also manipulated activation to provide evidence that anxiety and activation are independent constructs (one negative, the other positive). It is beyond the scope of this chapter to discuss activation at length, and for a review the reader is referred to Hardy and Whitehead (1984), Mackay *et al.* (1978) and Thayer (1978). Essentially, Hardy and Whitehead (1984) manipulated anxiety and activation by changing the environment in which subjects (experienced climbers) completed a four-dimensional self-report inventory and provided data on two physiological measures. The environments were very early in the morning, during the late evening, following a prolonged bouldering session, immediately prior to leading a pitch at two grades below their leading limit (LL–2), immediately prior to leading a pitch at one grade below their leading limit (LL–1), and immediately prior to leading a pitch at their leading limit (LL). The four-dimensional self-report inventory measured cognitive and somatic anxiety and cognitive and somatic activation, while the physiological measures were heart rate and oral temperature. Hardy and Whitehead's (1984) results confirmed that cognitive and somatic anxiety and cognitive and somatic activation function independently of each other: cognitive anxiety increased in the LL condition; cognitive activation increased in the LL–2 and bouldering conditions; somatic activation increased in all the climbing conditions; and somatic anxiety increased in the LL–1 and LL conditions. The physiological measures also increased in the LL–1 and LL conditions.

The alternative method for independently manipulating these two components of anxiety is by considering the temporal patterning of each of the components. As early as 1968 the two components identified in the test anxiety literature were shown to follow different temporal patterns prior to and immediately following an examination (Spiegler, Morris and Liebert, 1968). Emotionality was shown to peak late and fast immediately prior to the start of the examination, while worry remained stable throughout the pre- and post-examination periods. This paradigm was adopted by Martens *et al.* (1990) to dissociate the components of anxiety in their Competitive State Anxiety Inventory-2 (CSAI-2), further details of which will be provided in the next section.

Martens *et al.* (1990) administered the CSAI-1 to both wrestlers and gymnasts at various time intervals prior to important competitions (for example four days, one day, two hours, and five minutes before). The results they recorded were consistent with previous test anxiety research in the way the components varied: that is to say, cognitive anxiety remained stable prior to the competition, while somatic anxiety increased just before the competition (cf. Spiegler, Morris and Liebert, 1968).

The temporal patterning obtained by Martens *et al.* (1990) has been replicated on a number of occasions (see, for example, Jones and Cale, 1989a; Parfitt, 1988; Parfitt and Hardy, 1987; Ussher and Hardy, 1986). In all of these studies a control group was incorporated into the experimental design to provide comparative data between anxious and non-anxious subjects, while Parfitt (1988), Parfitt and Hardy (1987) and Ussher and Hardy (1986) also included an additional data collection after the competition. Figure 3.1 clarifies this in a stylized representation of the temporal patterning of the cognitive and somatic anxiety components obtained in these studies. It is worth noting, however, that the findings from a recent study by Jones and Cale (1989b) suggest that females may not conform to this patterning. Using a sample of university athletes during the week leading up to a prestigious competition, Jones and Cale reported that the patterning of cognitive and somatic anxiety did conform to the predictions represented in Figure 3.1 for the males. However, for the females, cognitive anxiety increased as the competition drew near and was higher than in the males immediately before the competition. Females also demonstrated an earlier increase in somatic anxiety than did the males. This differential temporal patterning of cognitive anxiety between males and females has received support from a recent study reported by Jones, Swain and Cale (in press), although they failed to find differences in the patterning of somatic anxiety. These findings imply that great caution needs to be exercised when using the time-to-event paradigm with female subjects.

Another variable which has been manipulated using this paradigm is heart rate. Heart rate has been used in a number of studies as a physiological indicator of anxiety (Hardy and Whitehead, 1984; Idzikowski and Baddeley, 1983; Ussher and Hardy, 1986). Furthermore, while physiological arousal was not assumed to be the same as somatic anxiety, both Parfitt (1988) and Parfitt and Hardy (1987) found that heart rate followed exactly the same temporal pattern as somatic anxiety.

Finally, one further component which has been measured in all of the research which has used Martens *et al.*'s (1990) CSAI-2 should also be described. Self-confidence was identified in the early construction of the CSAI-2 when an iterative factor analysis of the questionnaire split the hypothesized cognitive anxiety factor into two separate components, one consisting of negatively worded items (cognitive anxiety) and the other consisting of positively worded items (self-confidence). The notion of independent positive and negative dimensions to the anxiety response is not new and can be clearly identified in the work of Mackay *et al.* (1978), Thayer (1978) and Hardy and Whitehead (1984). However, the temporal patterning associated with the self-confidence components has not proved to be as reliable as the other two components. For example, Jones and Cale (1989a) and Martens *et al.* (1990) recorded no changes in self-confidence across the time-to-event paradigm; Ussher and Hardy (1986) recorded an elevation in self-confidence after the

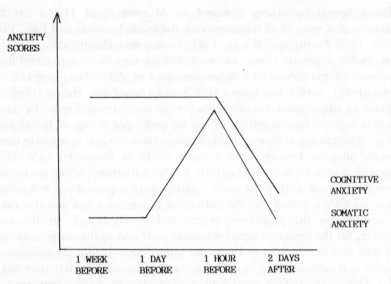

Figure 3.1. A stylized representation of the temporal patterning of cognitive and somatic anxiety in Parfitt and colleagues' design.

competition; Jones, Cale and Kerwin (1988) recorded a decrease in self-confidence immediately before their cricket subjects batted; Jones and Cale (1989b) recorded no change for men, but a decrease in self-confidence on the day of the competition for females; and Parfitt (1988) recorded either no change or a decrease in self-confidence on the day of the competition in her various experiments. The reasons for the variable results recorded are unclear, although it may be that self-confidence is more vulnerable to situational changes than cognitive anxiety.

The measurement of anxiety

As previously mentioned, anxiety has been measured using both self-report inventories and physiological measures. All of these can have shortcomings. On the one hand, considerable fractionation has almost always been observed between physiological measures (Lacey, 1967), while correlations between physiological and self-report measures have also been consistently poor (Thayer, 1970). On the other hand, the suitability of the self-report items used has been questioned (Magnusson, 1974), and several researchers (Mandler and Sarason, 1952; Sarason *et al.*, 1960; Watson and Friend, 1969; Magnusson and Ekehammar, 1975; Mellstrom, Cicala and Zuckerman, 1976) have suggested that anxiety is a learned response to situations, so that in order to predict behaviour, knowledge is required about how the individual reacts in the given situation. This line of reasoning led to the development of a number of situationally-specific anxiety inventories: for example, a fear of negative evaluation scale and a social avoidance and distress scale (Watson and Friend, 1969), a scale for measuring fear of snakes, heights and darkness (Mellstrom, Cicala and Zuckerman, 1976) and the Sport Competition Anxiety Test (SCAT) (Martens, 1977). During the development of SCAT, Martens (1977) also illustrated that situation-specific questionnaires were better predictors of state anxiety than were general inventories. When compared with the trait version of Spielberger's (1966) State–Trait Anxiety Inventory (STAI), the trait sport-specific questionnaire was a better predictor of state anxiety in sport situations than the STAI.

Bearing in mind the argument that state questionnaires should offer more worthwhile information regarding the anxiety–performance relationship (Spielberger, 1966), it is not surprising that Martens and his colleagues subsequently developed a state version of the SCAT; the Competitive State Anxiety Inventory (Martens, et al., 1980). However, this questionnaire did not incorporate the multidimensional nature of anxiety. As a result, Martens et al. (1990) developed the CSAI-2 as a sport-specific questionnaire which separately measured the cognitive and somatic components of state anxiety. The scale comprises 27 items, with nine items in each of the three subscales of cognitive anxiety, somatic anxiety and self-confidence. Examples of cognitive anxiety include 'I am concerned about performing poorly' and 'I am concerned that others will be disappointed with my performance', while somatic anxiety items include 'My heart is racing' and 'I feel nervous'. Finally, self-confidence items include 'I feel self-confident' and 'I am confident about performing well'. Responses to each item are on a Likert scale ranging from 1 (not at all) to 4 (very much so). Thus, possible scores on each of the three factors range from 9 to 36. The CSAI-2 has been shown to have good internal consistency and construct validity (Martens et al., 1990). Specifically, Gould, Petlichkoff and Weinberg (1984) reported that:

> Cronbach's alpha coefficients ranged from 0.70 to 0.90, revealing that the internal consistency of the various components was adequate, whereas concurrent validity was established by supporting predicted relationships between the CSAI-2 components and a variety of trait (e.g. Marten's Sport Competition Anxiety Test, 1977; Spielberger, Gorsuch & Lushene's Trait Anxiety Inventory, 1970) and state (e.g. Zuckerman's Affect Adjective Checklist, 1960; Schwartz, Davidson & Goleman's Cognitive–Somatic Anxiety Questionnaire, 1978) anxiety measures. . . (pp. 290–291)

Finally, recent research using the CSAI-2 (Jones and Cale, 1989b; Jones, Cale and Kerwin, 1988) has obtained similar intercorrelations between the

CSAI-2 subscales which were originally obtained by Martens *et al.* (1990), all of which indicate that the CSAI-2 is an appropriate tool for the study of multidimensional competitive state anxiety.

EFFECTS OF ANXIETY UPON PERFORMANCE

Four paradigms will be described which can be used to categorize research that has considered the effects of anxiety upon performance. The first of these will discuss research which has distinguished between components of anxiety and investigated their differential effects upon global performance. The second will discuss research which differentiates between subcomponents of performance but not the components of anxiety. The third describes research which considers both components of anxiety and subcomponents of performance. Finally, the fourth considers components of anxiety and their effects upon situationally relevant subcomponents of performance.

Effects of the anxiety components upon global performance measures

To date only a scant amount of research has considered the relationship between components of anxiety and global performance. Early correlational studies by Doctor and Altman (1969) and Morris and Liebert (1970) showed worry, but not emotionality, to be negatively related to academic test performance. Later, Morris *et al.* (1975) hypothesized that while worry might be the dominant influence upon cognitive performance in test situations, physiological arousal and the attendant emotionality might well interfere with motor performance. This was based upon Morris and Liebert's (1969) speculation that:

> whereas the cognitive component of anxiety (worry) interferes with cognitive performance, emotionality may be the component which interferes with motor performance (due to hands shaking, decreased muscular coordination etc.). (Cited by Morris *et al.*, 1975, p. 122)

However, in a correlational study involving typewriting skill, Morris *et al.* (1975) again obtained negative correlations between worry and performance, but no significant correlation between emotionality and performance. It is perhaps worth noting at this point that typing is a fairly 'fine' motor skill, requiring relatively little in the way of gross motor movements but a considerable amount in the way of cognitive processing. This distinction will become clearer later on in the chapter. More recently, Deffenbacher (1980) carried out an extensive re-analysis of test anxiety data and concluded that:

Partial correlations demonstrated that when the effects of emotionality were partialled out, worry continued to form a significant negative correlation with performance. However, when worry was partialled out, emotionality was not significantly correlated with performance. (Deffenbacher, 1980, p. 115)

The earliest work on sports performance in this area was conducted by Gould, Petlichkoff and Weinberg (1984). Gould, Petlichkoff and Weinberg used the CSAI-2 to collect data on levels of cognitive anxiety, somatic anxiety and self-confidence in wrestlers one week, two days, one day, two hours and 20 minutes before a match. These levels of anxiety were then compared with match outcome (win, lose), and points scored in the first period of two separate matches. Multivariate multiple regression analyses were conducted upon the data, with the match outcome and points scored as the dependent variables and the three CSAI-2 component scores at the 20-minute pre-match stage as the predictor variables. In the first of the matches there was no significant multivariate relationship, but in the second match the multivariate regression analysis was marginally significant. Follow-up univariate multiple regression analyses indicated that the match outcome, but not the points scored, regression was significant. Furthermore, the standardized beta coefficients showed that only cognitive anxiety (0.53) was a significant predictor of match outcome, with somatic anxiety (−0.12) and self-confidence (0.03) contributing little to the relationship.

Whilst Gould, Petlichkoff and Weinberg's (1984) experiment did obtain some significant findings, their results across the matches were inconsistent. A number of reasons can be proposed for this, including the way the scores of the CSAI-2 were used and the way performance was assessed. For example, past research has found that absolute levels of state anxiety measured across subjects have little relationship to performance (Sonstroem and Bernardo, 1982) but that variable levels of state anxiety around an individual's optimal level produce more consistent relationships. The research of Sonstroem and Bernardo (1982) implies that intra-individual relationships between CSAI-2 levels and performance might have been more appropriate and yielded more consistent results with regard to the way in which performance was assessed in Gould, Petlichkoff and Weinberg's (1984) study. A second weakness in Gould, Petlichkoff and Weinberg's (1984) paradigm was that the two matches used to assess performance were against different opponents, so that performance was not standardized and could have changed because of the opponent rather than the level of anxiety (Gould et al., 1987).

Research by Barnes et al. (1986) attempted to overcome this latter criticism by standardizing their performers' accomplishments against their own previous performance rather than against some other competitor's performance. Barnes et al. considered the effects of different components of anxiety (as measured by the CSAI-2) upon the competition performance of elite swimmers. They hypothesized that cognitive anxiety and self-confidence would both be related to competitive performance, but that somatic anxiety would not be. This prediction was based upon Fenz and Epstein's (1967, 1968) work with expert parachutists in which physiological arousal declined as experts approached the time to their parachute jump. Barnes *et al.* (1986) interpreted this finding as support for cognitive anxiety rather than somatic anxiety being the most likely predictor of performance. However, an alternative argument, not discussed by Barnes *et al.* (1986), but implied by Fenz and Epstein's results, is that the physiological arousal response was inhibited (controlled) by their experts immediately prior to jumping precisely because it was important.

Using a stepwise multiple linear regression analysis, Barnes *et al.* found that cognitive anxiety was a significant predictor of performance, but that self-confidence and somatic anxiety were not. This result surprised Barnes *et al.* as they were following Martens *et al.*'s (1990) suggestion that self-confidence and cognitive anxiety were opposite ends of a cognitive evaluation continuum. This suggestion originally arose as an explanation of the self-confidence component which was first identified by iterative factor analysis of the CSAI-2 items. However, since Martens *et al.'s* iterative factor analysis extracted these two factors *orthogonally*, they cannot logically be conceptualized as lying along the same continuum. Both Barnes *et al.* (1986) and Martens *et al.* (1990) seem to have overlooked this fact. Rather, Barnes *et al.* (1986) suggested that there was either a ceiling effect for self-confidence (mean = 28.13 with a standard deviation of 5.10) or, alternatively, that with cognitive anxiety already in the regression model, self-confidence could not be expected to add any further explained variance. However, precisely because the factors were extracted as orthogonal factors, one would in fact expect that each factor should contribute its own variance to the total model. Finally, Barnes *et al.*'s results may in fact simply be a reflection of the relatively unpredictable nature of self-confidence (cf. Jones and Cale, 1989b; Jones, Cale and Kerwin, 1988; Parfitt, 1988).

More recent research by Gould *et al.* (1987) on the effects of cognitive anxiety, somatic anxiety and self-confidence upon performance used Sonstroem and Bernardo's (1982) paradigm, together with polynomial trend analyses, to determine if there were significant linear or curvilinear relationships between the components of the CSAI-2 and competitive pistol shooting. Gould *et al.*'s results confirmed the independence of the three components (cognitive and somatic anxiety and self-confidence) and indicated a significant negative linear trend for performance and self-confidence, a significant inverted-U shaped quadratic trend for performance and somatic anxiety, but no significant trend for cognitive anxiety. Gould *et al.* were unable to explain the negative linear trend for self-confidence, but their results could be interpreted as a milestone in the literature, since it was the first time that somatic anxiety has accounted for more variance in performance than cognitive anxiety. For, as has already been indicated, the general consensus of the earlier test anxiety literature was that:

> Worry, the cognitive component of anxiety involving conscious concern about one's performance and its consequences, emerges consistently as the most important element of the anxiety experience when considering effects on performance. (Morris, Brown and Halbert, 1977, p. 155)

This lack of effects due to somatic anxiety or emotionality in the previous literature may have been due not only to the type of (linear) analysis employed, but also to the type of task and performance measure used. Gould et al.'s (1987) explanation of their results supports this latter point, as they suggested that because pistol shooting required very fine neuromuscular control, it would be particularly sensitive to changes in physiological arousal. Furthermore, in their concluding remarks Gould et al. stated that:

> In essence, there is a need to examine how various state anxiety components influence performance on tasks varying in specific neuromuscular and perceptual/ attentional characteristics. (p. 40)

This statement reflects the need to move towards considering the types of processes which underlie performance and reiterates Straub and Williams' (1984) argument for a more cognitive approach to research in sport psychology.

At a much more applied level, Landers and Boutcher (1986) have proposed a system for estimating the complexity of sports performance (see Chapter 2 in this book) which goes some way towards fulfilling Gould et al.'s suggestion. More precisely, Landers and Boutcher proposed that task complexity could be defined as the sum of the perceptual, decision-making and motor response demands of the task. Burton (1988) conducted a study on swimmers using the CSAI-2 and Landers and Boutcher's (1986) classification system. Burton's results suggested that cognitive anxiety was more strongly related to performance than somatic anxiety. An inverted-U shaped relationship was recorded between performance time and somatic anxiety, while positive linear and negative linear relationships were recorded between performance time and self-confidence, and performance time and cognitive anxiety, respectively. Finally, stronger relationships were recorded for somatic anxiety with short duration, and high and low complexity events, than with long duration or moderate complexity events. However, it is not clear whether Burton's (1988) subjective evaluation of the perceptual, decision-making and motor response characteristics of different swimming strokes can be used to determine a single continuum of task complexity (cf. Hockey and Hamilton, 1983). It could be argued that some way of objectively assessing each of the three characteristics is necessary, or that a more detailed breakdown of each characteristic into different aspects is required: for example whether the motor response is fine or gross, as well as simple or complex; whether the decision requirements are fast or slow, as well as high or low; and whether the perceptual needs are stable or variable. In any case, some tasks could have a complex motor response but simple (low) decision and perceptual needs (e.g. a gymnastic routine), while others could have a simple motor response but complex decision and perceptual needs (e.g. a badminton rally). In these cases, how would each sport be categorized? Are they low, high or moderate in complexity?

Finally, before discussing research which has adopted a subcomponents of performance approach, it is also worth considering the appropriateness of the statistical analyses which the above literature has used. It could be argued that rather than conducting between-subjects analyses of relative performance levels (which the above correlational analyses do), one should consider within-subject analyses of actual performance levels. For, it is the effect of changing anxiety levels upon an individual's actual performance that is important, not how scores vary between individuals with different (relative) anxiety levels. This statement is made with specific reference to research using the CSAI-2, but it could also be argued that the rationale behind it applies to all research considering the anxiety–performance relationship. This design issue, along with other design criticisms of the research described, will be discussed in much greater detail later.

Anxiety effects upon subcomponents of performance

Hockey, Coles and Gaillard's (1986) 'wet' model approach to studying the effects of stress upon performance was described in Chapter 2 in this book. To recap, the primary characteristic of 'wet' models is that they accommodate variability resulting from state changes, relationships between information processing and the typical underlying pattern of biological activity, and individual differences. Using this approach, Hockey and Hamilton (1983) argued that different stressors create qualitatively different cognitive activation states which then influence performance *via* different cognitive subcomponents or processes. Hockey and Hamilton's conclusions from their own experimentation were that noise increased attentional selectivity, speed of information transfer and recall of high association items, while impairing working memory and recall of low association items. However, while this approach may mark a cornerstone in stress research, a number of criticisms can be directed at its emphasis. For example, having suggested that different stressors differentially affect cognitive processes, Hockey and Hamilton's focus upon laboratory 'stressors' and verbal memory is notable. Indeed, if their loud noise experiments are considered in terms of their potential application to other settings, then it is worth noting that the type of performance which is required in such situations is unlikely to be a verbal recall task or a choice reaction test. It is much more likely to be a motor task of some sort, either gross or complex, such as working on a car assembly line, or working on an electronic interface. Furthermore, Adams (1983) has argued that it is unrealistic to expect to be able to infer effects on motor tasks from effects recorded upon verbal tasks, and suggested that research into the separate domains of motor and verbal memory is not yet sufficiently advanced to allow their integration. Therefore, for Hockey and Hamilton's paradigm to be applicable to many industrial situations, future research needs to focus on the effects of noise upon motor rather than verbal memory.

Some research has already considered ecologically valid stressors and tasks. Indeed, more than 20 years ago Baddeley (1966) used a manual dexterity task to compare diving performance in a pressure chamber with performance in the open sea. Manual dexterity performance was significantly worse in the open sea, which Baddeley interpreted as suggesting that there were other stressors in the open sea which were not replicated in the pressure chamber. Subsequent research studying the effect of depth upon diving performance has confirmed this finding for manual dexterity (see, for example, Mears and Cleary, 1980; Baddeley and Idzikowski, 1985). Furthermore, Lewis and Baddeley (1981) also reported negative effects upon a number of other tasks performed by divers including visual search and short-term memory (STM).

Similar effects have been reported with parachutists before their first jump. For example, Hammerton and Tickner (1968) reported decrements in a tracking task performed by novice parachutists just before they jumped, while Idzikowski and Baddeley (1987) found that performances on mannikin, letter search and digit span tasks were all significantly worse immediately before a jump compared with several hours before the jump. While it should be clear that the stressors in these situations are ecologically valid, it may not be as clear that the tasks are. However, a parachutist has to track and guide his descent, be able to orientate himself before his parachute opens, and pick out his landing target, all of which use short-term memory; so that the tasks could be argued to be very relevant, and ecologically valid, to jumping safely.

One of the most encouraging earlier studies which considered ecologically valid stressors and criterion tasks was carried out on public speakers by Idzikowski and Baddeley (1983). They included several verbal tasks and one motor task in their test battery, which consisted of digit span (with a verbal response), verbal fluency, logical reasoning, stroop, and tick length. Subjects' anxiety was measured using the self-report Visual Analogue Scale (Herbert, Johns and Dore, 1976) and ECG data. Both indicated a significant increase in anxiety on the day of the talk. Performance on the digit span and verbal fluency tasks was also significantly worse on the day of the talk compared with a control day, while performance on the other tasks was not significantly affected. These results were particularly encouraging because the tasks which were relevant to the situation (i.e. those requiring a verbal response) were affected, while those which were not relevant to the situation (i.e. did not require a verbal response) were unaffected. Such findings could be interpreted as evidence for anxiety exerting the same sort of patterning effect upon performance as had been previously reported by Hockey and Hamilton (1983) for noise. However, yet again, the example concerns verbal-type tasks, and although this cannot be criticized as the stressor was indeed 'real', there is still something of a gap in the literature with regard to the effects of environmental stressors upon the subcomponents of motor performance.

Differential effects of the components of anxiety upon the subcomponents of performance

While the above research findings have incorporated a research design which may be potentially very appropriate for studying how the different processes of performance may be affected by stressors, they have not considered the multidimensional nature of anxiety. The first research which considered the effects of different components of anxiety upon different subcomponents of performance was conducted by Ussher and Hardy (1986). Ussher and Hardy attempted to investigate whether or not the cognitive and somatic components of anxiety had differential effects upon some of the cognitive and motor processes involved in competitive rowing. Their experiment made use of the time-to-a-significant-event paradigm to manipulate cognitive and somatic anxiety. It was hypothesized that the components of anxiety would dissociate under a time-to-competition paradigm (see Figure 3.1). Furthermore, having manipulated the anxiety components in this way, if performance on any of the subcomponents of performance followed the same temporal patterning as one of the anxiety components, then it would be possible to infer that the effect was principally due to that anxiety component.

Ussher and Hardy's (1986) study incorporated control and experimental groups. The control group of subjects was tested across the same time intervals as the experimental group, but without any impending competitive event. This group was included to control for any learning effects across sessions on the experimental criterion tasks, and also to control for any task difficulty effects in parallel forms of tasks which could not be balanced across sessions. An additional purpose of the control group was to confirm that the experimental group's anxiety returned to baseline after the competition. The intervals for the data collections were determined by a pilot study to identify when the dissociation of anxiety components occurred for rowers. Based upon this, the first data collection was taken two weeks before, the second one day before, the third immediately before, and the fourth two weeks after the competition. Three familiarization sessions were conducted during the week before the first data collection; during these familiarization sessions the subjects performed all the experimental tasks.

The time of day for each testing session was set as close as possible to the starting time of the experimental group's regatta, as cognitive performance measures have been shown to fluctuate with time of day (Blake, 1967). Cognitive and somatic anxiety were measured using Martens *et al.*'s (1990) CSAI-2, with heart rate taken as a confirmatory measure of physiological arousal. As discussed in the first section of this chapter, physiological arousal follows the same temporal pattern as somatic anxiety. Consequently, using the time-to-event paradigm, it is not possible to differentiate between the effects of somatic anxiety upon performance and the effects of physiological arousal upon performance. Because of this, such effects will be referred to as physiological arousal/somatic anxiety effects—not because of any belief that these two constructs are the same, but simply because the paradigm does not distinguish between their effects.

Ussher and Hardy's results were encouraging in that they obtained a dissociation of cognitive and somatic anxiety under the time-to-event paradigm, and also some weak evidence in support of specific interference patterns for cognitive and somatic anxiety regarding different aspects of performance. More precisely, their results suggested that increases in somatic anxiety impaired learned hand grip, while increases in cognitive anxiety were not directly associated with the performance effects. Research by Jones, Cale and Kerwin (1988) further emphasized the importance of the somatic anxiety component when they showed that somatic anxiety accompanied by reduced self-confidence in cricket players immediately prior to batting was associated with an increase in errors in a choice reaction time task.

Parfitt (1988) suggested that it is possible to explain many of the anxiety– performance results in terms of motivational epiphenomena. For, suppose that subjects do not perceive the experimental tasks to be particularly relevant to the highly stressful situation in which they find themselves. Then it would appear to be a very reasonable cognitive strategy on their part to refuse to invest any attentional effort in them. Thus, while subjects might well be prepared to expend considerable effort on apparently meaningless tasks under control conditions, they might understandably refuse to do so under highly stressful experimental conditions. However, the associated performance decrements presumably represent a very appropriate coping strategy on the part of the subjects, rather than any reduction in the availability of resources.

This notion of perceived situational relevance is not necessarily a new one. As early as 1968, Spiegler, Morris and Liebert suggested that the inconsistencies which had occurred in the anxiety literature might have been due not only to the failure of researchers to consider the different components of anxiety, but also to factors such as experimental setting, type of task and instructions employed. The importance of employing situationally relevant criterion tasks is also implied by Idzikowski and Baddeley's (1983) findings with public speakers and has been further emphasized by Goolkasian (1982). Indeed, Goolkasian argued that it might be possible to identify stress effects only by considering situationally relevant criterion tasks.

Differential effects of the components of anxiety upon the subcomponents of situationally relevant performance

Parfitt and Hardy (1987) conducted several similar experiments to the one performed by Ussher and Hardy (1986) to investigate the effect that different anxiety components had upon subcomponents of hockey and basketball performance. However, there was one important difference in the design used by Parfitt and Hardy (1987): namely, that they deliberately emphasized the situational relevance to their subjects of each of the tasks which they asked them to perform. The tasks were critical flicker fusion (CFF) and pattern search for the hockey subjects, and letter span, Sargent jump and rebound shooting for the basketball subjects. The CFF test required subjects to indicate when a visual stimulus changed and measured the flicker speed at which this was achieved. The inclusion of this task was justified to subjects on the grounds that such discriminative ability is a fundamental aspect of any sport where decisions have to be made if and when something in the environment changes. The pattern search task was a sustained information transfer task which required subjects to identify when a specific pattern occurred. Its inclusion was justified on the grounds that team sports are structured around identifying patterns of play and reacting to them. The letter span task was included as a measure of working memory. Performance in 'major' games requires an ability to hold and recall salient strategic information for short periods of time. Sargent jump was included as a basic measure of leg power, an important ability in a sport like basketball where jumping height is crucial. Finally, rebound shooting was included as a fundamental ability in basketball which could be regarded as a long-term motor recall task.

Parfitt and Hardy again used the time-to-event paradigm to dissociate cognitive and somatic anxiety (see Figure 3.1), and tested subjects on three (basketball: two days before, one hour before, and one day after a major competition) or four (hockey: one week before, one day before, one hour before, and one day after a major competition) occasions. A familiarization session was included in both studies before the first testing session, and a control group was included in the basketball study. However, before performing each criterion task, subjects read priming instructions which specifically explained how the task was relevant to the actual sport which the subject was going to perform. As described in the previous section, this was to avoid genuine negative anxiety effects upon performance being confounded by perfectly appropriate motivational strategies whereby subjects choose to no longer invest effort in a task which they perceive to be extrinsic to their anxiety. On the basis of this reasoning, Parfitt and Hardy (1987) hypothesized that differential effects would be recorded upon the criterion tasks employed, rather than simply 'blanket' negative effects. Futhermore, the cognitive and somatic components of anxiety were hypothesized to affect these criterion tasks differently, as some of the tasks were largely physiological in nature, while others were cognitive (Morris and Liebert, 1969).

Parfitt and Hardy (1987) recorded positive effects associated with the temporal patterning of cognitive anxiety on critical flicker fusion (CFF), pattern search and rebound shooting; positive effects associated with physiological arousal/somatic anxiety on Sargent jump; and negative effects associated with physiological arousal/somatic anxiety on letter span (see Figure 3.2, 3.3, 3.4, 3.5 and 3.6). Cognitive anxiety was, therefore, shown to be associated with positive effects upon some subcomponents of performance, while physiological arousal, or somatic anxiety, was associated with both positive and negative effects (cf. Hockey and Hamilton's (1983) findings for loud noise). Furthermore, these differential effects recorded for physiological arousal/ somatic anxiety clearly support the argument that cognitive anxiety is not the only influence upon performance.

Jones and Cale (1989a) later carried out a similar study which examined the effects of competitive anxiety upon perceptuo-motor speed and digit span in hockey players. This study confirmed that somatic anxiety can have a positive effect upon performance by demonstrating that perceptuo-motor speed (as measured by a number cancellation task) was enhanced by somatic anxiety. A significant interaction between group and time-to-event was recorded for somatic anxiety and perceptuo-motor speed. For somatic anxiety, Tukey's follow-up tests showed that the only significant difference between the control and experimental groups was at 20 minutes prior to the match, when the experimental group was significantly higher than the control group. This pattern was replicated with the perceptuo-motor speed task, in which Tukey's follow-up test revealed that the experimental group's performance was significantly better at 20 minutes prior to the match than at any other stage in either group. The digit span data showed no significant changes.

Parfitt (1988) further investigated the importance of situationally relevant criterion tasks. A series of experiments was conducted using major basketball and volleyball competitions as the source of anxiety. The majority of these results are described in Parfitt and Hardy (1987). However, Parfitt (1988) replicated the positive Sargent jump effect and discussed at some length reasons for studying situationally relevant stressors and tasks. To recap, it was suggested that the significant patterning effects obtained in Parfitt (1988) and Parfitt and Hardy (1987) were due to subjects investing time and effort in performing tasks which they perceived to contain situationally relevant information, whereas in other research (Idzikowski and Baddeley, 1987) this might

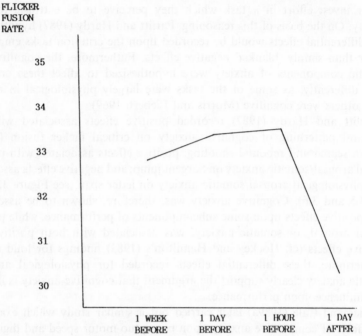

Figure 3.2. Mean critical flicker fusion scores of hockey players at various times before and after an important hockey match.

not have been the case. More precisely, if one assumes that the effects of cognitive and somatic anxiety depend upon the availability of processing resources (allocation and capacity), then it is not unreasonable to suggest that subjects who are aware of the situational relevance of a task will invest some of their resources in the task even when they are anxious. Conversely, subjects who are not aware of any situational relevance may well choose not to invest their resources in the task when they are anxious (Parfitt, 1988).

Theoretical implications

According to Morris and Liebert's (1969) arguments and Davidson and Schwartz' (1976) matching hypothesis, one would have predicted that cognitive anxiety should impair performance on the cognitively based tasks and physiological arousal/somatic anxiety should impair performance on the physiological and motor-based tasks. However, it is clear that the results which have been described in the preceding sections are not that straight-forward. This is illustrated by physiological arousal/somatic anxiety being associated with decrements in letter span (Parfitt and Hardy, 1987; Parfitt, 1988), a working memory task, while cognitive anxiety was associated with enhanced rebound

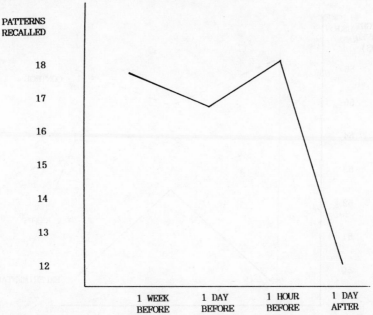

Figure 3.3. Mean pattern search scores of hockey players at various times before and after an important hockey match.

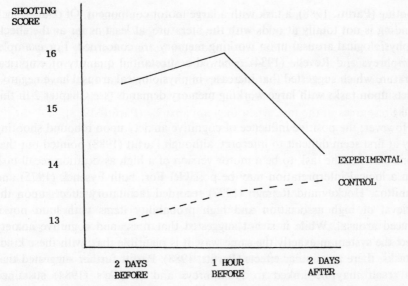

Figure 3.4. Mean rebound shooting scores for the control and experimental groups.

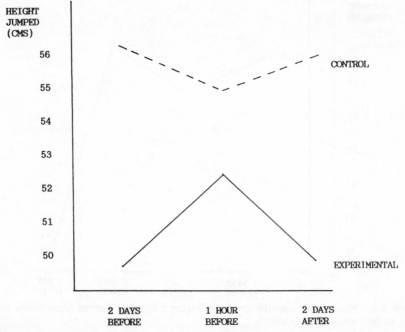

Figure 3.5.   Mean Sargent jump performance scores for the control and experimental groups.

shooting (Parfitt, 1988), a task with a large motor component. Of course, such a finding is not totally at odds with the literature, at least as far as the effects of physiological arousal upon working memory are concerned. For example, Humphreys and Revelle (1984) reviewed a substantial quantity of empirical literature which suggested that increases in physiological arousal have negative effects upon tasks with large working memory demands (see Chapter 2 in this book).

However, the positive influence of cognitive anxiety upon rebound shooting may at first seem difficult to interpret, although Parfitt (1988) pointed out that if one assumes the task to be a motor version of a high association recall task then a logical interpretation may be possible. For, both Eysenck (1975) and Hamilton, Hockey and Rejman (1977) recorded facilitatory effects upon the retrieval of high association and high probability items with loud noise-induced arousal. While it is not suggested that noise and cognitive anxiety affect the system in exactly the same way, it is plausible that, with these kinds of tasks, there are similar effects (Parfitt, 1988). Parfitt further suggested that this result may be linked to Humphreys and Revelle's (1984) sustained information transfer (SIT) tasks since rebound shooting, retrieval of high association items and retrieval of high probability items all have a substantial

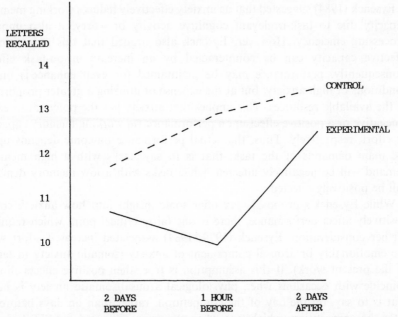

Figure 3.6. Mean letter span performance scores for the control and experimental groups.

element of information transfer. It is pointed out, however, that suggesting this link does oppose Humphreys and Revelle's prediction for negative effects of anxiety upon SIT performance. Perhaps achievement motivation and state anxiety should interact in Humphreys and Revelle's model in such a way that subjects who perceive the experimental task to be relevant to the source of the stress are motivated by anxiety to invest extra effort in it (cf. Dornic, 1977; Eysenck, 1979; Kahneman, 1973), thereby improving SIT performance on situationally relevant tasks. This argument is further supported by Parfitt and Hardy (1987), where situationally relevant SIT criterion tasks (critical flicker fusion and pattern search) were also reported to be positively affected by cognitive anxiety.

Eysenck (1979, 1984) has suggested that this type of positive anxiety effect is a result of effort serving as a compensatory factor that increases the attentional resources allocated to the task. The theoretical relationship proposed by Eysenck (1984) was described in Chapter 2 in this book. It is governed by two functions: 'processing effectiveness' and 'performance efficiency'. Eysenck used the term 'effectiveness' to refer to the quality of performance, and the term 'efficiency' to refer to the amount of effort required to achieve that quality of performance: that is to say, processing efficiency = performance effectiveness/effort.

Eysenck (1984) suggested that as anxiety effectively reduces working memory capacity due to task-irrelevant cognitive activity or worry, it also impairs processing efficiency. However, Eysenck also argued that this reduction in effective capacity can be counteracted by an increase in on-task effort. Consequently, performance may be maintained (or even enhanced) under conditions of high anxiety, but at the expense of utilizing a greater proportion of the available resources. This implies that anxiety has the potential to exert a negative or a positive effect upon performance *via* working memory capacity or effort, respectively. Thus, the actual performance outcome depends upon the main demands of the task: that is to say, tasks with a high memory demand will be negatively affected, while tasks with a low memory demand will be positively affected.

While Eysenck's proposal may offer some insight into how anxiety could positively affect performance, there is one fairly critical point which requires further consideration. Eysenck (1979, 1984) associated increased effort with the emotionality or arousal component of anxiety (somatic anxiety in terms of the present work). If this assumption is true, then positive effects should coincide with occasions when physiological arousal/somatic anxiety is high: that is to say, on the day of the competition, rather than on days before or after the competition, which was when they were recorded for SIT tasks in Parfitt and Hardy (1987) and Parfitt (1988).

Although the arguments which have been proposed here tend to implicate an attentional allocation explanation of the effects of cognitive anxiety upon performance, one can identify at least some evidence which suggests that somatic anxiety/physiological arousal may exert its influence upon perform-ance *via* capacity effects. For, in the letter span task (Parfitt and Hardy, 1987; Parfitt, 1988) performance was negatively affected by physiological arousal/ somatic anxiety even though the subjects were motivated to perform the task. Indeed, when Parfitt (1988) asked subjects to rate the relevance of each task prior to performing it, subjects indicated that immediately before the compe-tition they perceived the letter span task to be more relevant than at any other time. Thus, assuming that resources are allocated to tasks which are perceived to be relevant, subjects must have presumably reached the limit of their resources for the task to be negatively affected on this day.

Parfitt (1988) suggested that the argument for a capacity effect upon working memory is further enhanced by considering one of the components of working memory, the articulatory loop. Baddeley and Hitch (1974) described the articulatory loop as a transient store which facilitates the rehearsal of a limited amount of information, namely three chunks. Furthermore, the articulatory loop is thought to be a time-based system (Eysenck, 1982) which anxiety-induced arousal may speed up, thereby inducing a speed–accuracy trade-off (Baddeley, 1986, personal communication; Parfitt, 1988).

The above suggestion that the physiological arousal/somatic anxiety response exerts some effect upon attentional capacity can also be linked to Broadbent's (1971) model. As described earlier (Chapter 2 in this book), Broadbent's model comprises a lower mechanism which could be influenced by physiological arousal and which affects the availability of resources, together with an upper mechanism which controls the allocation of available resources based upon performance demands. Such a model could cope with the proposal that physiological arousal/somatic anxiety influences availability or capacity, while cognitive anxiety influences the allocation of resources based upon performance demands. In line with this, it would seem reasonable to suggest that when the time comes to allocate resources, those tasks which are perceived to be relevant have processing capacity invested in them, while those which are not perceived to be relevant do not. The results of the Sargent jump task (Parfitt, 1988) appear to provide an example of such an effect. In two experiments (one with basketball players and the other with volleyball players), Sargent jump was found to be significantly enhanced immediately before the competition when the subjects had been given priming instructions for the task. However, in a pilot experiment, when priming instructions were not given, basketball subject's performance did not change significantly (Parfitt, 1988). This would suggest that in the first two experiments resources were allocated to the task, whereas in the third experiment the resources were not allocated.

In summary, when the time-to-event paradigm has been used to investigate the effects of cognitive and somatic anxiety upon situationally relevant criterion tasks, positive effects have been associated with cognitive anxiety, while both positive and negative effects have been associated with somatic anxiety. It has also been argued that these results are best explained *via* resource allocation and attentional capacity effects.

A CRITIQUE OF ANXIETY–PERFORMANCE PARADIGMS

This section discusses the experimental designs and methods of analysis which have been used to examine the relationships that may exist between different components of anxiety and subcomponents of performance.

Criticisms of the manipulations and analyses used

One inherent weakness in the time-to-event design is that it does not differentiate between positive physiological arousal/somatic anxiety effects and interactions between cognitive anxiety and practice. For example, it is possible that cognitive anxiety and practice interact in such a way that performance is significantly improved immediately before the event. Using the present paradigm, such a change would be attributed to physiological arousal/somatic anxiety, rather than to cognitive anxiety and practice. The probability of this sort of confounding actually being responsible for observed effects is clearly much lower when one obtains negative effects upon performance on the day of a major event. Furthermore, the problem could be overcome by having subjects overlearn the task, but in most of the experiments reported above subjects received only one familiarization session at most. In spite of this shortcoming, the design could still be argued to be stronger than the correlational designs that have been traditionally used to investigate the effects of anxiety upon performance. It does at least manipulate the different components of anxiety, rather than simply measure whatever anxiety is present at the time of testing.

This criticism of correlation analysis was mentioned earlier in the chapter. To recap, the lack of agreement between research which has employed a correlational 'on the day' type of paradigm and that which has employed a time-to-event paradigm to manipulate anxiety was discussed as being partly due to the type of analysis used. For, as Parfitt (1988) has pointed out, correlational analysis provides information about the person-by-situation interaction, while analysis of variance, or other similar group effect analyses, provide information about situational main effects. A hypothetical description of the possible effects of cognitive anxiety upon performance may clarify the importance of this distinction. Suppose that small amounts of cognitive anxiety (worry) lead to concern about the task at hand and therefore motivate subjects to enhanced performance, while large amounts of cognitive anxiety lead to self-doubt and divided attention and therefore have an adverse effect upon performance. Then subjects with low or moderate levels of cognitive anxiety would be expected to show enhanced performance, while subjects with high levels of cognitive anxiety would be expected to get worse. Group performance could therefore improve overall (i.e. a positive effect), while a negative correlation could be simultaneously recorded. Figure 3.7 illustrates results which would lead to a negative correlation between cognitive anxiety and performance but a positive (main) effect for cognitive anxiety upon performance.

Such an explanation would suggest that these analyses offer complementary, rather than contradictory, information about the situation. Based upon this line of reasoning, Parfitt (1988) calculated partial correlation coefficients from her 'immediately before competition' data between cognitive anxiety and the criterion tasks (with somatic anxiety partialled out) and between somatic anxiety and the criterion tasks (with cognitive anxiety partialled out). Partial, rather than first-order, correlations were used in order to obtain a clearer indication of the influence of the different anxiety components upon performance (Deffenbacher, 1980).

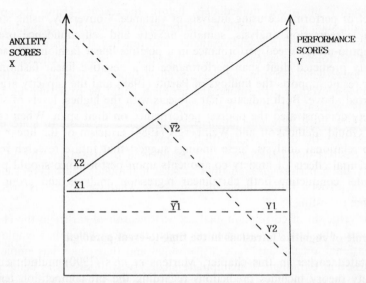

Figure 3.7. Performance results which could lead to the conclusion of cognitive anxiety having either a positive or a negative effect, depending on the analysis used. X1, cognitive anxiety baseline; X2, cognitive anxiety in a stressful environment; Y1, performance baseline; Y2, performance in a stressful environment; $\overline{Y1}$, mean performance in baseline condition; $\overline{Y2}$, mean performance in a stressful environment condition.

Perhaps the most striking thing about these partial correlations was their general lack of significance. One obvious reason for this lack of significance was the small number of subjects on which the correlations were based ($n = 16$). Furthermore, with such a large number of tests of significance there was also a considerable chance of committing a type I error. Consequently, even, significant correlations had to be interpreted with great caution. However, with one or two exceptions (notably letter span), the general trend of the correlations was not greatly at odds with those presented by Morris et al. (1975) in that the cognitive anxiety correlations were generally larger and more negative than the somatic anxiety correlations. Coupled with the positive group effects reported earlier for cognitive anxiety, this finding suggests that the 'explanation' shown in Figure 3.7 may well be a perfectly reasonable one which is worthy of further investigation.

Jones and Cale's (1989a) study also utilized two types of analysis: analysis of variance and stepwise multiple linear regression analysis. Their results support the argument that conducting different analyses can lead to different conclusions. For example, as described earlier, performance on a perceptuo-motor speed task significantly improved 20 minutes before the competition, and was accompanied by an increase in somatic anxiety. However, neither self-confidence nor cognitive anxiety could be shown to be related to any aspect of performance using analysis of variance. Conversely, using stepwise multiple regression analysis, somatic anxiety and self-confidence predicted perceptuo-motor speed performance in a positive linear fashion, and somatic anxiety predicted digit span performance in a negative linear fashion. This latter result supports the findings of Parfitt (1988) and the capacity argument reported above. Both indicate that subjects with the highest levels of somatic anxiety demonstrated the poorest performance on digit span. When coupled with Gould, Petlichkoff and Weinberg's (1984) criticism of the linear nature of correlational analysis, these findings suggest that future research into the differential effects of anxiety components upon performance should perhaps consider conducting both curvilinear regression analyses and group mean analyses.

The role of cognitive intrusions in the time-to-event paradigm

As stated earlier in this chapter, Martens *et al.*'s (1990) multidimensional anxiety theory includes predictions regarding the pre-competition temporal patterning of the anxiety components. Several studies (e.g. Jones and Cale, 1989a; Parfitt and Hardy, 1987) which have examined the relationship between the different components of anxiety and performance have used the time-to-event paradigm to manipulate cognitive and somatic anxiety. The time-to-event paradigm is, however, based on a somewhat limited measurement of anxiety. For example, consider cognitive anxiety, which is predicted to remain constant during the period leading up to competition. The items which comprise the cognitive anxiety subscale of the CSAI-2 include statements such as 'I am concerned about this competition', 'I am worried about reaching my goal' and 'I am concerned about performing poorly', with responses ranging from 'Not at all' to 'Very much so'. Predictions concerning the temporal patterning of cognitive anxiety suggest that responses should be the same on this subscale at, for example, both one week before and two hours before the competition in question. The responses to such items essentially represent the 'intensity' of cognitive anxiety symptoms, but another potential factor not considered is the 'frequency' with which the symptoms occur (Jones, in press). So the same score for cognitive anxiety on both occasions may represent the same intensity of the response, but does it actually represent the same cognitive state on both occasions? It is argued that cognitions regarding the upcoming competition may well be of the same intensity level but occur less frequently one week before than at two hours before. Consequently, even if cognitive anxiety intensity scores are the same on both occasions, the frequency of 'cognitive intrusions' (conceived of in terms of the proportion of time which such cognitions about the competition occupy an individual's thoughts) could well be much greater at two hours than at one week before the competition.

A further factor to consider concerns the 'direction' of the cognitive intrusions. In this context, direction refers to the nature of the competition-related cognitions: are they positively or negatively orientated? For example, one individual's cognitive intrusions might be positively orientated in the form of, say, anticipatory excitement, while another individual's cognitive intrusions might be negatively orientated in the form of images of failure. Yet another individual's cognitive intrusions might change from positive to negative, or *vice versa*, as the competition nears. Consequently, it is argued that the competitive state anxiety response may be much more complex than the sport psychology literature would suggest. The notions of intensity, frequency and direction of cognitive intrusions have potentially important implications for the use of the time-to-event paradigm. In particular, they raise a question about whether or not the same intensity of anxiety (reported on different occasions) can be assumed to represent the same state.

Practical implications

It would seem clear from the evidence which has been presented in this chapter that different components of anxiety are associated with differential effects upon certain subcomponents of performance. It is also clear from this research that, contrary to previous findings (e.g. Morris, Harris and Rovins, 1981), cognitive anxiety is not the only component of anxiety to influence performance. Neither is this influence always the negative one that is predicted by Wine's (1971) distraction hypothesis or Davidson and Schwartz's (1976) channel-blocking hypothesis. Nevertheless, it could still be argued that cognitive anxiety is the primary influence upon performance (Morris, Harris and Rovins, 1981) even though it is not the only influence, since it is possible that cognitive anxiety determines the effect which 'on-the-day' physiological arousal/somatic anxiety has upon performance. This statement will be clarified in Chapter 4 in this book in which Hardy and Fazey's (1987) catastrophe model of performance and anxiety is discussed. This model describes cognitive anxiety as a splitting factor which determines the precise nature of physiological arousal effects upon performance.

Clearly, ways of coping with either the cognitive or somatic components of anxiety are desirable if performance is detrimentally affected by them. Deffenbacher (1980) suggested that because cognitive anxiety:

> is elevated several days prior to examinations, cognitive restructuring programmes should be tailored to the pre-examination period as well as the task taking period itself;

while to accommodate physiological arousal:

relaxation might be cued most productively near the beginning of the exam. p. 125)

These recommendations were made with respect to coping with test anxiety, but the same principle could be applied to the sports context provided that it was established that performance was negatively affected by the anxiety component in question. Clearly, it would be inappropriate to reduce anxiety if it was having a positive effect upon performance. Indeed, it is worth noting that research which has employed the time-to-event paradigm has so far failed to find any negative group effects associated with cognitive anxiety.

In order to determine whether or not different aspects of a performer's 'game' were being disrupted by anxiety, it would clearly be necessary to perform some sort of 'match' analysis. Match analysis is a technique which provides coaches with objective data about different aspects of a player's performance during a competition. For example, a match analysis of a basketball match could include how many times a particular player drove at the basket, how many baskets the player scored, how many baskets the player missed, how many times the player 'stole' possession. Originally, paper and pencil techniques were used to record this information, but more recently sophisticated computer programmes which are operated by skilled analysts have been developed (Hughes, 1985).

Unfortunately, none of these match analysis systems seems to be based upon the cognitive and motor demands of performance. Rather, they tend to be construed somewhat atheoretically on the basis of coaches' intuitive requests. The present research would imply that it might be more meaningful to first of all identify the cognitive and motor subcomponents which underlie performance and then examine them in a match situation. While it is difficult to see how such fundamental aspects of performance could be measured objectively, match analysis does seem to provide a quasi-objective means of measuring them *in vivo*, or *via* video replay.

Although the present research suggests the possibility of patterns of dissociation across groups of subjects, it also seems likely that individual differences will play an important part in determining which aspects of performance are most likely to be disrupted. Table 3.1 illustrates some aspects of performance which the present and previous research (for example Baddeley and Idzikowski, 1985; Hammerton and Tickner, 1968; Humphreys and Revelle, 1984) suggests are likely to be disrupted by competitive anxiety in basketball performance. If these aspects of performance were scored for individual performers during a competition, it might be possible to obtain more specific information about precisely which aspects of their performance were negatively and positively affected. This technique would enable the specific strengths and weaknesses of

Table 3.1 The type of processes and their expected effects upon performance in basketball.

Process	Effect	Example
Perception	Attentional narrowing (Hammerton and Tickner, 1968), and selectivity leading to hyperdistractability (Deffenbacher, 1978)	Tunnel vision and ball watching leading to: failure to see free players (own and opposition); distraction by refereeing decisions niggling and self-distracting
Working memory or short-term memory	Impaired working memory with large memory loads (Humphreys and Revelle, 1984; Jones and Cale, 1989a; Parfitt, 1988)	Time penalties in attacking key. Slow to release early balls when there is a choice of passes. Failure to drive at the basket when there is a space
Long-term recall	Impaired for difficult tasks? Improved for easy tasks— rebound shooting (Parfitt, 1988)	Failed critical set shot. Accurate rebound shooting
Anaerobic power	Enhanced in simple tasks— Sargent jump (Parfitt, 1988)	Good height on backboard defending
Manual dexterity	Impaired (Baddeley and Idzikowski, 1985)	Poor ball handling under pressure
Fine control	Impaired, e.g. pursuit rotor (Matarazzo and Matarazzo, 1956)	Failed lay-ups. lack of touch
Dynamic balance	Unknown	Clumsy challenges in the air. 'Flat-footed' defending

an individual to be identified and, given appropriate technical support, suitable training programmes to be developed to overcome weaknesses.

The research which has been discussed in this chapter is still somewhat limited in scope, so that it is difficult to recommend specific intervention strategies. However, assuming that negative performance effects are caused by insufficient resources being allocated to the task, then one strategy could be to develop skills which would help to ensure that all available resources were being appropriately allocated. For example, as Jones and Hardy (1989) have indicated, in order to counter deficits in working memory one could use dual-task paradigms to train performers to make relevant decisions while under physical stress. Indeed, recent research by Guttman (1987) and Kuhn (1987) has shown that such paradigms do differentiate between elite and non-elite performers. Alternatively, distraction training (Schmid and Peper, 1983) or other attention control strategies (Hardy and Nelson, 1988) could be used to reduce the hyperdistractability which is often associated with high levels of anxiety (Eysenck, 1982). For example, relevant distractions such as other performers, bad refereeing decisions, 'niggling' opponents, etc., could be gradually introduced to desensitize performers to them. Other intervention strategies and psychological skills which could possibly be used to overcome such performance problems will be discussed in the second section of this book.

FUTURE DIRECTIONS FOR RESEARCH

This is clearly a very under-developed area of research which is in need of further exploration. Questions which are of theoretical interest abound, including the *in vivo* assessment of performance subcomponents in anxious subjects, as well as the roles of attentional capacity, effort, and the allocation of resources in any anxiety effects upon performance (see Chapter 4 in this book). However, underpinning all these questions and many others is the need to develop new paradigms for examining the effects of anxiety upon performance. Current research has undoubtedly been handicapped by the reluctance of researchers to explore beyond the inverted-U hypothesis in the field, or beyond verbal memory in the laboratory. What are needed are some radically new ways of looking at the problem. The following sections outline three areas which are particularly worthy of such investigation.

Antecedents of anxiety

Considering that a relatively large amount of research has been conducted using the CSAI-2, the detailed identification of factors which elicit cognitive anxiety, somatic anxiety and self-confidence responses during the pre-competition period has received relatively little research attention. This is particularly surprising in view of the fact that such information could prove valuable in the prevention and control of debilitating levels of anxiety. Martens *et al.* (1990) hypothesized that the antecedents of both cognitive anxiety and self-confidence are those factors in the environment which are related to the athlete's expectations of success. These include perception of one's own and opponent's ability (Gould, Petlichkoff and Weinberg, 1984; Martens *et al.*, 1990). Conversely, cues which elicit elevated somatic anxiety are thought to be non-evaluative, of shorter duration and consist mainly of conditioned responses to environmental stimuli (Morris, Harris and Rovins, 1981). In the sporting context, these might include changing room preparation and pre-competition warm-up routines (Gould, Petlichkoff and Weinberg, 1984; Martens *et al.*, 1990).

Gould, Petlichkoff and Weinberg (1984) reported that the CSAI-2 subscales were found to have different antecedents, although precise predictions by Martens *et al.* (1990) were not supported. Gould and colleagues' study involved 37 intercollegiate wrestlers who were administered the CSAI-2 immediately prior to two different competitions. The antecedents considered were competitive trait anxiety (as measured by SCAT; Martens, 1977), perceived ability, wrestling success and past experience. The results showed that no single antecedent was related to all three of the CSAI-2 components. However, the strongest predictor of cognitive anxiety was found to be 'years experience', which was established by ascertaining the competitors' intercollegiate varsity experience and the age at which they began wrestling. This relationship was negative in that performers with more experience reported less cognitive anxiety. On the other hand, perceived ability was strongly related to the CSAI-2 self-confidence component but showed little relationship to the cognitive and somatic anxiety components. The only significant predictor of somatic anxiety was SCAT.

More recently, Jones, Swain and Cale (1990) have investigated the antecedents of the CSAI-2 components in more detail. They developed a Pre-Race Questionnaire (PRQ) which they then administered to elite student middle-distance runners. When factor analysed, the PRQ was found to be composed of five different factors: perceived readiness, attitude towards previous performance, position goal, coach influence and external environment. The PRQ, along with the CSAI-2, was administered to a sample of 125 runners one hour before a race. Separate stepwise mutliple regression analyses were performed to ascertain which of the five PRQ factors best predicted each of the CSAI-2 components. The results showed cognitive anxiety to be predicted by perceived readiness, attitude towards previous performance and position goal. In the case of position goal as a predictor, cognitive anxiety was positively related to the difficulty of the goal which had been set and negatively related to the athlete's perception of whether he could achieve the goal. This finding indicates the possibility of an interesting relationship between goal setting and anxiety which has received very little research attention (see Hardy, Maiden and Sherry, 1986; and Chapter 6 in this book by Beggs). Furthermore, Cale and Jones (1989) have recently reported findings suggesting that goal difficulty is an important determinant of both cognitive anxiety and self-confidence, although position goal was not significantly related to self-confidence in Jones, Swain and Cale's (1990) study.

The major predictor of self-confidence was perceived readiness, with external environment also contributing significantly to this prediction. This helps to explain the results which have been recorded showing self-confidence to dissociate from cognitive anxiety some parts of the time but not others (Barnes *et al.*, 1986; Jones, Cale and Kerwin, 1988; Parfitt, 1988) as well as Martens and colleagues' proposal that performance expectations are antecedents of both cognitive anxiety and self-confidence. More precisely, the results suggest that cognitive anxiety and self-confidence share some common antecedents which contribute to performance expectations but that there are also factors which may be unique to each. Somatic anxiety was not predicted by any of the PRQ factors. This is perhaps not surprising since none of the PRQ factors related to conditioned pre-race stimuli. However, it is also worth noting that during the development of the questionnaire, runners did not identify such stimuli as contributing to how they felt one hour before a race.

At an applied level, these results clearly indicate the important role that the coach plays in the performer's competition preparation and, in particular, the performer's perceived readiness. The coach can either help to increase cognitive anxiety and reduce self-confidence by contributing to the performers' belief and perception that they are not 'ready', or else reduce cognitive anxiety and increase self-confidence by helping the performer perceive that he/she *is* 'ready'.

The study by Jones, Swain and Cale (1990) was exploratory in nature and investigated a specific population, but it is likely that further detailed studies of this nature with other populations would aid our understanding at a theoretical level, as well as providing knowledge of more practical significance, to enhance the mental preparation of sports performers. It is also worth noting that Jones, Swain and Cale (in press) have reported findings which indicate that different factors may predict multidimensional anxiety and self-confidence in males and females. This study examined predictors of CSAI-2 components in a sample of male and female athletes from a variety of sports one week, two days, one day, two hours and within 30 minutes prior to the start of the subjects' various matches. The results generally supported Gill's (1988) proposal that females focus more on personal goals and standards, whereas males focus more on interpersonal comparison and winning. The major predictors of cognitive anxiety and self-confidence in females were the importance of doing well personally in the match and perceived mental and physical readiness. On the other hand, in the males, cognitive anxiety and self-confidence were mainly predicted by the extent to which subjects thought that they would win, together with their perception of their opponents' ability in relation to their own. These are interesting differences and are, together with the whole anxiety antecedents area, worthy of greater research attention.

Intensity, frequency and direction of cognitive intrusions

The notion of cognitive intrusions relating to specific competitions raises several issues regarding the precise nature of the competitive state anxiety response. It is important to recognize that anxiety as measured by the CSAI-

2 represents only the intensity of the particular anxiety symptoms or cognitive intrusions. Although this approach has helped to advance knowledge of competitive state anxiety, it is very unlikely that it provides a complete picture. Rather, it can be argued that at least two other factors deserve careful consideration: frequency and direction of cognitive intrusions. To recap, these refer to the frequency with which cognitive intrusions occur and the nature of these intrusions, respectively. While consideration of these additional dimensions of the anxiety response is likely to create a much more detailed and complex theoretical and research framework, it also has great potential in the quest for greater knowledge and understanding of competitive state anxiety.

This approach clearly requires a re-examination of such measurement instruments as the CSAI-2 with a view to measuring not only the intensity, but also the frequency and direction of cognitive intrusions. Another possible approach is the study of athletes' experiences in a qualitative manner. In-depth interviews would provide valuable additional information when viewed in conjunction with quantitative data acquired *via* questionnaires. Indeed, Gould and Krane (in press) have commented on the lack of such an approach. In emphasizing the strengths of in-depth interviews with athletes, Gould and Krane advocated that anxiety–performance researchers would do well to use such an approach.

Perceptions of anxiety

As described earlier, some recent findings have shown that competitive anxiety does not necessarily debilitate performance and can actually facilitate it (e.g. Jones and Cale, 1989a; Parfitt, 1988; Parfitt and Hardy, 1987). Furthermore, Mahoney and Avener (1977) reported that successful gymnasts tended to use their anxiety as a stimulant to better performance, while less successful gymnasts seemed to arouse themselves to near panic states by self-doubting verbalization and images of failure. This suggests that anxiety may be perceived and labelled as either debilitative or facilitative to performance (see also Hollandsworth et al., 1979). As described earlier in this chapter, the notion of positive and negative dimensions of anxiety has received support from a number of studies (e.g. Hardy and Whitehead, 1984; Mackay et al., 1978; Thayer, 1978). It is perhaps rather surprising, therefore, that individuals' perceptions of their competitive state anxiety responses have received very little research attention within the sport psychology literature, and in the context of the CSAI-2 in particular. For example, do two individuals with the same score on the somatic anxiety subscale of the CSAI-2 perceive that 'anxiety' in the same way? And do individuals who perceive their anxiety differently perform differently? Clearly, in an age of 'cognitive sport psychology' this aspect of competitive anxiety almost demands research attention.

REFERENCES

Adams, A. J. (1983). On integration of the verbal and motor domains, in R. A. Magill (ed.) *Memory and the Control of Action.* Amsterdam: North Holland.

Baddeley, A. D. (1966). Influence of depth on the manual dexterity of free divers: a comparison between open sea and pressure chamber testing, *Journal of Applied Psychology*, **50**, 81–85.

Baddeley, A. D. and Hitch, G. (1974). Working memory, in G. H. Bower (ed.). *The Psychology of Learning and Motivation: Advances in Research and Theory.* London: Academic Press.

Baddeley, A. D. and Idzikowski, C. (1985). Anxiety, manual dexterity and diver performance, *Ergonomics*, **28**, 1475–1482.

Barnes, M. W., Sime, W., Dienstbier, R. and Plake, B. (1986). A test of construct validity of the CSAI-2 questionnaire on male elite college swimmers, *International Journal of Sport Psychology*, **17**, 364–74.

Blake, M. J. F. (1967). Time of day effects on performance in a range of tasks, *Psychonomic Science*, **9**, 349–350.

Borkovec, T. D. (1976). Physiological and cognitive processes in the regulation of anxiety, in G. E. Schwartz and D. Shapiro (eds). *Consciousness and Self-Regulation: Advances in Reserach I.* New York: Plenum Press.

Broadbent, D. E. (1971). *Decision and Stress.* London: Academic Press.

Burton, D. (1988). Do anxious swimmers swim slower? Reexamining the elusive anxiety–performance relationship, *Journal of Sport and Exercise Psychology*, **10**, 45–61.

Buss, A. H. (1962). Critique and notes: two anxiety factors in psychiatric patients, *Journal of Abnormal and Social Psychology*, **65**, 426–427.

Cale, A and Jones, J. G. (1989). Relationship between expectations of success, multidimensional anxiety and perceptuo-motor performance. Paper presented at the Annual Conference of the North American Society for the Psychology of Sport and Physical Activity, Kent State University, Ohio, USA, June.

Davidson, R. J. and Schwartz, G. E. (1976). The psychobiology of relaxation and related states: a multiprocess theory, in D. I. Mostofsky (ed.). *Behaviour Control and Modification of Physiological Activity.* Englewood Cliffs, NJ: Prentice Hall.

Deffenbacher, J. L. (1978). Worry, emotionality, and task-generated interference in test anxiety: an empirical test of attentional theory, *Journal of Educational Psychology*, **70**, 248–254.

Deffenbacher, J. L. (1980). Worry and emotionality in test anxiety, in I. G. Sarason (ed.). *Test Anxiety: Theory, Research and Applications.* Hillsdale, NJ: Erlbaum.

Doctor, R. M. and Altman, F. (1969). Worry and emotionality as components of test anxiety: replication and further data, *Psychological Reports*, **24**, 563–568.

Dornic, S. (1977). Mental load, effort, and individual differences. Report No. 509, Department of Psychology, University of Stockholm.

Eysenck, M. W. (1975). Effects of noise, activation level, and response dominance in retrieval from semantic memory, *Journal of Applied Psychology*, **69**, 69–78.

Eysenck, M. W. (1979). Anxiety, learning and memory: A reconceptualization, *Journal of Research in Personality*, **13**, 363–385.

Eysenck, M. W. (1982). *Attention and Arousal: Cognition and Performance.* Berlin: Springer-Verlag.

Eysenck, M. W. (1984). *A Handbook of Cognitive Psychology.* London: Erlbaum.

Fenz, W. D. and Epstein, S. (1967). Gradients of physiological arousal in parachutists as a funtion of an approaching jump, *Psychosomatic Medicine*, **29**, 33–51.

Fenz, W. D. and Epstein, S. (1968). Specific and general inhibitory reactions associated with mastery of stress, *Journal of Experimental Psychology*, **77**, 52–56.

Gill, D. L. (1988). Gender differences in competitive orientation and sport participation, *International Journal of Sport Psychology*, **19**, 145–159.

Goolkasian, P. (1982). Test anxiety and its effects on the speed–accuracy trade-off function, *Bulletin of the Psychonomic Society*, **19**, 133–136.

Gould, D. and Krane, V. (in press). The arousal–athletic performance relationship: current status and future direction, in T. Horn (ed.). *Advances in Sport Psychology*. Champaign, Illinois: Human Kinetics.

Gould, D., Petlichkoff, L. and Weinberg, R. S. (1984). Antecedents of, temporal changes in, and relationships between CSAI-2 subcomponents, *Journal of Sport Psychology*, **6**, 289–304.

Gould, D., Petlichkoff, L., Simons, J. and Vevera, M. (1987). Relationship between Competitive State Anxiety Inventory-2 subscale scores and pistol shooting performance, *Journal of Sport Psychology*, **9**, 33–42.

Guttman, G. (1987). Emotions and their correlations with cognitions and performance. Paper presented at the 7th European Congress on Sport Psychology, Badblankenburg, DDR, Spetember.

Hammerton, M. and Tickner, A. H. (1968). An investigation into the effects of stress upon skilled performance, *Ergonomics*, **12**, 851–855.

Hamilton, M. (1959). The assessment of anxiety states by rating, *British Journal of Medical Psychology*, **32**, 50–55.

Hamilton, P., Hockey, G. R. J. and Rejman, M. (1977). The place of the concept of activation in human information processing theory: an integrative approach, in S. Dornic (ed.). *Attention and Performance*: 6, Hillsdale, NJ: Erlbaum.

Hardy, L. and Fazey, J. F. (1987). The inverted-U hypothesis—a catastrophe for sport psychology. Paper presented at the Annual Conference of the North American Society for Psychology of Sport and Physical Activity, Vancouver, June.

Hardy, L., Maiden, D. and Sherry, K. (1986). Goal setting and performance anxiety, *Journal of Sports Sciences*, **4**, 233–234.

Hardy, L. and Nelson, D. (1988). Self-regulation training in sport and work, *Ergonomics*, **31**, 1573–1585.

Hardy, L. and Whitehead, R. (1984). Specific modes of anxiety and arousal, *Current Psychological Research and Reviews*, **3**, 14–24.

Herbert, M., Johns, W. and Dore, C. (1976). Factor analysis of the analogue scales measuring subjective feelings before and after sleep. *British Journal of Medical Psychology*, **49**, 373–379.

Hockey, G. R. J., Coles, M. G. H. and Gaillard, A. W. K. (1986). Energetical issues in research on human information processing, in G. R. J. Hockey, A. W. K. Gaillard and M. G. H. Coles (eds). *Energetics and Human Information Processing*. Dordrecht, The Netherlands: Martinus Nijhoff.

Hockey, G. R. J. and Hamilton, P. (1983). The cognitive patterning of stress states, in G. R. J. Hockey (ed.). *Stress and Fatigue in Human Performance*. Chichester: Wiley.

Hollandsworth, J. G., Glazeski, R. C., Kirkland, K., Jones, G. E. and Van Norman, L. R. (1979). An analysis of the nature and effects of test anxiety: cognitive, behavioural and physiological components, *Cognitive Therapy Research*, **3**, 165–180.

Holroyd, K. A., Westbrook, T., Wolf, M. and Badhorn, E. (1978). Performance, cognition, and physiological responding in test anxiety, *Journal of Abnormal Psychology*, **87**, 442–457.

Hughes, M. (1985). Using a microcomputer for notational analysis in squash, in D. Kidd *et al.* (eds). *Proceedings of Sport and Science Conference.* Bedford College of Higher Education.

Humphreys, M. S. and Revelle, W. (1984). Personality, motivation and performance: a theory of the relationship between individual differences and information processing, *Psychological Review,* **91,** 153–184.

Idzikowski, C. and Baddeley, A. D. (1983). Waiting in the wings: apprehension, public speaking and performance, *Ergonomics,* **26,** 575–583.

Idzikowski, C. and Baddeley, A. D. (1987). Fear and performance in novice parachutists, *Ergonomics,* **30,** 1463–1474.

Jones, J. G. (in press). Recent developments and current issues in competitive state anxiety research. *The Psychologist.*

Jones, J. G. and Cale, A. (1989a). Relationships between multidimensional competitive state anxiety and cognitive and motor subcomponents of performance, *Journal of Sports Sciences,* **7,** 129–140.

Jones, J. G. and Cale, A. (1989b). Precompetition temporal patterning of anxiety and self-confidence in males and females, *Journal of Sport Behavior,* **12,** 183–195.

Jones, J. G., Cale, A. and Kerwin, D. G. (1988). Multi-dimensional competitive state anxiety and psychomotor performance *Australian Journal of Science and Medicine in Sport,* **20,** 3–7.

Jones, J. G. and Hardy, L. (1989). Stress and cognitive functioning in sport. *Journal of Sports Sciences,* **6,** 41–63.

Jones, J. G., Swain, A. and Cale, A. (1990). Antecedents of multidimensional competitive state anxiety and self-confidence in elite intercollegiate middle-distance runners. *The Sport Psychologist,* **4,** 107–118.

Jones, J. G., Swain, A. and Cale, A. (in press). Gender differences in precompetition temporal patterning and antecedents of anxiety and self-confidence. *Journal of Sport and Exercise Psychology.*

Kahneman, D. (1973). *Attention and Effort.* Englewood Cliffs, NJ: Prentice Hall.

Kuhn, W. (1987). The dual task paradigm to diagnose tactical abilities in soccer. Paper presented at the International Conference on Sport, Leisure and Ergonomics, Burton Manor, Cheshire, UK, November.

Lacey, J. I. (1967). Somatic response patterning and stress: some revision of activation theory, in M. H. Appley and R. Trumbull (eds). *Psychological Stress: Issues in Research.* New York: Appleton-Century-Crofts.

Landers, D. M. and Boutcher, S. H. (1986). Arousal–performance relationships, in J. M. Williams (ed.). *Applied Sport Psychology: Personal Growth to Peak Performance.* Palo Alto, California: Mayfield.

Lewis, V. J. and Baddeley, A. D. (1981). Cognitive performance, sleep quality and mood during deep oxyhelium diving, *Ergonomics,* **24,** 773–793.

Liebert, R. M. and Morris, L. W. (1967). Cognitive and emotional components of test anxiety: A distinction and some initial data, *Psychological Reports,* **20,** 975–978.

Mackay, C., Cox, T., Burrows, G. and Lazzerini, T. (1978). An inventory for the measurement of self-reported stress and arousal, *British Journal of Social and Clinical Psychology,* **17,** 283–284.

Magnusson, D. (1974). The individual in the situation: some studies on individuals' perception of situations, *Studia Psychologica,* **16,** 124–132.

Magnusson, D. and Ekehammar, B. (1975). Perceptions of and reaction to stressful situations, *Journal of Personality and Social Psychology,* **31,** 1147–1154.

Mahoney, M. J. and Avener, M. (1977). Psychology of the elite athlete: an exploratory study, *Cognitive Research and Therapy,* **1,** 135–141.

Mandler, G. and Sarason, S. B. (1952). A study of anxiety and learning, *Journal of Abnormal Social Psychology*, **47**, 166–173.

Martens, R. (1977). *Sport Competition Anxiety Test*. Champaign, Illinois: Human Kinetics.

Martens, R., Burton, D., Rivkin, F. and Simon, J. (1980). Reliability and validity of the competitive state anxiety inventory (CSAI) in C. H. Nadeau, W. R. Halliwell, K. M. Newell and G. C. Roberts (eds). *Psychology of Motor Behavior and Sport— 1979*. Champaign, Illinois: Human Kinetics.

Martens, R., Burton, D., Vealey, R. S., Bump, L. A. and Smith, D. E. (1990). The Competitive State Anxiety Inventory-2 (CSAI-2), in R. Martens, R. S. Vealey and D. Burton (eds). *Competitive Anxiety in Sport*. Champaign, Illinois: Human Kinetics.

Matarazzo, R. G. and Matarazzo, J. D. (1956). Anxiety level and pursuitmeter performance, *Journal of Consulting Psychology*, **20**, 70.

Mears, J. D. and Cleary, P. J. (1980). Anxiety as a factor in underwater performance, *Ergonomics*, **23**, 549–557.

Mellstrom, M. Jr, Cicala, G. A. and Zuckerman, M. (1976). General versus specific trait anxiety measures in the prediction of fear of snakes, height, and darkness, *Journal of Consulting and Clinical Psychology*, **44**, 83–91.

Morris, L. W., Brown, N. R. and Halbert, B. (1977). Effects of symbolic modelling on the arousal of cognitive and affective components of anxiety in preschool children, in C. D. Spielberger and I. G. Sarason (eds). *Stress and Anxiety*, Vol 4. Washington, DC: Hemisphere.

Morris, L. W., Davis, M. A. and Hutchings, C. H. (1981). Cognitive and emotional components of anxiety: literature review and a revised worry–emotionality scale, *Journal of Educational Psychology*, **73**, 541–555.

Morris, L. W., Harris, E. W. and Rovins, D. S. (1981). Interactive effects of generalized and situational expectancies on the arousal of cognitive and emotional components of social anxiety, *Journal of Research in Personality*, **15**, 302–311.

Morris, L. W. and Liebert, R. N. (1969). The effects of anxiety on timed and untimed intelligence tests: another look, *Journal of Consulting and Clinical Psychology*, **33**, 240–244.

Morris, L. W. and Liebert, R. M. (1970). The relationship of cognitive and emotional components of test anxiety to physiological arousal and academic performance, *Journal of Consulting and Clinical Psychology*, **35**, 332–337.

Morris, L. W. and Liebert, R. M. (1973). Effects of negative feedback, threat of shock, and level of trait anxiety on the arousal of two components of anxiety, *Journal of Counseling Psychology*, **20**, 321–326.

Morris, L. W., Smith, L. R., Andrews, E. S. and Morris, N. C. (1975). The relationship of emotionality and worry components of anxiety to motor skill performance, *Journal of Motor Behaviour*, **7**, 121–130.

Parfitt, C. G. (1988). Interactions between models of stress and models of motor control. Unpublished PhD thesis, University of Wales, Bangor.

Parfitt, C. G. and Hardy, L. (1987). Further evidence for the differential effects of competitive anxiety upon a number of cognitive and motor sub-systems, *Journal of Sports Sciences*, **5**, 62–63.

Sarason, S. B., Davidson, K., Lighthall, F., Waite, F. and Ruebush, B. (1960). *Anxiety in Elementary School Children*. New York: Wiley.

Sassenrath, J. M. (1964). A factor analysis of rating-scale items on the test anxiety questionnaire, *Journal of Consulting Psychology*, **28**, 371–377.

Sassenrath, J. M., Kight, H. R. and Kaiser, H. F. (1965). Relating factors from anxiety scales between two samples, *Psychological Reports*, **17**, 407–416.

Schmid, A. B. and Peper, E. (1983). Do your thing when it counts, in L. E. Unestahl (ed.). *The Mental Aspects of Gymnastics*. Orebro, Sweden: Veje Publications.

Schwartz, G. E., Davidson, R. J. and Goleman, D. J. (1978). Patterning of cognitive and somatic processes in the self-regulation of anxiety: effects of meditation *versus* exercise, *Psychosomatic Medicine*, **40**, 321–328.

Segal, S. J. and Fusella, V. (1970). Influence of imaged pictures and sounds on detection of visual and auditory signals, *Journal of Experimental Psychology*, **83**, 458–464.

Smith, C. A. and Morris, L. W. (1977). Differential effects of stimulative and sedative music on two components of test anxiety, *Psychological Reports*, **41**, 1047–1053.

Sonstroem, R. J. and Bernardo, B. (1982). Intraindividual pregame state anxiety and basketball performance: a re-examination of the inverted-U curve, *Journal of Sport Psychology*, **4**, 235–245.

Spiegler, M. D., Morris, L. W. and Liebert, R. M. (1968). Cognitive and emotional components of test anxiety: temporal factors, *Psychological Reports*, **22**, 451–456.

Spielberger, C. D. (1966). The effects of anxiety on complex learning and academic achievement in C. D. Spielberger (ed.). *Anxiety and Behaviour*. London: Academic Press.

Straub, W. F. and Williams, J. H. (1984). Cognitive sport psychology: historical, contemporary and future issues, in W. F. Straub and J. M. Williams (eds). *Cognitive Sport Psychology*. Lansing, NY: Sport Science Associates.

Thayer, R. E. (1970). Activation states as assessed by verbal report and four psycho-physiological variables, *Psychophysiology*, **7**, 86–94.

Thayer, R. E. (1978). Toward a psychological theory of multidimensional activation (arousal), *Motivation and Emotion*, **2**, 1–34.

Ussher, M. H. and Hardy, L. (1986). The effect of competitive anxiety on a number of cognitive and motor sub-systems, *Journal of Sports Sciences*, **4**, 232–233.

Watson, D. and Friend, R. (1969). Social–evaluative anxiety, *Journal of Consulting and Clinical Psychology*, **33**, 448–457.

Wine, J. D. (1971). Test anxiety and direction of attention, *Psychological Bulletin*, **76**, 92–104.

Chapter 4

A catastrophe model of performance in sport

Lew Hardy
University of Wales, Bangor

Not unnaturally, the model of anxiety and performance that is presented in this chapter arose from a dissatisfaction with existing models of the anxiety–performance relationship. For example, the inverted-U hypothesis and multi-dimensional anxiety theory have already been criticized at several levels in this book (see Jones, Chapter 2, and Parfitt, Jones and Hardy, Chapter 3). However, it is perhaps worthwhile briefly reiterating some of these criticisms before proceeding.

THE INVERTED-U HYPOTHESIS AND AROUSAL THEORY

The inverted-U hypothesis originated from a study of habit strength formation in mice at different levels of punishment stimulus frequency (Yerkes and Dodson, 1908). However, following the work of Broadhurst (1957) and Oxendine (1970), it was commandeered to 'explain' the relationship between motivation (stress) and performance in terms of increases in 'arousal'. In this context, arousal was taken to be a unitary construct which embodied both the psychological and physiological response systems and reflected the potential energy available to the organism for release during subsequent behaviour. As has already been indicated (Jones, Chapter 2 in this book), this formulation of the inverted-U hypothesis can be criticized at several levels. First, there are difficulties with the basic concepts involved in the inverted-U hypothesis, since the hypothesis has on some occasions been described as *explaining* the relationship between arousal and performance, stress and performance, and anxiety and performance. On other occasions, the inverted-U hypothesis has simply been used as a *description* of the relationships which exist between these variables and performance. Furthermore, its use as a description of the

Stress and Performance in Sport. Edited by J. Graham Jones and Lew Hardy.
©1990 John Wiley & Sons Ltd.

nships between these variables and performance is clearly much less ntious than its use as an explanation of these relationships. Nevertheless, this use will still be criticized.

The sort of argument that is usually presented as an 'explanation' of the stress–performance relationship in terms of the inverted-U hypothesis is as follows. Moderate levels of stress lead to optimal levels of arousal which enhance performance, while high levels of stress lead to high levels of arousal which impede performance. While such a stimulus–response based 'explanation' may have been satisfactory in the halcyon days of behaviourism, it can hardly be considered appropriate in the post-cognitive revolution.

If the inverted-U hypothesis is to explain the stress–performance relationship, then supporting evidence needs to be produced which takes account of both the actual, and the perceived, demands of performance (Lazarus; 1966; Jones and Hardy, 1989). If it is to explain the relationship between anxiety and performance, then it should take at least some account of the different cognitive and somatic components of state anxiety which have been reported by several researchers (for example Hardy and Whitehead, 1984; Martens *et al.*, 1990; see Chapter 3 in this book by Parfitt, Jones and Hardy for a review). In both these cases, the arousal construct needs to be rigorously defined (Lacey, 1967; Eysenck, 1982) and causal evidence produced for any mediational role which it is assumed to play (Neiss, 1988). Furthermore, if arousal is assumed to mediate the stress–performance relationship, or the anxiety–performance relationship, then some explanation is also required about the role of cognition in these processes (see Chapter 2 by Jones in this book).

If the inverted-U hypothesis is simply a description of the relationship between stress and performance, then it does not seem to fit anecdotal evidence from the field of sport psychology which suggests that this relationship should not be symmetrical. As Hardy and Fazey (1987) pointed out, when performers 'go over the top' their performance usually drops dramatically rather than gradually; and once this has happened, it is very difficult to get performance back up to even a mediocre level. This seems to suggest that small reductions in stress/arousal/anxiety do not really make any difference to performance once this stage has been reached. However, the inverted-U hypothesis implies that performance should return to its optimal level with such an intervention.

MULTIDIMENSIONAL ANXIETY THEORY

Essentially, multidimensional anxiety theory (Martens *et al.*, 1990; Burton, 1988) argues that at least two different components can be distinguished in the anxiety response: a cognitive component associated with fear about the consequences of failure and a somatic component reflecting perceptions of the physiological response. The theory also argues that these different components have different antecedents and can be independently manipulated. For example, both Morris, Davis and Hutchings (1981) and Martens *et al.* (1990) have argued that somatic anxiety is a conditioned response to entering the performing environment, which should therefore dissipate once performance commences. They have also argued that since cognitive anxiety reflects concerns about the consequences of failure, it should only change when the subjective probability of success changes.

On the basis of these arguments, Martens *et al.* (1990) predicted that cognitive anxiety should remain stable and high throughout the period preceding an important event, while somatic anxiety should peak late and fast on arrival at the site of the competition. Furthermore, Martens *et al.* produced results which supported both of these predictions, although it should be pointed out that this finding had been previously obtained in the context of test anxiety by Spiegler, Morris and Liebert in 1968. Nevertheless, the finding appears to be a very reliable one and has now been replicated on a number of occasions. Later studies have also shown that physiological arousal (as measured by heart rate) follows the same time course as somatic anxiety (see Chapter 3 in this book for a review).

Martens *et al.*'s other prediction was that cognitive anxiety would be the principal influence upon performance, because somatic anxiety should dissipate once performance actually commences, while the subjective probability of a successful outcome might fluctuate throughout the competitive event. The only evidence which at present exists to support the contention that somatic anxiety dissipates once performance commences is based on test anxiety (see Morris, Davis and Hutchings, 1981) and weak retrospective self-report in a sports setting (Martens *et al.*, 1990). However, there are clearly differences between academic examinations and sports competitions which may limit the generalizability of findings between test anxiety and competitive sports anxiety. Furthermore, there is also a considerable quantity of research which suggests that the physiological response associated with anxiety continues to fluctuate during performance in many sports-like situations (for example Baddeley and Idzikowski, 1985; Idzikowski and Baddeley, 1987).

Although early correlational studies of test anxiety did show that cognitive anxiety was negatively related to performance while somatic anxiety was uncorrelated with it (Morris *et al.*, 1975), these relationships were demonstrated on the day of the test, when physiological arousal (and somatic anxiety) were presumably high. Subsequent studies employing the same paradigm, but using polynomial regression analyses, have obtained a negative linear relationship between cognitive anxiety and sports performance (Burton, 1988), but an inverted-U shaped relationship between somatic anxiety and sports performance (Gould *et al.*, 1987; Burton, 1988). Unfortunately, the situation is even further complicated by the fact that other studies which have employed the 'time-to-event' paradigm have produced results which appear to contradict even these findings. For example, Parfitt and Hardy (1987) have reported positive effects for cognitive anxiety on the days leading up to an important competition when physiological arousal was low, and mixed positive and negative effects for physiological arousal upon different aspects of performance on the day of the competition when cognitive anxiety was high (see Chapter 3 in this book for a review).

These apparent contradictions are interpreted by this author as being a direct consequence of the different paradigms and analyses which have been used. For example, Burton's (1988) inverted-U shaped somatic anxiety–performance relationship could not have been demonstrated by Morris et al.'s (1975) *linear* correlational analysis. Similarly, Parfitt and Hardy's (1987) within-subjects analysis of group performance across the days leading up to an important competition conveys qualitatively different information to that contained in Burton's (1988) curvilinear regression analysis of the between-subjects relationship between anxiety and performance. In particular, the combination of positive group effects for cognitive anxiety, coupled with a negative linear relationship across subjects, seems to suggest that small amounts of cognitive anxiety on the day of an important event exert a beneficial effect upon performance, while large amounts of cognitive anxiety have a detrimental effect upon performance. This finding has been replicated by Jones and Cale (1989a). Furthermore, this sort of interpretation of the literature is perfectly plausible. Mild concern about the outcome of a competitive event might well motivate performers to greater effort and higher levels of performance (Kahneman, 1973; Eysenck, 1982) while uncontrollable fear about the consequences of failure would almost certainly constitute a very powerful source of distraction (Wine, 1971). However, this interpretation, and the research findings from which it is derived, definitely do not support multidimensional anxiety theory.

One final problem with Martens et al.'s (1990) multidimensional anxiety theory is that it attempts to explain the relationship between cognitive anxiety, somatic anxiety and performance in terms of a series of two-dimensional effects. More precisely, it makes predictions about the separate effects of cognitive anxiety and somatic anxiety upon performance, when what is really required is an explanation of how cognitive and somatic anxiety *interact* to influence performance. This seems to imply that any satisfactory model of anxiety and performance must be at least three-dimensional.

As a result of their general dissatisfaction with these existing models of the anxiety–performance relationship, Hardy and Fazey (1987) proposed a catastrophe model of anxiety and performance which attempted to clarify the relationship between cognitive anxiety, physiological arousal and performance. This paper was subsequently published as Fazey and Hardy (1988).

It is perhaps appropriate at this stage, to say something about the term *'physiological arousal'* as it was used by Fazey and Hardy (1988). Physiologcal arousal was regarded as part of the organism's natural physiological respo to anxiety-inducing situations (Cannon, 1953). Furthermore, Fazey and Hardy (1988) argued that this response may be reflected (at least partially) by self-reports of somatic anxiety (Morris, Davis and Hutchings, 1981; Hardy and Whitehead, 1984; Martens *et al.*, 1990), or any physiological indicator. Of course, the individual idiosyncrasies of different situations, physiological systems and task demands could superimpose variations between any two physiological indicators, and if the overall physiological response demanded by the situation were small, then these individual differences in particular physiological systems could swamp the generalized trend of the physiological arousal response (Lacey, 1967; Neiss, 1988). Nevertheless, Fazey and Hardy (1988) argued that the physiological response to performance anxiety was sufficiently well established (Selye, 1979; Frankenhauser, 1980) for it to be meaningful to talk about physiological arousal as a generalized response within this context.

CATASTROPHE MODELS OF BEHAVIOUR

Catastrophe theory was first developed by the French mathematician Rene Thom (1975) as a means of modelling discontinuities in functions which were normally continuous. Thom's central theorem was that, with certain qualifications, all naturally occurring discontinuities could be classified as being of the 'same type' as (i.e. topologically equivalent to) one of seven fundamental catastrophes. Catastrophe theory was subsequently popularized by Zeeman (1976), who drew attention to some of the possible applications of the theory to both the behavioural and the natural sciences. Other applications of catastrophe theory to the behavioural sciences quickly followed (Isnard and Zeeman, 1977; Poston and Stewart, 1978), although this early enthusiasm was not without its critics and Sussman and Zahler (1978) even went so far as to suggest that catastophe models could never be formally tested by experimental methodologies. This criticism was fiercely contested by Woodcock and Davis (1978), Stewart and Peregoy (1983) and others, but was eventually laid to rest by the development of several statistical catastrophe theories which enabled experimental designs to be constructed to explicitly test catastrophe models of behaviour (Cobb, 1981; Guastello, 1981, 1987; Oliva *et al.*, 1987).

The most commonly applied of Thom's seven fundamental catastrophes is the 'cusp catastrophe'. This catastrophe is perhaps most easily understood by considering the physical machine which Zeeman (1976) designed to demonstrate it. Zeeman's machine comprises a circular disc which is pivoted at its centre and which has two rubber bands attached to a point near the perimeter of the disk. The opposite end of one of these rubber bands is attached to a fixed point outside the disk, while the opposite end of the other rubber band

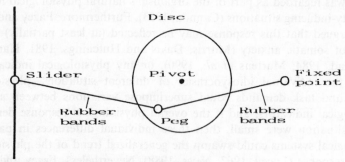

Figure 4.1. Zeeman's (1976) catastrophe machine.

is free to slide up and down a rod that is in the same plane as the disk but at right angles to the line which passes from the fixed point through the centre of the disk (see Figure 4.1).

The machine has two input variables, the height of the slider on the rod and the distance between the fixed point and the rod. Moving the slider slowly up the rod one can demonstrate that the disk gradually rotates until it reaches some critical point, at which it suddenly 'flips' to a new point of stability before continuing its gradual rotation. Furthermore, by moving the rod and fixed point closer together or further apart to change the tension in the rubber bands, two more phenomena can be demonstrated:

1. The point at which the disk flips and the amount by which it jumps vary as a function of the tension in the rubber bands. As the tension increases (up to a certain point) the catastrophic jump of the disk occurs later and is bigger. Conversely, as the tension decreases the catastrophic jump becomes smaller and eventually disappears;

2. The point of discontinuity at which the jump occurs for any given tension level is different when the slider is moved up the rod to when it is moved down. This phenomenon is known as 'hysteresis'.

In fact, if the height of the attachment point for the two rubber bands to the disk is plotted against the tension in the rubber bands and the height of the slider on the rod, a three-dimensional behaviour surface is obtained which looks something like Figure 4.2, except that the middle sheet of the fold is inaccessible.

At one extreme, when the tension in the rubber bands (Y) is very small, gradual changes in the height of the slider (X) lead to gradual changes in the height of the attachment point on the disk (Z). At the other extreme, when the tension in the rubber bands (Y) is very high, gradual changes in X lead to

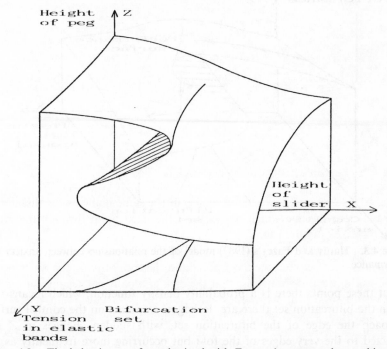

Figure 4.2.   The behaviour surface obtained with Zeeman's catastrophe machine.

a sudden jump in Z at one of two points, dependent upon whether X is increasing or decreasing at that moment. In this sort of situation, the effect of X upon Z is clearly at least partially determined by the value of Y. In such a catastrophe model, the variable arranged along the Y axis is called a 'splitting factor' and the variable arranged along the X axis is called the 'normal factor'. The X–Y plane is called the 'control surface', and the set of points on the X–Y plane for which there are two possible values of Z on the behavioural surface is known as the 'bifurcation set.' It is the set of (X, Y) values which lies beneath the folded part of the behaviour surface.

  Zeeman's machine is, of course, a deterministic one: that is to say, the mechanics of the system are such that the disk *necessarily* assumes a position of minimum potential energy (Cobb, 1978). In the behavioural sciences, models are usually more statistical in nature, so that changes in one variable do not *necessarily* cause changes in another. Rather, changes in independent variables *increase the likelihood* that the dependent variable will change in some predicted direction. Consequently, the upper and lower behaviour sheets of behavioural science catastrophes become the set of points of maximum likelihood rather than minimum energy, while the middle (inaccessible) sheet becomes the set of points of minimum likelihood instead of maximum energy.

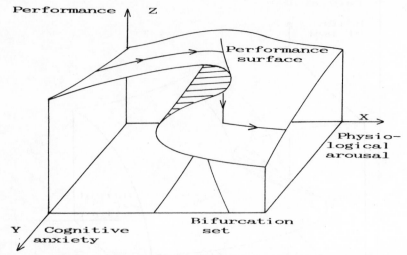

Figure 4.3. Hardy and Fazey's (1987) model of the relationship between anxiety and performance.

About these points there is a probability density function, which means that within the bifurcation set there are 'leakages' as points on the control surface approach the edge of the bifurcation set, with sudden changes in Z not restricted to the very edges of the fold but occurring more frequently as the edges are approached (Oliva *et al.*, 1987).

HARDY AND FAZEY'S CATASTROPHE MODEL OF ANXIETY AND PERFORMANCE

Hardy and Fazey's (1987) model assumes that anxiety has at least two components, cognitive anxiety and a physiological arousal response. The model proposes that cognitive anxiety acts as a splitting factor which determines whether the effect of physiological arousal (the normal factor) will be smooth and small, large and catastrophic, or somewhere in between these two extremes (see Figure 4.3).

These roles were chosen so that the model would possess four characteristics of the anxiety–performance literature. When cognitive anxiety is low (for example in most laboratory situations), the model predicts that the relationship between physiological arousal and performance should be the uniform or mildly inverted-U shaped curve which is given by the back face of Figure 4.3 (see, for example, Davey, 1973). When physiological arousal is high on the day of a competition, the model predicts a negative correlation between cognitive anxiety and performance as shown by the right-hand face of Figure 4.4 (cf. Morris *et al.* 1975; Gould, Petlichkoff and Weinberg, 1984; Burton,

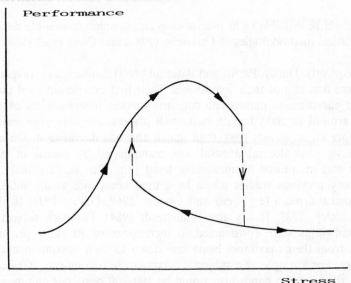

Figure 4.4.   The hysteresis predicted under conditions of high cognitive anxiety.

1988). When physiological arousal is low during the days prior to a competition, the model predicts that cognitive anxiety should lead to enhanced performance (cf. Parfitt and Hardy, 1987; Parfitt, 1988). Finally, when cognitive anxiety is elevated as in the time-to-event paradigm, the model predicts that the effect of physiological arousal upon group performance could be either positive or negative, depending upon exactly how high cognitive anxiety is. This manipulation represents a slice through Figure 4.3, parallel to the physiological arousal by performance plane (cf. Parfitt and Hardy, 1987; Parfitt, 1988; Jones and Cale, 1989a).

Fazey and Hardy (1988) proposed four further testable hypotheses from the model:

1. Physiological arousal, and the associated somatic anxiety, are not necessarily detrimental to performance. However, they will be associated with catastrophic effects when cognitive anxiety is high;
2. Under conditions of high cognitive anxiety, hysteresis will occur: that is to say, performance will follow a different path when physiological arousal is increasing compared to the path it follows when physiological arousal is decreasing (see Figures 4.3 and 4.4). Under conditions of low cognitive anxiety hysteresis will not occur;
3. Intermediate levels of performance are most unlikely in conditions of high cognitive anxiety. More precisely, performance should be bimodal under conditions of high cognitive anxiety and unimodal under conditions of low cognitive anxiety (see Zeeman, 1976);

4. It should be possible to fit precise cusp catastrophes to real-life data using the statistical methodologies of Guastello (1987) and Oliva *et al.* (1987).

Subsequently, Hardy, Parfitt and Pates (in press) conducted two experiments to test the first two of these hypotheses. Their first experiment used the time-to-event paradigm to manipulate cognitive anxiety independently of physiological arousal in eight female basketball players. Subjects were tested one day before an important basketball match and one day after it. On each of these days, physiological arousal was manipulated by means of physical exercise and monitored by measuring heart rate. This is, of course, in line with many previous studies which have used heart rate as an indicator of physiological arousal (e.g. Fenz and Epstein, 1969; Davey, 1973; Idzikowski and Baddeley, 1987; Hardy and Whitehead, 1984). For each subject, heart rate bandwidths were constructed in increments of 10 beats per minute, ranging from their maximum heart rate down to their maximum heart rate minus 40. For example, if a subject's maximum heart rate was 200 beats per minute, then the top bandwidth would be 190–200 beats per minute and the bottom bandwidth 150–160 beats per minute. Subjects' physiological arousal levels were increased by requiring them to perform shuttle runs until the required bandwidth was reached, or decreased by allowing them to rest until the required bandwidth was reached.

The performance task used to test the hysteresis hypothesis was a basketball set shot. This is a 'pressure' shot in basketball which any player can be called upon to make at any stage in the game. It was therefore considered to be a relevant and appropriate task to ask basketball players to perform under conditions of elevated cognitive anxiety and physiological arousal.

Prior to the first data collection, two familiarization sessions were completed by all subjects. In the first of these, each subject's maximum heart rate was obtained by the subject performing repeated shuttle runs to exhaustion. This was crucial to the experimental design, as subjects were required to perform the criterion task while working up to their maximum heart rate and then back down, or *vice versa*. In the second session, subjects were required to perform shuttle runs until they reached certain heart rate bandwidths, at which they were then required to perform five set shots. This was not a complete run through of a data collection session because such a session would have taken over one hour per subject to complete and the experimenters were concerned about losing subjects by making excessive time demands upon them. Instead, each subject completed approximately one-third of a testing session to ensure that the procedure and situation were not novel.

Data collections took place one day before the first ever North Wales Ladies Basketball Tournament and one day after it, as these days had been repeatedly shown to produce high and low cognitive anxiety in basketball players (Parfitt and Hardy, 1987; Parfitt, 1988). Testing on the day of the tournament in order to evaluate the effects of somatic anxiety upon performance was neither necessary nor possible because physiological arousal was independently manipulated on both the high and low cognitive anxiety days.

Cognitive and somatic anxiety were measured using Martens et al.'s (1990) Competitive State Anxiety Inventory-2 (CSAI-2), while heart rate was monitored using a Polar Electro Sport Tester (PE 3000). This comprised a small transmitter, which was strapped to the subject's chest, and a receiver, which was worn on the wrist.

After completing the CSAI-2, subjects had 20 practice set shots before being given a task description sheet explaining the experimental procedure and what was required of them. In order to control for fatigue effects, the subjects were then randomly divided into two groups. One group performed the criterion task with heart rate bandwidths increasing to a maximum (M) and then decreasing to maximum minus 40 (M–40), while the other group performed the task with heart rate bandwidths decreasing from maximum down to M–40 and then increasing back up to maximum. Subjects who started from their maximum heart rate bandwidth in the first data session started from their lowest heart rate bandwidth in the second data session, and vice versa.

The heart rate apparatus allowed the required bandwidths to be specified so that the apparatus would 'bleep' if the heart rate was outside that bandwidth. An aural signal was therefore available to indicate when some action was required either to increase or decrease heart rate. Once the 20 practice shots had been completed the apparatus was set at the specified bandwidth, which was either subjects' maximum heart rate bandwidth M or M–40, depending upon which group they were in. The subjects then had to perform shuttle runs until the 'bleeping' stopped: that is, until their heart rate reached the required bandwidth. Once the bandwidth was achieved, the subject performed five shots. Subjects' heart rates always remained within the required bandwidth while they completed these five shots. Following the five shots, the heart rate bandwidth was either increased or decreased by 10 beats per minute and the procedure repeated.

In total, subjects performed 70 set shots: 20 practice and two sets of five at each bandwidth (five going down and five going up). The experimeter recorded each set shot, using a scoring system of 5 for a 'clean' basket; 4 for a rim and in; 3 for backboard and in; 2 for a rim and out; 1 for backboard and out; and 0 for a complete miss. Performance was measured by summating the scores for the five shots at each bandwidth.

Correlated t-tests indicated that both cognitive and somatic anxiety were significantly elevated on the day before the tournament relative to the day after it. This result was not anticipated. In previous studies which had used the time-to-event paradigm, significant increases in somatic anxiety had generally occurred only on the day of the event, and not the day before it (see Chapter 3 in this book). However, most of these studies had used male subjects and it is possible that female subjects do not demonstrate the same temporal dissociation of cognitive and somatic anxiety as men (see Jones and Cale, 1989b; Jones, Swain and Cale, in press; Swain, Jones and Cale, 1990). It is also possible that the increases in somatic anxiety which Hardy, Parfitt and Pates (in press) obtained in their first data collection session were due to the requirements of the experiment itself. For, as Hardy *et al.* pointed out, in the familiarization session subjects completed only about one-third of an actual data collection session. Consequently, in the first full data session (before the event) subjects knew that the experiment would be very physically demanding, but were unaware of exactly how physically demanding it was going to be. The elevated somatic anxiety may, therefore, have been in response to the impending experimental treatment, rather than the subsequent tournament. By the second data session the subjects were aware of the physical demands of the experiment, and were also aware of their ability to cope with them. As a result, they may not have been as somatically anxious about the experiment on this day.

Whatever the reason for it, Hardy *et al.* argued that this finding did not invalidate their test of Hardy and Fazey's (1987) model. They based this argument on three facts. First, the independent variable in question in Hardy and Fazey's model is physiological arousal, not somatic anxiety. Secondly, while one could present a fairly resonable argument to support the view that increases in physiological arousal generally lead to increases in somatic anxiety, the converse is not true. Increased somatic anxiety does not necessarily imply that physiological arousal has changed (see, for example, Borkovec, 1976). Finally, physiological arousal was independently manipulated on both days of the experiment, so that even if the somatic anxiety results did reflect a global decrease in *baseline* physiological arousal from one day to the other, the independent variables in Hardy and Fazey's catastrophe model were still manipulated independently of each other. Because of these arguments, Hardy *et al.* considered it appropriate to proceed to an analysis of their performance data.

This produced much clearer results. On the basis of Hardy and Fazey's hysteresis hypothesis, Hardy, Parfitt and Pates (in press) predicted that this analysis should reveal a significant three-way interaction, whereby performance by heart rate would follow a different path with heart rate increasing compared to when heart rate was decreasing under conditions of high cognitive anxiety; but that this dissociation would not occur under conditions of low cognitive anxiety. Trend analysis of the performance data confirmed this prediction (see Figures 4.5 and 4.6).

In their second experiment, Hardy, Parfitt and Pates (1990) used neutral and ego-threatening instructional sets to manipulate cognitive anxiety in experienced crown green bowlers (cf. Morris and Liebert, 1973; Morris, Harris and Rovins, 1981). Otherwise the experiment followed a similar paradigm to

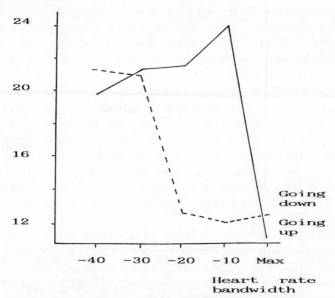

Figure 4.5. Set shot performance in the high cognitive anxiety condition.

their first experiment. In this experiment, cognitive anxiety was manipulated independently of somatic anxiety, and the performance data again demonstrated the hypothesized three-way interaction between cognitive anxiety, heart rate and direction of heart rate change (see Figures 4.7 and 4.8). Hardy *et al.* interpreted these findings as offering strong support for Hardy and Fazey's hysteresis hypothesis.

It could be argued that Hardy *et al.*'s findings contradict previous studies of the relationship between somatic anxiety and performance under conditions of high cognitive anxiety (for example Gould *et al.*, 1987; Burton, 1988) which have reported quadratic relationships between somatic anxiety and performance. However, these studies have not measured physiological arousal, and have not taken any account of the direction of change of somatic anxiety. Furthermore, it seems highly likely that the direction of change for somatic anxiety would be upwards for the vast majority of performers on the day of a major competition. Consequently, it is perfectly reasonable that a quadratic curve should fit these data.

Hardy *et al.* also performed two other supplementary analyses on their data. These indicated that in both experiments the highest levels of performance achieved in the high cognitive anxiety condition were significantly higher than the highest levels of performance achieved in the low cognitive anxiety

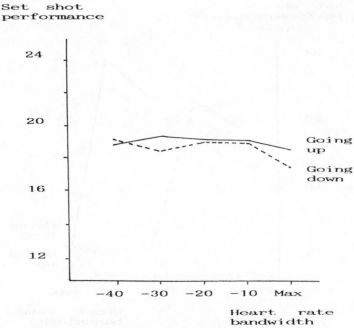

Figure 4.6. Set shot performance in the low cognitive anxiety condition.

condition. Conversely, the lowest levels of performance achieved in the high cognitive anxiety condition were significantly lower than the lowest levels of performance achieved in the low cognitive anxiety condition. These results were interpreted as indicating the potential gains and catastrophic drops which can occur in performance under conditions of high cognitive anxiety. While it is clear that other predictions from Hardy and Fazey's catastrophe model still need to be tested, it is equally clear that Hardy *et al.*'s results offer quite strong support for the model.

This is not the first time that an attempt has been made to use catastrophes to model the effects of anxiety upon performance. Kirkcaldy (1983) attempted to describe the effects of stress upon sports performance in terms of cortical arousal and anxiety, while Booth (1985) attempted to model the effects of test anxiety upon examination performance in terms of worry (cognitive anxiety) and emotionality (somatic anxiety). However, both these models contained serious theoretical flaws, which are discussed in much more detail by Fazey and Hardy (1988), so that empirical support for them was not forthcoming.

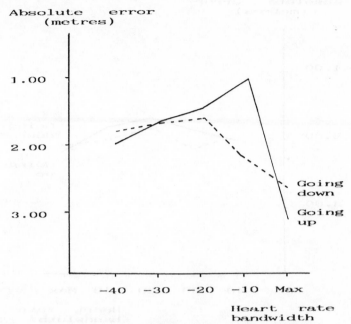

Figure 4.7.   Bowls performance in the high cognitive anxiety condition.

THEORETICAL IMPLICATIONS AND SPECULATIONS

While Hardy and Fazey's (1987) catastrophe model may offer a reasonable description of the anxiety–performance relationship, there are much more interesting questions concerned with how cognitive anxiety and physiological arousal interact to influence performance.

Eysenck (1979, 1982) argued that the difference between present aspirations and previous levels of performance is greater in high-anxiety performers. He consequently went on to argue that this greater goal discrepancy should enhance motivation and effort in high-anxiety subjects, provided that there is at least a moderate probability of success. Conversely, he argued that if the task was very difficult or impossible, then the greater goal discrepancy of highly anxious performers should lead to reduced motivation. In support of this position, Eysenck (1979) cited Revelle and Michaels' (1976) use of two popular proverbs to explain these relationships: 'The tough get going when the going gets tough', but 'Wise men do not beat their heads against brick walls'.

Furthermore, it is possible that in Hardy *et al.*'s experiments physiological arousal was simply a reflection of the effort which was required to cope with the demands of the experimental tasks which were used (Naatanen, 1973). If

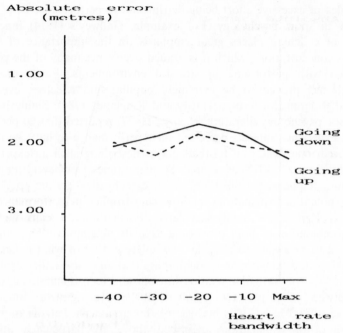

Figure 4.8.   Bowls performance in the low cognitive anxiety condition.

this was the case, then Eysenck's (1982) motivation explanation would fit Hardy *et al.*'s results perfectly, since one might reasonably expect that following a catastrophic fall-off in performance, physiological arousal would have to be quite considerably reduced before subjects would perceive themselves able to cope well enough to justify investing the extra effort required to regain the upper performance surface. This theory could be empirically tested by examining what happens to subjects' effort on the task at critical points. According to this explanation, subjects' problem-focused attempts at coping should decrease at a downward critical point, while the opposite should be true at an upward critical point.

Alternatively, it may be that performers do not actually give up trying to cope with the task when they are both cognitively anxious and physiologically aroused. Nevertheless, their level of physiological arousal might well interfere with performance, either by distraction (Deffenbacher, 1980), a reduction in processing capacity (Humphreys and Revelle, 1984), or by leading performers to believe that they should selectively attend to maintaining effort rather than their performance on the task at hand (Naatanen, 1973). To put this latter possibility crudely, performers may waste valuable resources telling themselves to 'try hard' instead of focusing all of their attention on the task that they need to perform.

The idea of excessive effort being detrimental to performance is, of course, not new in sport psychology. For example, Gallwey's (1974) inner game method of coaching places great emphasis on the importance of 'relaxed effortless concentration', which it is argued overcomes many of the problems associated with performing in stressful environments. Furthermore, this approach has proved to be extremely popular and effective, even when subjected to empirical testing (Hardy and Ringland, 1984). Similarly, in the humanistic psychology literature, Ravizza (1977) reported that 90 per cent of all peak experience subjects perceived their performance to have been effortless. Indeed, one American football player describing such an experience is quoted by Ravizza (1977) as saying: 'So many times I put everything into it but nothing happens, but this time . . . it was effortless for me' (p. 38).

These potential explanations of how catastrophes in performance might occur are all, of course, highly speculative. Furthermore, it seems most likely that a combination of both processing capacity and motivational allocation effects will be necessary to provide a complete picture of what is happening. Nevertheless, the catastrophe model implies that any satisfactory explanation of the anxiety–performance relationship must include qualitatively different states between which performers shift when they are cognitively anxious and physiologically aroused. It is because of this argument that the motivation-based allocation explanations described above are particularly attractive. Continuous changes in attentional capacity can only account for the discontinuous changes in performance which Hardy and Fazey's catastrophe model predicts if it is assumed that the catastrophic change in performance occurs at some critical level of capacity after which performance completely breaks down. However, even this sort of explanation would still require something to be said about why the cut-off point is never reached under conditions of low cognitive anxiety.

Further examination of the processes by which performance catastrophes occur is clearly an area of great importance and interest to theoreticians and practitioners alike.

PRACTICAL IMPLICATIONS OF THE CATASTROPHE MODEL

In view of the relatively small amount of validatory research which has been performed upon Hardy and Fazey's (1987) catastrophe model, it is perhaps a little premature to consider the practical implications of the model. Nevertheless, this section does present just two of them.

The first and most obvious implication of Hardy and Fazey's catastrophe model is that when cognitive anxiety is high, the penalty for physiological overarousal is very severe. Since performers are already highly cognitively anxious and physiologically aroused on the day of important competitions (Jones and Cale, 1989a,b; Martens *et al.*, 1990; Ussher and Hardy, 1986; Parfitt and Hardy, 1987), the catastrophe model would implicate a most conservative and controlled approach to any pre-match 'psyching up' strategies which a coach might employ.

The second implication of the catastrophe model is that the choice of preferred intervention for a given performer will depend upon exactly where on the performance surface the performer is at the time of the intervention. Strategies are required which can independently modify cognitive anxiety or physiological arousal as appropriate. If Davidson and Schwartz's (1976) matching hypothesis is correct, then this implies that performers should be taught both cognitive and somatic strategies rather than just one or the other (see Chapter 7 in this book). Alternatively, performers might be taught integrated strategies which can be fine-tuned to the particular requirements of each situation, for example stress inoculation training (see Chapters 7 and 8 in this book).

IMPLICATIONS FOR FUTURE RESEARCH

While Hardy and Fazey's (1987) catastrophe model may be intuitively attractive, two experiments testing the same hypothesis definitely do not constitute a proof. Consequently, one of the most pressing needs is for further empirical tests to be performed upon the model. In particular, two of Hardy and Fazey's other hypotheses would seem to merit some attention:

1. The probability distribution of performance scores should be unimodal under conditions of low cognitive anxiety and bimodal under conditions of high cognitive anxiety (see also Zeeman, 1976);
2. It should be possible to fit precise catastrophe curves to real-life data using the methodologies of Guastello (1987) or Oliva *et al.* (1987). Because of its (relative) simplicity, Guastello's method of direct differences is particularly attractive in this respect.

Another feature of the model which is of interest is the notion of shifts between qualitatively different (motivational?) states when performers are both cognitively anxious and physiologically aroused. This prediction seems to bear a distinct resemblance to the reversal theory (Apter, 1982) prediction of reversals between telic and paratelic states under conditions of high arousal (see Chapter 5 in this book). In particular, Kerr (1985) has suggested that such switches between states of great anxiety and states of high excitement may be an important determinant of some performers' games (for example John McEnroe). It would clearly be interesting to explore any common ground which exists between reversal theory and Hardy and Fazey's catastrophe model of anxiety and performance.

On a rather different tack, even if supporting evidence for Hardy and Fazey's catastrophe model was forthcoming, this model would still only represent a very tentative start to the problem of describing and explaining how metacognitive variables such as anxiety influence performance in sports. In particular, the model ignores several other potentially important metacognitive variables, such as perceived control (Fisher, 1986), self-image (Gal-Or and Tenenbaum, 1986) and self-confidence (Bandura, 1977). Fazey and Hardy (1988) did propose an extension of their basic catastrophe model which included self-confidence as a predictor variable, but this model is something of a 'shot in the dark' and, as will be seen, it can be criticized on several grounds.

HIGHER DIMENSIONAL CATASTROPHES

The cusp catastrophe model which has been discussed so far is a three-dimensional model of anxiety and performance. It has two control parameters and one behavioural parameter and can be represented by the equation $Z = X + YZ^3$. The next most commonly used of Zeeman's catastrophes is the 'butterfly catastrophe'. This is a five-dimensional catastrophe which can be obtained from the cusp catastrophe by adding two further control dimensions. The first of these is the 'bias factor' which has the effect of swinging the 'front' S-shaped curve of the cusp to the left or right, while at the same time raising or lowering the behaviour surface as bias increases or decreases. The second additional control factor is called the 'butterfly factor', and is rather more difficult to describe. Essentially, the butterfly factor promotes the growth of a pocket containing a new fold in the behaviour surface. This pocket gradually evolves between the two stable surfaces of the cusp catastrophe, so producing a third stable behaviour surface in between the upper and lower surfaces of the cusp catastrophe (see Zeeman, 1976 for further details).

In order to draw the butterfly catastrophe it is necessary to suppress two of the dimensions, and usually the bias and butterfly factors are chosen. It is worth noting that the butterfly catastrophe contains three cusp catastrophes joined together (see the bifurcation set in Figures 4.9 and 4.10). Furthermore, the pocket in the behaviour surface which is produced by the butterfly factor allows the possibility of a third mode of compromise stable behaviour which can lead back to the smooth area of stable behaviour at the back of the behaviour surface.

In a piece of wildly optimistic speculation, Fazey and Hardy (1988) proposed that their cusp catastrophe model of anxiety and performance could be extended to a butterfly catastrophe model which included task difficulty as a

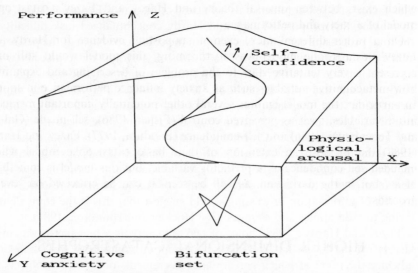

Figure 4.9. Fazey and Hardy's (1988) butterfly catastrophe model of the effects of cognitive anxiety, physiological arousal, task difficulty and self-confidence upon performance-low task difficulty (bias).

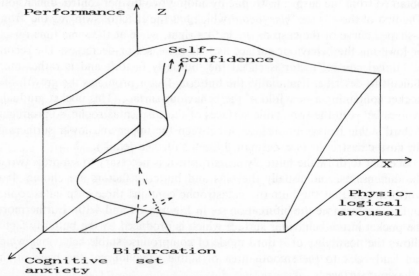

Figure 4.10. Fazey and Hardy's (1988) butterfly catastrophe model of the effects of cognitive anxiety, physiological arousal, task difficulty and self-confidence upon performance—high task difficulty (bias).

bias factor and self-confidence as a butterfly factor (see Figures 4.9 and 4.10). In making this proposal, Fazey and Hardy conceptualized task difficulty as the total processing demands placed upon the cognitive system of the performer. While this operationalization of task difficulty avoids the criticisms which have been made of earlier purely perceptual conceptualizations of task difficulty (by, for example, Easterbook, 1959), it still suffers from the implicit assumption that the information-processing system has a single pool of resources. More precisely, it attempts to describe the differences in perceptual demand and differences in memory demand in terms of a single dimension. Such a definition attempts to equate the processing demands of such gymnastic movements as a full twisting double back somersault with the processing demands of selecting which shot to 'kill' at squash. Multiple resource-based models of information processing would suggest that this is the equivalent of trying to 'add apples and oranges' (see Hockey and Hamilton, 1983).

Fazey and Hardy's 1988 choice of task difficulty as a bias factor was made largely on the basis that increases in perceptual complexity were known to advance the point at which performance decrements occur when subjects are required to perform tasks under high levels of stress. Furthermore, their attempt to include self-confidence in the model is also laudable in view of the quantity of research which indicates that self-confidence is an important predictor of performance (Bandura, 1977; Mahoney and Avener, 1977) that is, at least partially, independent of cognitive anxiety (Burrows, Cox and Simpson, 1977; Thayer, 1978; Hardy and Whitehead, 1984; Martens et al., 1990). However, quite apart from the task difficulty definition problem, Fazey and Hardy's choice of roles for task difficulty and self-confidence as bias and butterfly factors, respectively, can be criticized on several grounds.

The first criticism is as much heuristic as theoretical. Essentially, Hardy and Fazey's (1987) cusp catastrophe model attempts to describe the relationship between certain metacognitive and physiological variables, and motor (or cognitive) performance. However, the inclusion of task difficulty in their butterfly catastrophe model involves a different level of cognition to the other variables that are included. Task difficulty is a 'true' cognitive variable concerned with 'lower-level' information processing, while cognitive anxiety and self-confidence are metacognitive variables concerned with 'higher-level' affective states.

The second criticism concerns the role which Fazey and Hardy (1988) assigned to self-confidence. If self-confidence is a butterfly factor then, as Fazey and Hardy pointed out, it should be associated with trimodal performance at moderate levels of cognitive anxiety. In simple terms, this implies that, at moderate levels of cognitive anxiety, highly confident performers are allowed the possibility of intermediate levels of performance rather than performance always being either brilliant or dismal under such conditions. While there has as yet been no empirical test of this prediction, it does not sit very comfortably with findings that high self-confidence is associated with both actual and retrospectively reported peak performance (Mahoney and Avener, 1977; Ravizza, 1977; Privette, 1981). Such findings would seem to suggest that self-confidence might be better included as a bias factor rather than a butterfly factor.

The third criticism is that one might reasonably expect that any model of the influence of metacognitive variables, such as cognitive anxiety and self-confidence, upon performance would say something about the role of self-control in this process. Furthermore, one could present quite a strong argument that such metacognitive skills would be highly likely to allow the possibility of intermediate levels of performance, and should therefore be included as a bias factor in the model. Of course, all this is simply speculation about the precise form which any higher-order catastrophe model of metacognitive variables and performance should take.

SUMMARY AND CONCLUSION

Not surprisingly, the cusp catastrophe model which has been reviewed in this chapter arose as a result of Hardy and Fazey's (1987) dissatisfaction with both the inverted-U and existing multidimensional anxiety explanations of the anxiety–performance relationship. Dissatisfaction with the inverted-U explanation included both theoretical and practical criticisms, while dissatisfaction with Martens et al.'s (1990) multidimensional anxiety theory approach centred around the theory's inability to cope with the empirical evidence generated by different paradigms (Jones and Cale, 1989a; Parfitt and Hardy, 1987; Parfitt, 1988). The means by which Hardy and Fazey's (1987) cusp catastrophe model attempts to cope with these criticisms were discussed, together with Hardy, Parfitt and Pates' (in press) empirical evidence in support of the model. Furthermore, while it is clear that the model requires considerably more validation work before it can be accepted, it was concluded that the available evidence does seem to fit it fairly well.

Despite its early developmental stage, Hardy and Fazey's cusp catastrophe model raises some interesting theoretical questions. Perhaps the most fundamental prediction of the model is the notion that, under conditions of high cognitive anxiety and physiological arousal, performance is determined by qualitively different states between which the performer may shift. However, once performance has degenerated to the lower performance surface, a considerable reduction in physiological arousal or cognitive anxiety may be necessary for the upper performance surface to be regained. On the basis that physiological arousal is a reflection of the effort which is being invested in the task, it is possible to identify several potential 'causes' of such performance shifts in the literature. These include: policy decisions to stop investing effort in the task (Revelle and Michaels, 1976); 'trying too hard' (Gallwey, 1974); reductions in memory capacity as a result of physiological arousal (Humphreys and Revelle, 1984); and distraction by excessive physiological arousal (Morris, Harris and Rovins, 1981). However, the 'qualitatively different states' notion gives the allocation-based explanations a rather higher profile than the capacity-based explanations.

Practically, the cusp catastrophe model points to the need for great caution in the use of 'psyching up' strategies on the day of competitions. It also points to the need for performers to have multiple relaxation strategies so as to adjust their position on the cognitive anxiety by physiological arousal control surface as necessary.

This is clearly an area which would benefit from further research, and future work might consider at least three issues. First, Hardy and Fazey's (1987) cusp catastrophe model requires further validatory work. In particular, Guastello's (1987) method for fitting catastrophe surfaces to real-life data seems to offer much potential in this direction. Secondly, it would be interesting to explore the possible links which may exist between the cusp catastrophe model and Apter's (1982) theory of reversals. Finally, if the cusp catastrophe model does prove to be a useful model of cognitive anxiety, physiological arousal and performance, then it would be interesting to attempt to include other metacognitive variables such as self-confidence in higher-order catastrophe models. Conversely, if Parfitt, Jones and Hardy's (see Chapter 3 in this book) doubts regarding the conceptualization of cognitive anxiety are confirmed, then the very foundations of all this work will need to be reexamined. These are exciting times in sport psychology research!

REFERENCES

Apter, M. J. (1982). *The Experience of Motivation: The Theory of Psychological Reversals*. London: Academic Press.

Baddeley, A. and Idzikowski, C. (1985). Anxiety, manual dexterity and diver performance, *Ergonomics*, **28**, 1475–1482.

Bandura, A. (1977). Self-efficacy: toward a unifying theory of behavioural change, *Psychological Review*, **84**, 191–215.

Booth, P. I. (1985). Geometric models of the effects of test anxiety upon performance, *Mathematical Intelligencer*, **7**, 56–63.

Borkovec, T. D. (1976). Physiological and cognitive processes in the regulation of anxiety, in G. E. Schwartz and D. Shapiro (eds). *Consciousness and Self-regulation: Advances in Research I*. New York: Plenum Press.

Broadhurst, P. L. (1957). Emotionality and the Yerkes–Dodson law, *Journal of Experimental Psychology*, **54**, 345–352.

Burrows, G. C., Cox, T. and Simpson, G. C. (1977). The measurement of stress in a sales training situation, *Journal of Occupational Psychology*, **50**, 45–51.

Burton, D. (1988). Do anxious swimmers swim slower? Re-examining the elusive anxiety–performance relationship, *Journal of Sport Psychology*, **10**, 45–61.

Cannon, W. B. (1953). *Bodily Change in Pain, Hunger, Fear, and Rage*, Boston: Branford.

Cobb, L. (1978). Stochastic catastrophe models and multimodal distributions, *Behavioural Science*, **23**, 360–416.

Cobb, L. (1981). Parameter estimation for the cusp catastrophe model, *Behavioural Science*, **26**, 75–78.

Davey, C. P. (1973) Physical exertion and mental performance, *Ergonomics*, **16**, 595–599.

Davidson, R. J. and Schwartz, G. E. (1976). The psychobiology of relaxation and related states: a multi-process theory, in D. Mostofsky (ed.). *Behavioural Control and Modification of Physiological Activity*. Englewood Cliffs, New Jersey: Prentice-Hall.

Deffenbacher, J. L. (1980). Worry and emotionality in test anxiety, in I. G. Sarason (ed.). *Test Anxiety: Theory, Research and Applications*. Hillsdale: Erlbaum.

Easterbrook, J. A. (1959). The effect of emotion on cue utilization and the organization of behaviour, *Psychological Review*, **66**, 183–201.

Eysenck, M. W. (1979). Anxiety, learning and memory: a reconceptualization, *Journal of Research in Personality*, **13**, 363–385.

Eysenck, M. W. (1982). *Attention and Arousal: Cognition and Performance*. Berlin: Springer-Verlag.

Fazey, J. A. and Hardy, L. (1988). The inverted-U hypothesis: catastrophe for sport psychology. *British Association of Sports Sciences Monograph No 1*. Leeds: The National Coaching Foundation.

Fenz, W. D. and Epstein, S. (1969). Stress in the air, *Psychology Today*, Sept., 27.

Fisher, S. (1986). *Stress and Strategy*. London: Lawrence Erlbaum.

Frankenhauser, M. (1980). Psychoneuroendocrine approaches to the study of stressful person–environment transactions, in H. Selye (ed.). *Selye's Guide to Stress Research*. New York: Van Nostrand, Reinhold.

Gallwey, T. (1974). *The Inner Game of Tennis*. New York: Random House.

Gal-Or, Y. and Tenenbaum G. (1986). Psychological determinants of performance under threat, *International Journal of Sport Psychology*, **17**, 199–214.

Gould, D., Petlichkoff, L., Simons, J. and Vevera, M. (1987). Relationship between Competitive State Anxiety Inventory-2 subscale scores and pistol shooting performance, *Journal of Sport Psychology*, **9**, 33–42.

Gould, D., Petlichkoff, L. and Weinberg, R. S. (1984). Antecedents of, temporal changes in, and relationships between CSA1-2 subcomponents, *Journal of Sport Psychology*, **6**, 289–304.

Guastello, S. (1981). Catastrophe modelling of equity in organisations, *Behavioural Science*, **23**, 63–74.

Guastello, S. J. (1987). A butterfly catastrophe model of motivation in organizations: academic performance, *Journal of Applied Psychology*, **72**, 161–182.

Hardy, L. and Fazey, J. (1987). The inverted-U hypothesis: a catastrophe for sport psychology? Paper presented at the Annual Conference of the North American Society for the Psychology of Sport and Physical Activity, Vancouver, June.

Hardy, L., Parfitt, C. G. and Pates, J. (in press). A catastrophe model of anxiety and performance. Manuscript submitted for publication.

Hardy, L. and Ringland, A. (1984). Mental training and the Inner Game, *Human Learning*, **3**, 203–207.

Hardy, L. and Whitehead, R. (1984). Specific modes of anxiety and arousal, *Current Psychological Research and Reviews*, **3**, 14–24.

Hockey, G. R. J. and Hamilton, P. (1983). The cognitive patterning of stress states, in G. R. J. Hockey (ed.). *Stress and Fatigue in Human Performance*. Chichester: Wiley.

Humphreys, M. S. and Revelle, W. (1984). Personality, motivation and performance: a theory of the relationship between individual differences and information processing, *Psychological Review*, **91**, 153–184.

Idzikowski, C. and Baddeley, A. (1987). Fear and performance in novice parachutists, *Ergonomics*, **30**, 1463–1474.

Isnard, C. A. and Zeeman, E. C. (1977). Some models from catastrophe theory in the social sciences, in E. C. Zeeman (ed.) *Catastrophe Theory: Selected papers, 1972–1977*. Reading, Mass: Addison-Wesley.

Jones, J. G. and Cale, A. (1989a). Relationships between multidimensional competitive state anxiety and cognitive and motor subcomponents of performance, *Journal of Sports Sciences*, **7**, 229–240.

Jones, J. G. and Cale, A. (1989b). Precompetition temporal patterning of anxiety and self-confidence in males and females, *Journal of Sport Behavior*, **12**, 183–195.

Jones, J. G. and Hardy, L. (1989). Stress and cognitive functioning in sport, *Journal of Sports Sciences*, **7**, 41–63.

Jones, J. G., Swain, A. and Cale A. (in press). Gender differences in precompetition temporal patterning and antecedents of anxiety and self-confidence. *Journal of Sport and Exercise Psychology*.

Kahneman, D. (1973). *Attention and Effort*. Englewood Cliffs: Prentice-Hall.

Kerr, J. (1985). A new perspective for sports psychology, in M. J. Apter, D. Fontana and S. Murgaroyd (eds). *Reversal Theory: Applications and Developments*. Cardiff: University College Cardiff Press.

Kirkcaldy, B. D. (1983). Catastrophic performances, *Sportswissenschaft*, **13**, 46–53.

Lacey, J. I. (1967). Somatic response patterning and stress: some revisions of activation theory, in M. H. Appley and R. Trumbull (eds). *Psychological Stress: Issues in Research*. New York: Appleton-Century-Crofts.

Lazarus, R. S. (1966). *Psychological Stress and the Coping Process*. New York: McGraw-Hill.

Mahoney, M. J. and Avener, M. (1977). Psychology of the elite athlete: an exploratory study, *Cognitive Research and Therapy*, **1**, 135–141.

Martens, R., Burton, D., Vealey, R. S., Bump, L. A. and Smith, D. E. (1990). The Competitive State Anxiety Inventory-2, in R. Martens, R. S. Vealey and D. Burton (eds). *Competitive Anxiety in Sport*. Champaign, Illinois: Human Kinetics.

Morris, L. W., Davis, M. A. and Hutchings, C. H. (1981). Cognitive and emotional components of anxiety: literature review and a revised worry–emotionality scale, *Journal of Educational Psychology*, **73**, 541–555.

Morris, L. W., Harris, E. W. and Rovins, D. S. (1981). Interactive effects of generalised and situational expectancies on cognitive and emotional components of anxiety, *Journal of Research in Personality*, **15**, 302–311.

Morris, L. W. and Liebert, R. M. (1973). Effects of negative feedback, threat of shock, and trait anxiety on the arousal of two components of anxiety, *Journal of Counselling Psychology*, **20**, 321–326.

Morris, L. W., Smith, L. R., Andrews, E. S. and Morris, N. C. (1975). The relationship of emotionality and worry components of anxiety to motor skills performance, *Journal of Motor Behavior*, **7**, 121–30.

Naatanen, R. (1973). The inverted-U relationship between activation and performance: a critical review, in S. Kornblum (ed.) *Attention and Performance IV*. New York: Academic Press.

Neiss, R. (1988). Reconceptualizing arousal: psychobiological states in motor perform-ance, *Psychological Bulletin*, **103**, 345–366.

Oliva, T. A., Descarbo, W. S., Day, D. L. and Jedidi, K. (1987). Gemcat: a general multivariate methodology for estimating catastrophe models, *Behavioural Science*, **32**, 121–137.

Oxendine, J. B. (1970). Emotional arousal and motor performance, *Quest*, **13**, 23–32.

Parfitt, C. G. (1988). Interactions between models of stress and models of motor control. Unpublished PhD thesis, University of Wales, Bangor.

Parfitt, C. G. and Hardy, L. (1987). Further evidence for the differential effects of competitive anxiety upon a number of cognitive and motor sub-components, *Journal of Sports Science*, **5**, 62–63.

Poston, T. and Stewart, I. N. (1978). *Catastrophe Theory and its Applications*. London: Pitman.

Privette, G. (1981). Dynamics of peak performance, *Journal of Humanistic Psychology*, **21**, 57–67.

Ravizza, K. (1977). Peak experience in sport, *Journal of Humanistic Psychology*, **17**, 35–40.

Revelle, W. and Michaels, E. J. (1976). The theory of achievement motivation revisited: the implication of inertial tendencies, *Psychological Review*, **83**, 394–404.

Selye, H. (1979). The stress concept and some of its implications, in V. Hamilton and D. M. Warburton (eds). *Human Stress and Cognition*. Chichester: Wiley.

Spiegler, M. D., Morris, L. W. and Liebert, R. M. (1968). Cognitive and emotional components of test anxiety: temporal factors, *Psychological Reports*, **22**, 451–456.

Stewart, I. and Peregoy, P. (1983). Catastrophe theory modelling in psychology, *Psychological Bulletin*, **94**, 336–362.

Sussman, H. and Zahler, R. (1978). A critique of applied catastrophe theory in the behavioural sciences, *Behavioural Science*, **23**, 28–39.

Swain, A. B. J., Jones, J. G. and Cale, A. (1989). Temporal patterning and antecedents of competitive state anxiety in males and females. *Journal of Sports Sciences*, **8**, 84–85.

Thayer, R. E. (1978). Toward a psychological theory of multidimensional activation (arousal), *Motivation and Emotion*, **2**, 1–34.

Thom, R. (1975). *Structural Stability and Morphogenesis*, trans. D. H. Fowler. New York: Benjamin–Addison Wesley.

Ussher, M. H. and Hardy, L. (1986). The effects of competitive anxiety on a number of cognitive and motor sub-systems, *Journal of Sports Sciences*, **4**, 232–233.

Wine, J. D. (1971). Test anxiety and direction of attention, *Psychological Bulletin*, **76**, 92–104.

Woodcock, A. and Davis, M. (1978). *Catastrophe Theory*, New York: E. P. Dutton.

Yerkes, R. M. and Dodson, J. D. (1908). The relation of strength of stimulus to rapidity of habit formation, *Journal of Comparative and Neurological Psychology*, **18**, 459–482.

Zeeman, E. C. (1976). Catastrophe theory, *Scientific American*, **234**, 65–82.

Chapter 5

Stress and sport: reversal theory

John H. Kerr
Netherlands School of Business

As might be implied from its name, 'reversal theory' (Apter, 1982) explores psychological reversals and, more specifically, reversals in the motivational orientation of the individual. It is a general theory of motivation and personality which has been applied to a variety of areas in psychology and has recently received increased attention in the study of psychological effects in sport. Although the term 'stress' was barely mentioned in Apter's (1982) text, the study of stress has been a major focus of reversal theory work in the intervening period.

This chapter will attempt to outline the theoretical position of reversal theory, describing some of the consistent models which have been generated within it. Particular attention will be focused on the reversal theory account of stress, and its relevance for understanding psychological stress effects in sport will be underlined. In doing so, reference will be made to empirical findings. In addition, a number of theoretical and practical implications for stress management, including cognitive intervention possibilities for use with sports performers experiencing stress, will be discussed.

A glossary will be found at the end of the chapter.

REVERSAL THEORY: A STRUCTURAL PHENOMENOLOGICAL APPROACH

The theory of psychological reversals (Apter, 1982), or reversal theory as it is usually known, gives priority to the individual's experience of his or her own motivation. It is a unique phenomenological theory of motivation, emotion, personality and psychopathology based on structural phenomenology (see Apter, 1981). Structural phenomenology, considerably different to other phenomenological approaches, attempts to provide a systematic structure to

Stress and Performance in Sport. Edited by J. Graham Jones and Lew Hardy.
©1990 John Wiley & Sons Ltd.

the way in which the individual's own motivation is experienced. It is defined within the theory as 'the study of the structure of experience, and the way which the nature of this structure changes over time. It primarily concerns the structure of experience itself, rather than the particular structures which occur within experience' (Apter, 1982, pp. 368–369). Given this theoretical perspective, cognitive and emotional factors are obviously important, as is an underlying principle of the theory—the inconsistency of human behaviour. A number of novel concepts have been put forward by reversal theory which allow it to accommodate a conceptual base which incorporates such inherently difficult notions as the inconsistency of behaviour and the provision of a structure to the individual's experience of motivation. For clarification purposes, a glossary of reversal theory terms is included at the end of this chapter.

In psychology, the term 'state' is generally a statement about or description of something about a person at any one moment in time. As such, states are temporary and subject to change, sometimes quite rapid change. In reversal theory, 'metamotivational states', thought to exist together in opposite pairs, are also subject to change, more specifically change in one of two directions or 'reversals'. Four sets, or pairs, of metamotivational states (telic–paratelic, negativism–conformity, autic–alloic, sympathy–mastery) have been postulated by reversal theory. Of these four pairs of phenomenological states, the telic–paratelic pair has been the focus of much of the work carried out on reversal theory to date. In the paratelic state, behaviour tends to be spontaneous, playful and present-oriented, with a preference for high arousal and the pleasure of immediate sensation. By way of contrast, in the telic state, behaviour tends to be serious and planning-oriented, with a preference for low arousal.

Linked with the concepts of metamotivational state and reversal is the notion of 'bistability', from cybernetics. A bistable system is one type of multistable system which has two alternative preferred stable states, in one of which the system finds itself operating at any one time. The simplest example of a bistable system, often referred to in the reversal theory literature, is a light switch. Either the 'on' or 'off' position is stable, but any position in between these two is unstable. In reversal theory, bistability is concerned with which of the two metamotivational states (e.g. telic or paratelic) is operative. This is thought to be governed by the particular conditions pertaining at the time, such as aspects of the environment or biological functioning. The limitations of homeostatic system constructs which argue that organisms have only one preferred stable state have been avoided by the use of this concept. The currently popular homeostatic system conceptualization is a fundamental element in a number of other theoretical approaches in theories of motivation, for example optimal arousal theory (e.g. Fiske and Maddi, 1961). More complete descriptions of the bistable system approach and its advantages over

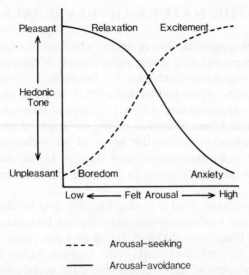

Figure 5.1. The relationship between arousal and hedonic tone for the telic state (solid line) and the paratelic state (dashed line)(reproduced by permission of Academic Press from Apter, 1982).

homeostatic systems, especially optimal arousal theory, have been given by Apter (1982). Murgatroyd (1985) and this author (Kerr, 1989).

Metamotivational states are phenomenological states which are characterized by the manner in which an individual interprets some aspect(s) of his or her motivation. Consequently, the telic and paratelic pair, as the pair concerned with the individual's experience of felt arousal and hedonic tone, are especially relevant to performance in sport. Felt arousal is the degree to which an individual feels himself to be 'worked up' at a given time. The interaction between felt arousal and hedonic tone (experienced pleasure) and the way arousal levels are interpreted have been represented graphically by Apter (1982) (see Figure 5.1).

Individuals have preferences for different levels of arousal in the telic and paratelic states. Consequently, levels of arousal in particular metamotivational states will be interpreted in different ways. The feelings associated with the experience of high or low felt arousal in the telic and paratelic states are 'excitement', 'anxiety', 'boredom' and 'relaxation'. In the telic state, low arousal is preferred and experienced as pleasant relaxation, whereas high arousal in this state would be experienced as unpleasant anxiety. In the paratelic state, high arousal is pleasant and experienced as excitement, while low arousal is unpleasant and will result in feelings of boredom.

THE NATURE OF REVERSALS

It is now clear from research that reversals, which are thought to be involuntary, can take place frequently within short periods of time and that they may well be sudden and unexpected (see, for example, Lafreniere, Cowles and Apter, 1988; Walters, Apter and Svebak, 1982). Reversal theory posits three different sets of circumstances which can induce reversals: (1) contingent events, for example where a feature of the environment changes; (2) under conditions of frustration, where the needs of an individual are not being satisfied in a particular metamotivational state; or (3) satiation, where as the period of time an individual spends in one state increases, reversal is increasingly likely.

Some simple examples from everyday life may help to illustrate how these changes or reversals in metamotivational state can take place. Jumping off a five-metre diving board into the pool, riding as a passenger on a motor bike, or performing in a competitive sports event, perhaps for the first time in front of a large audience, are all experiences which, for many people, are likely to be accompanied by anxiety. The very nature of these events, as described, means that they are likely to be characterized by high arousal, which in the telic state is experienced as unpleasant anxiety. After a few jumps off the board, a reversal may take place (telic to paratelic) and the previously unpleasant anxiety is now experienced as pleasant excitement. Similarly, once the journey on the motor bike is completed, the experienced feelings of anxiety may change to feelings of exhilaration. A telic to paratelic reversal has again taken place. One has to be careful of generalizations in using these examples, because some people may not reverse. They will always experience anxiety in these hypothetical situations and so, because their experience has continued to be unpleasant, they will probably avoid them in the future. Of course, reversals in the other direction, paratelic to telic, are also possible and other examples might have been used to illustrate reversals at low levels of arousal.

METAMOTIVATIONAL DOMINANCE: THE TELIC–PARATELIC PAIR

Individuals are thought to be biased in their experience of metamotivational states. In other words, they are likely to spend more time in one metamotivational state than the other. This is known as metamotivational 'dominance'. This applies to all the metamotivational states, but in this case, where the telic and paratelic states have been under discussion, individuals are said to be telic dominant or paratelic dominant (see Murgatroyd, 1985). The Telic Dominance Scale (TDS), developed by Murgatroyd *et al.* (1978), allows this bias to be measured. Research carried out since its development has shown the TDS to be a valid and reliable instrument and it has, in the intervening years, been used in a wide variety of settings, including sport (e.g. Kerr, 1987a). The fact that a psychometric scale has been developed may suggest to the reader that telic dominance is really the same type of concept as the traditional personality trait. However, it should be remembered that, in reversal theory, it is the inconsistency of the processes which is of importance. Thus, although the individual has a predisposition to be in a certain metamotivational state under certain conditions, he or she will switch or 'reverse' to the opposite paired state. Dominance reflects the ascendancy of one metamotivational state over another. This is fundamentally different to the notion of personality traits, which considers behaviour to be consistent, with individuals having an enduring predisposition to act in a particular way. For example, when an individual is classified as an 'extravert' (Eysenck and Eysenck, 1975), it indicates that extraverted behaviour is a regular and stable characteristic of that individual's personality.

A state version of the TDS (the Telic State Measure (TSM); Svebak and Murgatroyd, 1985) has been developed. The measure is composed of four questions which ask subjects to estimate (1) how serious or playful they felt, (2) how far they would have preferred to plan ahead or be spontaneous, (3) how aroused they felt, and (4) the level of arousal which they would have preferred. Each of the four questions is followed by a six-point rating scale with defining adjectives at each end (serious–playful, preferred planned–preferred spontaneous, low arousal–high arousal, preferred low arousal–preferred high arousal). Low scores on this six-point scale indicate that the telic state is operative and, conversely, high scores indicate that the paratelic state is operative. A fifth item, the discrepancy between preferred and actual levels of arousal, is computed by subtracting felt arousal from preferred arousal (i.e. score on item (4) minus the score on item (3)) and can therefore be positive or negative. The TSM, often used in combination with other types of measure, such as psychophysiological measures (e.g. Svebak, 1984) or structured interviews conducted blind to the TSM results (e.g. Svebak and Murgatroyd, 1985), provides a measure of the extent to which individuals remain in their dominant state during a particular event.

Reversal theory's phenomenological/cybernetic theoretical framework, supported by a series of innovative concepts, forms a novel approach to human action and especially motivation. Of special relevance to the study of sport, and, in particular, performance in sport, is the interaction between metamotivational dominance, states, felt arousal and hedonic tone in the individual's experience of his or her own motivation. Reversal theory's approach to the understanding of stress provides a systematic conceptual framework in which other theoretical explanations can be encompassed and from which a number of important practical implications for stress management and cognitive intervention, in both the general and sports contexts, become manifest. Before a discussion of these implications for sport can be undertaken, the reversal theory approach to stress should be clarified.

STRESS FROM THE REVERSAL THEORY PERSPECTIVE

Two types of stress, 'tension-stress' and 'effort-stress', are recognized in reversal theory (Apter and Svebak, 1990). Tension-stress is concerned with the experience of unpleasant emotions and occurs when there is a discrepancy between preferred and actual levels of some variable (e.g. felt arousal or felt transactional outcome). 'Effort-stress', on the other hand, occurs as a response to tension-stress, as a result of the individual's attempts to cope with some threat or challenge, i.e. efforts aimed at reducing tension-stress. A somewhat similar conceptualization of stress, based on the discrepancy between levels of self-reported arousal and required levels of arousal, has been described by Cox, Thirlaway and Cox (1982), the required level of arousal being determined by situational and internal factors. Using a self-report measure, the Stress/ Arousal Checklist (SACL) (Mackay et al., 1978), they investigated stress and arousal in repetitive work situations. They argued that any marked discrepancy between actual and required arousal might lead to 'compensatory' behaviour. This in turn was thought to lead to negative emotional experience (self-reported stress) brought about by the threat of inappropriate levels of arousal and the effort of compensating (see also Kerr, 1985a).

Returning to the discussion of the telic–paratelic pair, there are two possible forms of tension-stress, telic tension-stress and paratelic tension-stress. The latter is more likely to arise from conditions of low arousal experienced as unpleasant boredom. Telic tension-stress is thought to arise when conditions of high arousal are experienced by the individual in the telic state, resulting in unpleasant feelings of anxiety.

Likewise, there are two forms of effort-stress. The paratelic form is concerned with increasing levels of arousal to a preferred level, often by means of pleasant present-oriented coping activities (see Baker, 1988). Telic effort-stress is experienced during coping efforts aimed at reducing tension. This may well involve performing an activity which one does not wish to perform. Apter and Svebak (1990) claim that:

> . . . telic effort-stress comes closest to what is known as 'stress' in the medical and physiological literature. . . . telic tension-stress comes closest to the way in which the term 'stress' is used in certain parts of the counselling and psychotherapy literature. The present analysis shows not only how these two stress concepts are related, but also shows that there are other types of experience and behaviour which can also be labelled as forms of 'stress'.

Examining just one example, the consequences of unsuccessful coping for individuals who experience prolonged tension-stress while the telic state is operative are likely to be severe. They may well be subject to, for example, neurotic symptoms of chronic anxiety and phobias, but are also likely to be subject to psychosomatic complaints. By way of contrast, paratelic dominant individuals, or individuals for whom the paratelic state is operative for an extended period, perceive and respond to stress in a different way. This is the subject of the next section, which highlights some of the intriguing findings of recent reversal theory stress research.

REVERSAL THEORY STRESS RESEARCH

This section concentrates on the research work of Martin and his colleagues (see Martin, Kuiper and Olinger, 1988 for a review) at the University of Western Ontario in Canada, which has done much to establish the importance of telic and paratelic dominance in the moderation of stress. Reversal theory, in contrast to other theoretical explanations of stress effects, predicts that increases in the frequency or severity of stressful events can bring about improvements in some individuals' emotional and physical functioning. In support of reversal theory's apparently paradoxical prediction, research findings from three different studies (reported in Martin, 1985; Martin et al., 1987) indicated that paratelic dominant individuals were adversely affected by the absence of stressors in their everyday lives and actually thrived on moderate amounts of stress.

The first of these studies (Martin, 1985) examined the responses of telic and paratelic dominant subjects to increasing levels of arousal. Reversal theory argues that, for telic dominant individuals, hedonic tone should become increasingly unpleasant as arousal increases. In addition to the TDS, the Profile of Mood States (POMS) (McNair, Lorr and Droppleman, 1971), the Daily Hassles Scale (DHS) (Kanner et al., 1981) and the Life Events of College Students (LECS) (Sandler and Lakey, 1982) were included. Here, the POMS provided a measure of prevailing hedonic tone while the latter two scales (DHS, LECS) provided measures of enduring stress-related arousal levels. Following correlation analysis of subjects' scores on all the scales, no significant correlations between TDS scores and mood disturbance were identified, thus indicating that telic and paratelic subjects did not differ in their moods overall. However, as can be seen graphically in Figures 5.2 and 5.3, hierarchical multiple regression analysis (see Cohen and Cohen, 1983) revealed the important nature of the interaction between telic dominance, stress and moods. In Figure 5.2, the expected linear relationship between life events and moods for telic dominant subjects is represented by the dashed line.

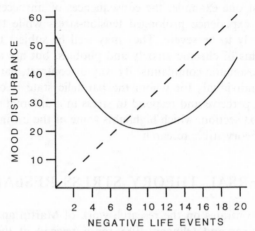

Figure 5.2. Regression curves showing the relationship between negative life events and mood disturbance for telic dominant and paratelic dominant subjects. Solid line, paratelic dominant; dashed line, telic dominant (from Martin, 1985).

The curvilinear relationship, represented by the solid line, confirms the researcher's pre-experiment reversal theory-based predictions about the response of paratelic dominant subjects. Initially, for paratelic dominant subjects, as the frequency of negative life events increased, a corresponding *decrease* in mood disturbance was experienced (i.e. the negative life events were experienced as pleasant). Further increases in the frequency of negative life events, however, resulted in a change. Mood disturbance then *increased* as a function of the negative life events so that, as with the telic subjects, these events were experienced as increasingly unpleasant as their frequency increased. In other words, it was low arousal conditions which were experienced as stressful by paratelic dominant individuals, at least up to a certain level of stress, at which point, it might be assumed, they tended to reverse to the telic state and show the same pattern as telic dominant subjects. The important point is that, over a certain range of stress/arousal, the effects were opposite in telic and paratelic dominant individuals. Similar regression curves computed from subjects' scores on the DHS, illustrated in Figure 5.3, provided further support for the reversal theory telic/paratelic distinction in stress response.

Findings from this first study showed that differences between telic and paratelic dominant individuals are most pronounced when levels of stress are low to moderate. Two subsequent studies (both reported in Martin *et al.*, 1987) have concentrated on this low to moderate range. In the second study, ongoing stressors in 48 subjects' lives were investigated by means of the Recent Stressful Event Questionnaire, constructed by the researchers. As a part of this questionnaire, subjects were required to describe the most stressful event they had experienced during the preceding month and then rate the event as

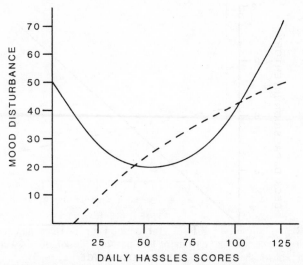

Figure 5.3. Regression curves showing the relationship between daily hassles and mood disturbance for telic dominant and paratelic dominant subjects. Solid line, paratelic dominant, dashed line, telic dominant (from Martin, 1985).

ongoing or resolved. In addition to completing the TDS, subjects also completed the Beck Depression Inventory (BDI) (Beck *et al.*, 1961) as a measure of mood. Scores on this scale (mean 5.7, SD 5.21) were reported as being well below the clinically depressed range, and the results were therefore discussed in terms of dysphoria rather than clinical depression. Pre-experiment hypotheses predicted that, if recent life stressors were ongoing rather than resolved, telic dominant subjects would be more dysphoric; paratelic dominant subjects, on the other hand, would be more dysphoric if recent stressors were resolved rather than ongoing.

Data were again treated using hierarchical multiple regression analysis, and the predicted interaction ($F_{1,\,38} = 4.07$; $p < 0.05$); shown graphically in Figure 5.4), between the dichotomously coded resolved/unresolved variable and metamotivational dominance upon dysphoria was obtained. Two main conclusions could be drawn from these results. First, for subjects who reported their most stressful recent event as ongoing, a positive linear relationship between telic dominance and dysphoria was found. For subjects who reported their most stressful recent event as resolved, a negative, but statistically non-significant, relationship between telic dominance and dysphoria was identified. Secondly, subjects' dysphoria scores became increasingly divergent, as a function of whether the stressful event had been resolved or remained unresolved, as telic dominance scores became more extreme. Consequently, if the most stressful event reported by telic dominant subjects during the past

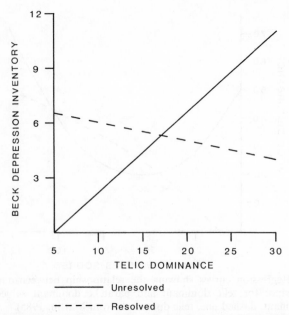

Figure 5.4. Relationship between Beck Depression Inventory (BDI) and Telic Dominance Scale (TDS) for subjects with resolved *versus* unresolved events (reproduced by permission of Elsevier Science Publishers from Martin, Kuiper and Olinger, 1988).

month remained unresolved, then, in comparison with paratelic subjects, higher levels of dysphoria were experienced. If, however, their most stressful event had been resolved, then the levels of dysphoria experienced were similar to those reported by paratelic subjects.

The findings from this second study underline the earlier findings that telic and paratelic dominant individuals differ in their response to stress. Once again, paradoxically, paratelic dominant individuals were found to experience greater dysphoria in the absence rather than the presence of ongoing stressors.

A third study (see also Martin *et al.*, 1987), perhaps of more direct relevance to the sports context, compared telic and paratelic dominant subjects performing a video game in the laboratory under two different levels of social evaluation stress. Under the two conditions, subjects were instructed either to play the game simply for fun (non-stressful) or to try to do their best, as their performance would be evaluated by the experimenter and compared to that of other subjects (moderately stressful). Subjects' heart rate and skin conductance were monitored on a polygraph during play and, following each 10-minute task period, they were asked to rate how they had been feeling while engaged in the task. This involved rating, on a seven-point scale, such items as how pleasant or unpleasant they felt, how satisfied or dissatisfied they were with their performance, how much they liked or disliked the experience, and the degree to which they perceived the experimenter as being friendly and supportive *versus* hostile and critical. Subjects were divided into telic ($N = 13$) and paratelic dominant ($N = 14$) groups and the order of stressful conditions during performance on the video game was randomized across groups.

The variable of particular interest to the researchers was the subjects' performance on the video task. Univariate ANOVA for this variable produced a significant interaction ($F_{1,25} = 8.22$; $p < 0.009$). Examination of the cell means revealed that paratelic dominant subjects obtained significantly higher task performance scores in the stressful condition than they did in the non-stressful condition. By comparison, the telic dominant subjects obtained higher, although not significantly higher, scores in the non-stressful than in the moderately stressful condition. Furthermore, the paratelic dominant group's mean performance score under the moderately stressful condition was significantly higher than the telic dominant group's mean scores for both the non-stressful and the moderately stressful conditions.

Following univariate analysis, the self-report data results indicated no differences in group means for paratelic dominant subjects between the two conditions, but group means for the telic dominant subjects between the non-stressful and moderately stressful conditions were found to be significantly different. Specifically, members of the telic dominant group reported feeling more unpleasant and more dissatisfied with their performance, perceived the experimenter as being more hostile, critical, and disapproving, and revealed a higher mean frequency of spontaneous skin responses (an index of autonomic emotional arousal) in the moderately stressful condition in comparison with the non-stressful condition. While paratelic dominant subjects remained relatively unaffected by the moderately stressful condition, telic dominant subjects were more adversely affected by the moderately stressful condition than they were by the non-stressful condition. The researchers suggested that increased social evaluation stress might have tended to interfere with the performance of the telic dominant subjects but might have enhanced the performance of the paratelic dominant subjects. The results of this study, especially those from the self-report and psychophysiological data, add further support for the stress-moderating effect of paratelic dominance.

The positive nature of the results of this preliminary series of experiments has done much to provide general supportive evidence (see also Dobbin and Martin, 1988) for the reversal theory explanation of stress. As Martin, Kuiper and Olinger (1988) pointed out:

> Of particular interest to us is the fact that a reversal theory account suggests that stress is not always deleterious or noxious, but may in fact be invigorating for some people, providing them with an enhanced sense of challenge and excitement. In this regard, some researchers in the stress area have suggested

that a distinction may be made between 'good stress' and 'bad stress' (e.g. Frankenhaeuser, 1980; Ursin and Murison, 1983) or between 'eustress' and 'distress' (Selye, 1976). Reversal theory suggests that the differences between the two reside not so much in the nature of the actual events but rather in the metamotivational state of the individual who is experiencing the stressors. (p. 102)

Kerr (1985b; see also Kerr and Svebak, 1989) has drawn attention to participation by some individuals in sports activities in which the 'positive' aspects of stress (sometimes called 'eustress') are experienced as pleasant.

In addition, there are a number of important implications for stress management in sport arising out of the findings described above. For example, in dealing with competitors experiencing difficulty in optimizing their level of arousal prior to performance, the choice of particular intervention techniques (see Kerr, 1987b, 1989) or advice on the development of coping strategies may well be inappropriate for some competitors if their metamotivational dominance characteristics are ignored. Additional research (Baker, 1988), not reported above, has shown that telic and paratelic dominance plays an important role in stress appraisals and coping style. Other preliminary research work (Kerr, 1987a; Kerr and van Lienden, 1987; Svebak and Kerr, 1989) has already identified differences in the metamotivational dominance characteristics of performers of different sports.

OPTIONS FOR COGNITIVE INTERVENTION

In spite of a number of recent publications (e.g. Kirschenbaum and Bale, 1984) commending the use of cognitive interventions in sport, some caution is required in advocating the use of such techniques until a good deal more research has been carried out. Other writers (Heyman, 1984; Mahoney, 1984) have expressed concern at the difficulty of determining whether a sports performer's problems are only related to sport or are more comprehensive clinical conditions requiring a therapeutic approach to psychological and behavioural change. As a result, the application, in the sports context, of intervention techniques derived from clinical psychology should be regarded as a possibility rather than a confident recommendation. However, keeping these concerns in mind, Kerr (1987b) has outlined a number of possible options for cognitive intervention with sports performers based on the reversal theory approach. These options are especially important with regard to affecting arousal levels prior to and during performance in sport. It is the control and influencing of sports performers' pre-performance arousal levels, thought to be crucial for the enhancement of subsequent competitive performance, which has been a major concern of sport psychologists. For example, Rushall (1982) has advocated the formulation of detailed strategies and competition-specific plans and the use of 'on-site' intervention techniques aimed at the enhancement of competitive performance.

The search for the most appropriate level of arousal prior to performance has been strongly influenced by optimal arousal theory (e.g. Hebb, 1955). Consequently, much of the work has concentrated on preventing sports performers from becoming 'overaroused', with a resultant emphasis on the use of arousal reduction techniques from clinical psychology. Treatment in the clinical setting, based on the reduction of arousal levels, has been effective for patients who have problems controlling anxiety levels (see also Mace, Chapter 8 in this book). Optimal arousal theory, of course, argues that performance will improve with increases in arousal up to a maximal point, beyond which further increases in arousal produce decrements in performance. However, some research studies (Heide and Borkovec, 1983; Budzinski, Stoyva and Peffer, 1980) have shown that some subjects are unable to achieve a state of low arousal and that, for others, relaxation training can paradoxically induce anxiety. As well as arousal reduction, reversal theory (see Svebak and Stoyva, 1980; Kerr, 1987b, 1989) argues that there are other equally effective options for intervention.

Three alternative strategies or options which could be used to change or cause a reinterpretation of arousal levels are proposed. These are outlined in Figure 5.5. For the sports performer in the telic state experiencing an unpleasantly high arousal level, arousal could be reduced by utilizing one of the arousal-reducing techniques from clinical psychology, for example progressive relaxation (option 1). Where the level of arousal is unpleasantly low for a competitor in the paratelic state, it could be increased by, for example, utilizing biofeedback techniques in an innovative way (option 3). Subjects could learn to voluntarily increase arousal rather than decrease it (Svebak and Stoyva, 1980).

By bringing about a metamotivational reversal, a reinterpretation of how the individual experiences either high or low arousal, in terms of hedonic tone (pleasantness), can be effected. For instance, for a performer in the telic state experiencing tension-stress, inducing a telic to paratelic reversal would result in unpleasant high arousal (anxiety) being reinterpreted as pleasant (option 2). The situation, or the particular activity, would then be perceived by the individual as an enjoyable challenge to be undertaken with enthusiasm. For a sports competitor with the paratelic state operative, experiencing paratelic tension-stress, a paratelic to telic reversal would result in unpleasant low arousal (feelings of boredom) being reinterpreted as pleasant relaxation (option 4). Conversely, in this case (as shown in option 3), arousal levels could be increased to more preferable levels by means of pleasant present-oriented coping activities (see Baker, 1988).

It should be obvious, however, that before any attempt at intervention is carried out by a sport psychologist, coach or perhaps the performers themselves,

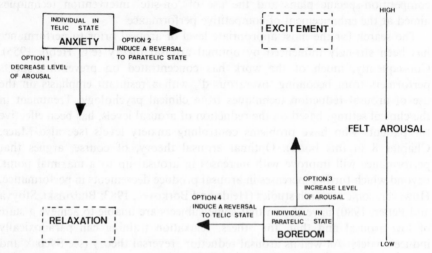

Figure 5.5. Possible options for affecting felt arousal (from Kerr, 1987b).

a crucial requirement is to be able to recognize when inappropriate metamotivational states are operative. Many sports performers learn through experience
which operative mental state is most appropriate for them prior to, or even
during, performance. Indeed, some are able, and others could perhaps be
taught, to recognize when something is amiss and an inappropriate metamotivational state is operative. The close relationship sport psychologists or
coaches have with their performers may also allow them to recognize when
the operative mental state of their sports performers is not consistent with
their normal pre-competitive metamotivational state. In addition, the TSM
(Svebak and Murgatroyd, 1985), the self-report state version of the TDS, is
currently being used in sport (as well as a number of other settings) and it
seems likely that it could also be used to assist in the recognition of operative
metamotivational states. Once an inappropriate pre-competitive metamotivational state has been identified, one of the options described above could be
utilized. Although, under the terms of reversal theory, individuals are thought
not to be able to bring about reversals voluntarily, reversals can be triggered
by a change in the environment. In addition to environmental change, it has
also been suggested (Kerr, 1987b) that top sports performers could, after the
correct training, induce the necessary reversal by means of a cognitive
restructuring or imaging strategy (i.e. mental change).

Much of what has been said above is theoretical, and certainly little work
with sports competitors has been undertaken to date. All of this depends on
knowing a good deal more about which metamotivational state is most
appropriate for a particular sport and for a particular individual. The relationships would appear to be complex. A crucial element is the interplay between

metamotivational dominance and state. It has also been shown that participation in at least some sports is linked to dominance (Svebak and Kerr, 1989; Kerr and Svebak, 1989) and that 'professional' (Kerr, 1987a) and 'masters' (Kerr and van Lienden, 1987) performers are more telic dominant then 'serious amateurs' or 'recreational' performers. One suggestion (e.g. Kerr, 1987c) was that a matching of dominance and state might provide the most appropriate condition for maximum performance in the sports context.

SPORTS-SPECIFIC RESEARCH: PRELIMINARY FINDINGS

Kerr (1988) designed a research strategy for the study of psychological effects in squash which incorporated reversal theory measures. A major objective of this series of studies was to attempt to overcome the limitations of single research paradigm investigations. Laux and Vossel (1982), for example, have criticized laboratory experiments as an inadequate strategy for stress research. They pointed out that studying stress effects under artificial conditions produces results of only limited generalizability. Several authors (e.g. Lazarus and Launier, 1978) have advocated abandoning laboratory-based research in favour of field investigations which study stress in real-life settings. However, Laux and Vossel (1982) and McGrath (1972) have argued that combining laboratory and field research has a number of potential benefits.

A 'laboratory type' squash study examined the effects of telic dominance and metamotivational state on squash task performance (Kerr and Cox, 1988; see also Kerr and Cox, 1990). No significant differences in telic dominance between 'skilled', 'average' and 'novice' players were found. Data from the TSM, which was administered before and after performance on the squash task, revealed no significant differences between groups on all five items, but significant telic increases were found in the planning–spontaneous and felt arousal item scores. Telic increases in scores on the serious–playful item, pre- to post-task, approached significance ($p = 0.06$). Also, a significant decrease in discrepancy scores (preferred arousal minus felt arousal) before and after task performance was obtained. In all cases, trends were least for the skilled group. This result suggests that levels of tension-stress were decreased and that skilled players would have experienced less tension-stress than the other ability groups.

This was supported to some extent by the results obtained in the same study from the Stress/Arousal Checklist (SACL) (Mackay et al., 1978; Cox and Mackay, 1985). The SACL is a 30-item adjective self-report checklist containing 18 stress and 12 arousal adjectives and originally developed from the work of Thayer (1967). The results showed that the skilled group reported low stress accompanied by high levels of arousal throughout the experiment, while the

Table 5.1. Numbers of subjects pre- and post-task performance in telic and paratelic states and experiencing high levels of felt arousal.

	N	Telic	Paratelic	Chi square (actual compared to equal distribution of scores)	High arousal
Total pre-task	39 (20:19)	31	8	12.42, $df=1$ $p<0.001$	25 (63%)
Total post-task	39 (20:19)	32	7	14.78, $df=1$ $p<0.001$	30 (75%)

average and novice players reported constantly high levels of arousal along with high levels of stress. Further analysis of the subject responses on the TSM revealed that the majority of subjects from all three ability groups were in the telic state both before and after completion of the squash tasks. In addition, a large proportion of subjects in both the telic and paratelic states reported that they were experiencing high levels of arousal (see Table 5.1). This observation again suggests that a large number of players with the telic state operative would have been subject to tension-stress. Those players with the paratelic state operative would have experienced high levels of arousal as pleasant and would not have experienced tension-stress.

A second study (Kerr, 1988; Cox and Kerr, 1990) set out to examine psychological responses in squash under ecologically valid conditions. Three, simulated, squash tournaments were built into the research design so that differences in psychological states and responses between successful and unsuccessful male players could be measured under 'real' competitive tournament conditions. Included, with a number of other measures, were the TDS (Murgatroyd *et al.*, 1978) and the TSM (Svebak and Murgatroyd, 1985), again in combination with the SACL (Mackay *et al.*, 1978). These were administered to players during the tournament.

Following statistical analysis, no significant differences between initial (ability-based) subject groups in the three tournaments were obtained on telic dominance or any of the initial mood measure scores. The most successful ('winners'; $N=7$) and least successful players ('losers'; $N=7$) were then identified on the basis of their final points score in each tournament. Each tournament had consisted of two leagues of five players with each player playing the other four members of his particular league (i.e. four games). When the TSM responses of winners and losers were compared, non-significant differences on the serious–playful (with the exception of post-game 2 scores), planning–spontaneous and level of felt arousal items were obtained. Of more

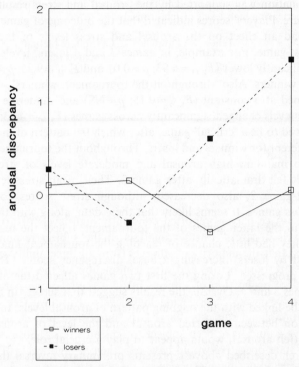

Figure 5.6. Mean arousal discrepancy scores for winners and losers at the four games of the squash tournament (reproduced by permission of Hemisphere Publishing Corporation from Kerr, 1989).

specific interest, perhaps, with regard to stress were winners' and losers' scores on the discrepancy item (preferred minus felt arousal), which indicated that winners' scores did not change significantly across games but the losers' scores did ($F_{3, 36} = 3.84$; $p = 0.017$), as shown in Figure 5.6.

In general, discrepancy scores of winners were smaller and more consistent than those of losers. Tension-stress experienced by winners was, therefore, likely to have been minimal and the consequent effort-stress not realized. The discrepancy scores of losers after game 2 were positive, indicating that after game 2 losers would have preferred much higher levels of arousal than they actually experienced. This discrepancy in losers' preferred and felt arousal scores increased as the tournament proceeded, probably bringing about increased feelings of negative hedonic tone and the likely experience of tension-stress. A probable outcome was that losers were also likely to have experienced effort-stress brought about by their attempts to cope (Apter and Svebak, 1990).

This explanation was supported by the arousal and stress results from the SACL measure. Players' scores indicated that the outcome of game 2 (winning or losing) had an effect on the arousal and stress levels of the losers, as recorded post-game. For example, in games 3 and 4 losers' levels of arousal became significantly lower ($F_{1, 12} = 6.93$; $p = 0.02$ and $F_{1, 12} = 9.25$; $p = 0.01$) than those of the winners. Also, throughout the tournament, winners' self-reported stress remained at a constant ($F_{3, 36} = 0.15$; $p = NS$) and moderate level while losers' stress levels changed significantly across games ($F_{3, 36} = 4.73$; $p = 0.007$). Game 2 proved to be a 'crucial' game, after which the pattern of mood change was very different for winners and losers. Throughout the tournament, winners continued to maintain high arousal and moderate levels of stress. Losers' arousal levels fell dramatically after game 2. Their mean stress levels, which peaked post-game 2, also decreased, although stress scores continued to increase across games. It seems likely that these data, along with the performance scores in the latter games of the tournament, reflect the realization by losers that they had little chance of reaching the tournament final. This was also reflected by losers' increasing arousal discrepancy scores (TSM) as the tournament progressed. Losing the first two games affected the mood of the losers in games 3 and 4. Overall, the results suggest that success in tournament squash may be linked with the ongoing pattern of arousal levels. In particular, the interaction between preferred arousal and the level of arousal actually experienced (felt arousal) would appear to play a crucial role.

The research described above represents preliminary reversal theory-based experimental work in sport. The findings of these studies are of interest, but a comprehensive programme of sports-specific research designed to test reversal theory constructs is required. As work in reversal theory continues to make progress, a number of challenges have to be faced, not the least of which is to shed more light on the current debate focused on optimal performance in sport. It may be worth pointing out that, at this point, reversal theory deals with arousal in relation to hedonic tone and not performance. The research which has been carried out asks, among other questions, whether preferred levels of arousal (i.e. optimal), as defined in reversal theory, determine performance as well as hedonic tone. In other words, reversal theory provides a new approach to performance and it is a reasonable hypothesis that hedonic tone relates to performance.

CONCLUDING COMMENTS

It should be pointed out that the discussion in this chapter has concentrated on the telic–paratelic metamotivational pair. Likewise, the explanation offered above has only taken into account possible stress effects concerned with mismatches in levels of felt arousal. Under the terms of reversal theory, felt arousal is only one of the variables which can lead to the experience of tension and resulting tension-stress. For example, no mention has been made here of 'self-tone' or 'felt transactional outcome' (Apter and Smith, 1985), experiences associated more closely with the mastery–sympathy metamotivational pair. The squash studies summarized above were concerned with telic–paratelic pair, but individuals involved in competitive sports situations may well also be in the mastery state while competing, thus bringing into consideration possible discrepancies in felt transactional outcome. No reversal theory research examining changes or discrepancies in felt transactional outcome has yet been attempted. Undoubtedly, it will become a focus of investigation in other 'real-life' situations, as well as competitive sports contexts, in the future.

From the beginning, and unlike some other approaches or theories in psychology, reversal theory has involved itself with sport. Many of the examples and illustrations used to explain concepts and arguments from the theory are taken from sport. This, of course, is not the only reason why reversal theory is attractive to psychologists. There are already quite a number of theoretical approaches which attempt to provide a basis for the understanding of stress. What is it about reversal theory that is so special? Why should it warrant special attention from sport psychologists?

As Apter and Svebak (1990) point out, the theory has, within its systematic conceptual framework, the potential of integrating a number of other recent approaches to stress. In addition, the reversal theory perspective on stress helps to explain the relationship between stress and psychopathology, psychosomatic disorders and stress symptoms. Thirdly, it has important practical implications for stress management. Given the advantages listed above, the theory should be of interest to all psychologists working in the area of stress and of particular interest to those working with competitive sports performers, who may well have to perform under potentially stressful circumstances. Reversal theory could prove to be a valuable tool in the business of stress in sport, especially in unravelling the intriguing relationship between arousal, hedonic tone and sports performance.

REFERENCES

Apter, M. J. (1981). The possibility of a structural phenomenology: the case of reversal theory, *Journal of Phenomenological Psychology*, **12**(2), 173–187.

Apter, M. J. (1982). *The Experience of Motivation: The Theory of Psychological Reversals*. London and New York: Academic Press.

Apter, M. J. and Smith, K. C. P. (1985). Experiencing personal relationships, in M. J. Apter, D. Fontana and S. Murgatroyd (eds). *Reversal Theory: Applications and Developments*. Cardiff, Wales; University College Cardiff Press.

Apter, M. J. and Svebak, S. (1990). Stress from the reversal theory perspective, in C. D. Spielberger and J. Strelau (eds). *Stress and Anxiety 12*. New York: Hemisphere/ McGraw Hill.

Baker, J. (1988). Stress appraisals and coping with everyday hassles, in M. J. Apter, J. H. Kerr and M. P. Cowles (eds). *Progress in Reversal Theory*. Advances in Psychology Series, 51. Amsterdam: North-Holland.

Beck, A., Ward, C., Mendelson, M., Mock, J. and Erbaugh, J. (1961). An inventory for measuring depression, *Archives of General Psychiatry*, **4**, 53–63.

Budzinski, T. H., Stoyva, J. M. and Peffer, K. E. (1980). Biofeedback techniques in psychosomatic disorders, in A. Goldstein and E. Foa (eds). *Handbook of Behavioural Interventions: A Clinical Guide*. New York: Wiley.

Cohen, J. and Cohen, P. (1983). *Applied Multiple Regression/Correlational Analysis for the Behavioural Sciences*. Hillsdale, New Jersey: Erlbaum.

Cox, T. and Kerr, J. H. (1990). Self-reported mood in competitive squash, *Personality and Individual Differences*, **11** (2), 199–203.

Cox, T. and Mackay, C. J. (1985). The measurement of self-reported stress and arousal, *British Journal of Psychology*, **76**, 183–186.

Cox, T. Thirlaway, M. and Cox, S. (1982). Repetitive work, well-being and arousal, in H. Ursin and R. Murison (eds.) *Biological and Psychological Basis of Psychosomatic Disease*. Advances in the Biosciences, 42. Oxford: Pergamon Press.

Dobbin, J. P. and Martin, R. A. (1988). Telic versus paratelic dominance: personality moderator of biochemical responses to stress, in M. J. Apter, J. H. Kerr and M. P. Cowles (eds). *Progress in Reversal Theory*. Advances in Psychology Series, 51. Amsterdam: North-Holland.

Eysenck, H. J. and Eysenck, S. B. G. (1975). *Manual of the Eysenck Personality Questionnaire*. London: Hodder and Stoughton.

Fiske, D. W. and Maddi, S. R. (1961). A conceptual framework, in D. W. Fiske and S. R. Maddi (eds). *Functions of Varied Experience*. Homewood, Illinois: Dorsey.

Frankenhauser, M. (1980). Psychobiological aspects of life stress, in S. Levine and H. Ursin (eds). *Coping and Health*. New York: Plenum.

Hebb, D. O. (1955). Drives and the CNS (Conceptual Nervous System), *Psychological Review*, **62**, 243–254.

Heide, F. J. and Borkovec, T. D. (1983). Relaxation and induced anxiety–paradoxical anxiety enhancement due to relaxation training, *Journal of Consulting and Clinical Psychology*, **51**, 171–182.

Heyman, S. R. (1984). Cognitive interventions: theories, applications and cautions, in W. F. Straub and J. M. Williams (eds). *Cognitive Sport Psychology*. New York: Sport Science Associates.

Kanner, A. D., Coyne, J. C., Schaefer, C. and Lazarus, R. S. (1981). Comparison of two modes of stress management: daily hassles and uplifts versus major life events, *Journal of Behavioural Medicine*, **4**, 1–39.

Kerr, J. H. (1985a). The experience of arousal: a new basis for studying arousal effects in sport, *Journal of Sports Sciences*, **3**, 169–179.

Kerr, J. H. (1985b). A new perspective for sports psychology, in M. J. Apter, D. Fontana and S. Murgatroyd (eds). *Reversal theory: Applications and Developments*. Cardiff, Wales: University College Cardiff Press.

Kerr, J. H. (1987a). Differences in the motivational characteristics of 'professional', 'serious amateur' and 'recreational' sports performers, *Perceptual and Motor Skills*, **64**, 379–382.

Kerr, J. H. (1987b). Cognitive intervention with elite performers: reversal theory, *British Journal of Sports Medicine*, **21** (2), 29–33.

Kerr, J. H. (1987c). Structural phenomenology, arousal and performance, *Journal of Human Movement Studies*, **13**, 211–229.

Kerr, J. H. (1988). Arousal mechanisms, attention and sports performance. Unpublished PhD thesis, University of Nottingham, England.

Kerr, J. H. (1989). Anxiety, arousal and sport performance: an application of reversal theory, in D. Hackfort and C. D. Spielberger (eds). *Anxiety in Sports: An International Perspective*. Series in Health and Behavioural Medicine. New York: Hemisphere.

Kerr, J. H. and Cox, T. (1988). Effects of telic dominance and metamotivational state on squash task performance, *Perceptual and Motor Skills*, **67**, 171–174.

Kerr, J. H. and Cox, T. (1990). Cognition and mood in relation to the performance of a squash task, *Acta Psychologica*, **73**, 1, 103–114.

Kerr, J. H. and Van Lienden, H. J. (1987). Telic dominance in masters swimmers, *Scandinavian Journal of Sports Sciences*, **9** (3), 85–88.

Kerr, J. H. and Svebak, S. (1989). Motivational aspects of preference for and participation in 'risk' and 'safe' sports, *Personality and Individual Differences*, **10** (7), 797–800.

Kirschenbaum, D. S. and Bale, R. M. (1984). Cognitive-behavioral skills in sports, in W. F. Straub and J. M. Williams (Eds). *Cognitive Sport Psychology*. Lansing, New York: Sports Science Associates.

Lafreniere, K., Cowles, M. P. and Apter, M. J. (1988). The reversal phenomenon: reflections on a laboratory study, in M. J. Apter, J. H. Kerr and M. P. Cowles (eds). *Progress in Reversal Theory*. Advances in Psychology series, 51. Amsterdam: North-Holland.

Laux, L. and Vossel, G. (1982). Paradigms in stress research: laboratory versus field and traits versus processes, in L. Goldberger and S. Breznitz (eds). *Handbook of Stress: Theoretical and Clinical Aspects*. London: Free Press.

Lazarus, R. S. and Launier, R. (1978). Stress-related transactions between person and the environment, in L. A. Pervin and M. Lewis (eds). *Perspectives in Interactional Psychology*. New York: Plenum Press.

Mackay, C. J., Cox, T., Burrows, G. C. and Lazzerini, A. J. (1978). An inventory for the measurement of self-reported stress and arousal, *British Journal of Social and Clinical Psychology*, **17**, 283–284.

Mahoney, M. J. (1984). Cognitive skills and athletic performance, in W. F. Straub and J. M. Williams (eds). *Cognitive Sport Psychology*. Lansing, New York: Sports Science Associates.

Martin, R. A. (1985). Telic dominance, stress and moods in M. J. Apter, D. Fontana and S. Murgatroyd (eds). *Reversal Theory: Applications and Developments*. Cardiff, Wales: University College Cardiff Press and New Jersey: Lawrence Erlbaum.

Martin, R. A., Kuiper, N. A. and Olinger, L. J. (1988). Telic versus paratelic dominance as a moderator of stress, in M. J. Apter, J. H. Kerr and M. P. Cowles (eds). *Progress in Reversal Theory*. Advances in Psychology series, 51. Amsterdam: North-Holland.

Martin, R. A., Kuiper, N. A., Olinger, L. J. and Dobbin, J. P. (1987). Is stress always bad?: Telic versus paratelic dominance as a stress moderating variable, *Journal of Personality and Social Psychology*. **53**, 970–982.

McGrath, J. E. (1972). Major methodological issues, in J. E. McGrath (ed.). *Social and Psychological Factors in Stress*. New York: Holt.

McNair, D. M., Lorr, M. and Droppleman, L. F. (1971). *The Profile of Mood States*. San Diego, California: EDITS.

Murgatroyd, S. (1985). The nature of telic dominance, in M. J. Apter, D. Fontana and S. Murgatroyd (eds). *Reversal theory: Applications and Developments*. Cardiff, Wales: University College Cardiff Press and New Jersey: Lawrence Erlbaum.

Murgatroyd, S., Rushton, C., Apter, M. J. and Ray, C. (1978). The development of the Telic Dominance Scale, *Journal of Personality Assessment*, **42**, 519–528.

Rushall, B. S. (1982). On-site psychological preparation for athletes, in T. Orlick, J. Partington and J. H. Salmela (eds). *Mental Training for Coaches and Athletes*. Ottawa, Canada: Sport in Perspective Inc. and Coaching Association of Canada.

Sandler, I. N. and Lakey, B. (1982). Locus of control as a stress moderator: the role of control perceptions and social support, *American Journal of Community Psychology*, **10**, 65–80.

Selye, H. (1976). *The Stress of Life*. New York: McGraw-Hill.

Svebak, S. (1984). Active forearm flexor tension patterns in the continuous perceptual motor task paradigm: the significance of motivation, *International Journal of Psychophysiology*, **2**, 167–176.

Svebak, S. and Kerr, J. H. (1989). The role of impulsivity in preference for sports, *Personality and Individual Differences*, **10**, 51–58.

Svebak, S. and Murgatroyd, S. (1985). Metamotivational dominance: a multi-method validation of reversal theory constructs, *Journal of Personality and Social Psychology*, **48** (1), 107–116.

Svebak, S. and Stoyva, J. (1980). High arousal can be pleasant and exciting. The theory of psychological reversals, *Biofeedback and Self-Regulation*, **5** (4), 439–444.

Thayer, R. E. (1967). Measurement of activation through self-report, *Psychological Reports*, **20**, 663–678.

Ursin, H. and Murison, R. (1983). The stress concept, in H. Ursin and R. Murison (eds). *Biological and Psychological Basis of Psychosomatic Disease*. Advances in the Biosciences, 42. Oxford: Pergamon.

Walters, J., Apter, M. J. and Svebak, S. (1982). Colour preference, arousal and the theory of psychological reversals, *Motivation and Emotion*, **6** (3), 193–215.

GLOSSARY OF REVERSAL THEORY TERMS USED IN THIS CHAPTER

Alloic state—A metamotivational state in which pleasure and displeasure derive primarily from what happens to someone else rather than what happens to oneself at the time in question. It forms a pair with the autic state.

Arousal, felt—The degree to which an individual feels himself to be 'worked up' at a given time, and in this sense the degree of intensity of his feelings of motivation. The felt arousal dimension defined in this way is different from the sleep–wakefulness dimension. Felt arousal should also be distinguished from tension.

Autic state—A metamotivational state in which pleasure and displeasure derive primarily from what happens to oneself rather than what happens to someone else at the time in question. It forms a pair with the alloic state.

Bistability—A system exhibits bistability if it tends to maintain a specified variable, despite external disturbance, within one or another of two ranges of values of the variable concerned. (This contrasts with homeostasis, in which only one range of values is involved.)

Conformist state—A metamotivational state in which the individual wants, or feels compelled to comply with, some requirement. It forms a pair with the negativistic state.

Dominance—A metamotivational state is said to be dominant, or 'state-dominant', if the individual is predisposed to spend longer periods in this state than in the other member of the pair which they together constitute. It implies that there is an innate bias in the individual in favour of one state rather than its opposite, although this may be obscured by environmental influences. It is measured by the Telic Dominance Scale.

Effort-stress—The stress experienced as a concomitant of the expenditure of effort in order to reduce tension-stress; the effort expended to overcome some cause of anxiety or to avoid boredom.

Mastery state—A metamotivational state in which the individual seeks to master (dominate, control, etc.) the other with whom he is interacting at the time. In this state, transactions with the other are seen as involving taking or yielding up. It forms a pair with the sympathy state.

Metamotivational state—A phenomenological state which is characterized by a certain way of interpreting some aspect(s) of one's own motivation. Such metamotivational states as have been identified in reversal theory go in pairs of opposites, only one member of each pair being operative at a given time but reversal always being possible between members of a pair.

Multistability—A system exhibits multistability if it tends to maintain a specified variable, despite external disturbance, within one or another of a specifiable set of ranges of values of the variable concerned. The simplest case is that of bistability.

Negativistic state—A metamotivational state in which the individual wants, or feels compelled to act against, some requirement (whether or not this action is actually carried out). It forms a pair with the conformist state.

Paratelic state—A metamotivational state in which the individual is oriented towards, or feels the need to be oriented towards, some aspect of his continuing behaviour and its related sensations. It forms a pair with the telic state. It tends to be associated with an interest in activity for its own sake, playfulness, spontaneity and a preference for high-intensity experiences.

Reversal—In its strictest sense in reversal theory, a reversal is a switch from one metamotivational state being operative to the other member of the pair of states which they together constitute being operative. The term is also used to refer to other kinds of sudden switches between opposites within experience, such as switches between opposite meanings of a given identity.

Satiation—In the reversal theory sense this refers to the way in which, as one member of a pair of metamotivational states remains operative over time, so some innate force for change builds up in such a way as to facilitate a reversal to the opposite member of the pair of states. Eventually, this process of satiation of the operative state may lead to reversal, even in the absence of any other factors which might tend to induce a reversal.

Self-tone—A type of hedonic tone which arises from one's perception of oneself and one's own identity, especially in relation to others.

Significance, felt—The degree to which one sees one's actions at a given time in a context which extends beyond the immediate effects of these actions. In particular, the degree to which one sees a goal one is pursuing as nested within a hierarchy of superordinate goals—also known as 'goal coherence'.

Structural phenomenology—The study of the structure of experience, and the way in which the nature of this structure changes over time. It primarily concerns the structure of experience itself, rather than particular structures which occur within experience.

Sympathy state—A metamotivational state in which the individual seeks to be liked by the other with whom he is interacting at the time. In this state, transactions with the other are seen as involving giving or being given. It forms a pair with the mastery state.

Telic Dominance Scale (TDS)—A 42-item multiple-choice paper-and-pencil test designed to measure the testee's bias towards the telic or paratelic state, i.e. the strength of the testee's underlying tendency to be predominantly in one state or the other over time. It consists of three subscales: seriousmindedness, planning orientation and arousal–avoidance.

Telic state—A metamotivational state in which the individual is oriented towards, or feels the need to be oriented towards, some essential goal or goals. It forms a pair with the paratelic state. It tends to be associated with seriousmindedness, planning ahead and a preference for low-intensity experiences.

Telic State Measure (TSM)—A short paper-and-pencil test designed principally to disclose whether the testee is in the telic or paratelic state of mind at a given moment of time.

Tension—In reversal theory, a feeling that accompanies, and is proportional to, any discrepancy between a preferred and actual level of some variable, the preferred level of which characterizes a metamotivational state. Unlike arousal, tension is always unpleasant (cf. Arousal, felt).

Tension-stress—The stress experienced as a concomitant of tension. For example, both anxiety and boredom would be experienced as forms of tension-stress. It contrasts with effort-stress.

Transactional outcome, felt—The perceived outcome of an interaction in terms of the degree of gain or loss which it is felt to represent.

2

STRESS MANAGEMENT AND SELF-REGULATION IN SPORT

Chapter 6

Goal setting in sport

W. D. Alan Beggs
Nottingham University

The purpose of this chapter is threefold: first, to give the reader a grasp of the techniques of effective goal setting which have been established in laboratory and industrial/organizational settings; secondly, to discuss the possible processes by which goal setting may motivate people and lead to improvements in their performance; and finally, to try to relate these ideas and findings, together with the available literature on goal setting in sport, to the somewhat different question of stress in competitive sport. Much of the theoretical and practical work done on goal setting to date has focused neither on sport nor stress, and some readers may be wondering why the topic has been included in a book on stress in sport. In fact, goal setting in sport is a very new, and potentially exciting, development, taking the technique into a completely different area. Unlike most tasks in areas where goal setting has already been used, in competitive sport the task to be performed is usually very difficult, complex or threatening. As a result, the athlete may suffer from anxiety, lack of confidence, or both. Recent advances in understanding the relationships between anxiety and performance were discussed by Parfitt, Jones and Hardy in Chapter 3 in this book; when applied to sport, the technique of goal setting seems to offer both coach and athlete a practical way to gain leverage on these problems.

Goal setting itself is not new. Psychologists have been trying to develop a theory of goals and refine the practice of goal setting for a very long time. Work on the topic started at the very beginnings of psychology—at the Wurzburg school of Ach, Kulpe and Watt—and was continued by the Gestalt psychologists, such as Lewin (1921, 1922). These early psychologists were concerned with something which has once again become a contemporary issue, intentionality. Intention, of course, is another word for goal—the knowledge or representation of the to-be-performed action.

The story, however, is perhaps best taken up about 20 years ago. Around that time, Ryan (1970) published an influential review of his own and others' work on the role of intention in motivation. He described the work of the

Stress and Performance in Sport. Edited by J. Graham Jones and Lew Hardy.
©1990 John Wiley & Sons Ltd.

early European psychologists and discussed the seminal ideas of Tolman (1932) and Miller, Galanter and Pribram (1960), all of whom focused on the now fashionable concept of cognitive mediation. Ryan presented his own closely argued view that intentions are causally linked to actions, and was scathing in his attack on the reductionist ideas of the behaviourists. More recently, psychologists such as Shotter (1980, 1984) have advanced these ideas; goal setting is one of the few empirical techniques which can be used to test this line of psychological theory, something which Ryan (1970) recognized as vital.

At about the same time, Locke (1968) described his goal-directed model of motivation in an organizational setting. This was a bid to apply the 'new' ideas to a real-life scenario, and drew on both those early views and more contemporary restatements of them; task completion was regarded as being directed by an intention to do just that. What Locke succeeded in doing was making a clear theoretical statement about the importance of cognitive mediation in task performance. For Locke, 'the basic (implicit or explicit) premise . . . is that man's conscious ideas affect what he does, i.e. that one of the (biological) functions of consciousness is the regulation of action' (p. 158); there are few these days who would disgaree with the basic concepts of the cognitive revolution.

Pure and applied psychology have not always advanced hand-in-hand, and this is certainly the case as far as goals and goal setting are concerned. The search for management techniques which would power the American industrial machine at the turn of the century spawned the work of Taylor (1911/1967). He studied and analysed industrial processes (better known as time and motion study) and developed his scientific management techniques. In Taylor's view, each worker was to be assigned a task (or goal) which was a component in the larger production process. The almost universally employed 'management by objectives' philosophy (e.g. Odiorne, 1978) is the end result of Taylor's early efforts—in other words, goal setting in an industrial context. It is salutary to note that well worked out theoretical explanations for the success of these techniques had to wait for over half a century.

It is hardly surprising, therefore, that virtually all of the literature on goal setting is based on research in an industrial/organizational setting, or an analogue of it. The enterprise, however, has produced some very clear findings, and the transfer to the sports context is just beginning (e.g. Danish, 1983; Larsen, 1983). Already, strong recommendations are being made about how goal setting should be applied in sport, mainly by drawing on work from the industrial and organizational contexts (e.g. Botterill, 1978, 1980; Gould, 1986). As Locke and Latham (1985) pointed out, however, much of this has been developed at an intuitive and anecdotal level. Relatively little empirical research has been undertaken to determine the degree of transferability of goal setting techniques to sport. It therefore seems timely to review the literature on goals and goal setting, and to attempt to evaluate the extent to which both theory and practice transfer to the sports context.

GOAL-SETTING RESEARCH

The dominant concern in much of goal-setting research seems to have been to show how effective (and cost-effective) goal-setting techniques in industry can be. Frequently, the data have been transformed into pounds or dollars, as the improvements in performance are turned into percentage increases in productivity. This reflects the tradition of management involvement in goal setting, which has been promoted as a tool to improve worker output.

It is only relatively recently that the techniques have been tried in other settings—in schools (e.g. Bandura and Schunk, 1981), in clinical practice (see, for example, Ahrens (1987) for a review of the role of goals in depression, and Ward and Eisler (1987) on the relationship between type A personality and ineffective goal-setting skills) and in sport. There is a corresponding dearth of reported findings in these areas, and some confusion about how to explain the sometimes differing results which are beginning to come from these varied contexts.

Perhaps the most useful starting point is with the extensive review of goal setting research undertaken by Locke et al. (1981). They presented a traditional narrative review of over 100 studies of goal setting done between 1969 and 1980, excluding only those concerned with the clinical and social psychology areas. The results of their review were conclusive in respect of the benefits of goal setting, and they identified a number of variables which affect goal setting's effects. More recent literature has done little more than clarify a few of the empirical inconsistencies which they identified, but has succeeded in moving the theoretical ideas ahead.

Locke and Latham had been working on goal setting for some years before they published their literature review in 1985. During that time, they had identified four mechanisms by which goals seem to affect performance. These are:

(a) goals direct attention and action (Locke and Bryan, 1969);
(b) goals mobilize and regulate the amount of effort that a person is prepared to put into a given task (Locke, 1966);
(c) they also result in this effort being prolonged until the goal is reached; this may be called persistence (Latham and Locke, 1975);
(d) finally, goal setting motivates people to develop alternative strategies in their attempts to reach the goal (Latham and Baldes, 1975).

On the face of it, this catalogue of desirable outcomes would seem to have
as much relevance to the sports context as it has in an industrial or organizational setting, as Locke and Latham (1985) pointed out.

In fact, perceptive readers will note that all of the research findings reported
above are concerned with maximizing output—what management scientists
call employee motivation. Locke and Latham (1984) called this the 'most
mysterious and difficult (of human resource problems) to comprehend' (p. 2);
motivation is something which can appear equally impenetrable to the coach
or an athlete in training or competition. It is to be hoped that an understanding
of the concept of goals, a grasp of effective goal setting techniques, and a
passing acquaintance with the role of the coach and athlete in goal setting
may be of as much help in motivation in sport as it seems to have been in the
industrial/organizational sphere.

It is likely, however, that the several differences between work and sport
will have important effects, and that the transferal of goal-setting techniques
to sport will not necessarily be as direct as early proponents claimed. For
example, while there is no doubt that the workplace can often be stressful,
many sporting activities take place in an overtly competitive context. This,
accompanied by the fact that some sports have high levels of arousal or
danger associated with them, can lead to performance anxiety. The relationships between anxiety and goal setting are only beginning to be explored in
the sports context; some of the major issues which concern goal setting will
be explored later in the chapter.

Secondly, in interpreting results from studies done in the American industrial setting, a curious power relationship has to be taken into account.
American management seem able to tell the workforce what to do, and expect,
and get, compliance. It is clear that this is not the case in other cultures, such
as Israel (Erez and Earley, 1987) or Japan (Matsui et al., 1985), and it is
questionable that such a situation exists in sports or other arenas. Nevertheless,
several important parameters of goals and the goal setting process have
emerged from studies carried out in other contexts: these suggest clear
guidelines for research, and possibly practice, in goal setting in sport in the
future. The two most widely researched parameters are those of goal difficulty
and goal specificity.

Goal difficulty

Locke et al. (1981) considered a total of 57 studies which had varied the
difficulty of goals and measured the performance of subjects who had attempted
to reach these goals. The studies were conducted either in the laboratory,
using familiar tasks such as reaction time, card-sorting and anagram-solving,
amongst others, or in real-life settings, using, for example, typists, lumberjacks
or soft drinks salesmen. Of the 57, a total of 48 studies showed that hard

goals led to better performance than medium or easy goals; only nine studies failed to confirm this. In other words the harder the goal, the better the performance; indeed, this relationship has sometimes been presented as a linear one (Locke, 1968), a position which may seem to the reader to be ultimately untenable. Common sense tells us that setting a goal which lies so far outside a person's ability as to appear to be completely unreachable (such as a sub-four minute mile for a ten-year-old schoolgirl) is unlikely to produce a truly great performance. We will return to this conundrum later; for now, we will have to accept the evidence which seems to suggest that, on the whole, people do try harder when they have a difficult goal to try to reach.

Goal specificity

In all, 53 studies about the effects of specific (and challenging) goals, 'do your best' goals and no goals on performance were reviewed by Locke *et al.* (1981). The areas of interest of researchers varied widely, and studies covered topics as diverse as dieting, loading trucks and ships, card-sorting and arithmetic. Only two of these studies failed to show that specific and challenging goals produced the best performances. It would seem that giving people a very clear idea of what is required of them is helpful, even if this means that they will have to try very hard to reach such a goal.

These goal difficulty–performance and goal specificity–performance relationships have been replicated many times—later reviews by Latham and Lee (1985) and meta-analyses of the literature by Tubbs (1986) and Mento, Steel and Karren (1987) showed that the effects are extremely robust. Tubbs ended by saying that 'there appears to be little need to continue conducting studies solely concerned with testing the effects of goal difficulty and goal specificity on performance' (p. 480); Mento *et al.* echoed this, and added 'If there ever is to be a viable candidate from the organizational sciences for elevation to the lofty status of a scientific law of nature, then the relationships between goal difficulty, specificity/difficulty and task performance are worthy of our serious consideration' (p. 74).

This is heady stuff; on the face of it, results and statements like these might suggest to a coach or athlete that all that needs to be done is to set difficult, but clearly defined, goals sit back, and watch for steady, inevitable improvements in performance. Sadly, life is not like that. The situation with respect to sporting endeavour and sports performers may be somewhat different, and possibly more complicated, than this simple picture would suggest.

Nevertheless, early work in sports-related goal setting seemed to be encouraging. Locke and Bryan (1966) found that when subjects were given specific, challenging goals in a psychomotor task, they performed better than when they were simply asked to 'do their best'. Botterill (1977) found similar effects in an endurance task, while Barnett and Stanicek (1979) showed that specific, numerical goals led to higher scores in archery than a goal-free control condition. Training subjects to use goal-setting skills for themselves seemed to result both in better swimming performances and the development of better, more positive thoughts about their abilities, compared with an untrained group (Burton, 1983). It therefore seems likely that at least some of the benefits of goal setting may accrue to some of the users of the technique in sports.

There are, however, a number of studies where the usual goal setting results have apparently failed to transfer to sports. For example, Hollingsworth (1975) and Barnett (1977) failed to find differences in juggling performances between groups with specific goals and groups where no goals were set. It may be, however, that in the latter groups, covert goal setting occurred, as it did in a study by Weinberg et al. (1987). In this study, covert goals (which were ascertained by questionnaire) accounted for between 70 per cent and 85 per cent of the variance of performance in a sit-up task. In other words, sports performers do not appear to respond to challenges in exactly the same way as workers in industrial settings. It might be speculated that they are so familiar with the idea of implicit or covert goal setting that manipulations by a coach or experimenter have, at best, an indirect effect. They may use assigned goals, if there are any, as ball-park figures; if there are no stated goals, then they may simply make some up.

Failure to confirm the goal specificity–performance relationship seems fairly common in sports settings, but covert goal setting may not be the only mechanism responsible. Recently, Hall, Weinberg and Jackson (1983) using a circuit training task, Weinberg, Bruya and Jackson (1985) using sit-ups, and Hall, Weinberg and Jackson (1987) using an endurance task with a dynamometer failed to demonstrate the usual goal specificity–performance relationship. It may be that in these studies competition between subjects in the control groups masked the effects of assigned goals, a result which has been reported before in the industrial/organizational literature (e.g. Latham and Baldes, 1975; Komacki, Barwick and Scott, 1978). That being the case, future research in sports settings will need to take account of factors such as competitiveness, high levels of achievement motivation and the presence of existing self-management skills which may make sports performers a very different population from either working people or the usual subjects in psychological laboratories.

Moderating factors

A number of other factors have been identified which appear to affect, or moderate, the relationship between goals and performance in industrial/ organizational settings. It may be that these effects extend into sports situations. Some of these factors can be seen as internal to the subject; some are factors which are related to differences in the interaction between the goal setter and subject; and others are concerned with the context in which the whole exercise takes place.

Internal factors

Two factors which may be called internal, or intrapersonal, appear to have been identified. These are related to the way a person perceives the goal, and himself.

Acceptance or commitment?

Locke (1968) regarded goal acceptance or commitment as a crucial variable in goal setting. If a person decides that a goal is impossible to reach, he may abandon his efforts to reach it. Clearly, one of the most important things to achieve, if you are a superior of some sort, is acceptance of, and commitment to, goals by a subordinate. These two are not necessarily the same, as Locke *et al.* (1981) and Hollenbeck and Klein (1987) pointed out. Goal commitment is an inclusive concept which refers to one's attachment to, or determination to reach, a goal, whether self-set, participatively set, or assigned. Acceptance, on the other hand, refers only to assigned goals. Logically, an assigned goal may be accepted initially but the person may not remain committed to it for very long: for example, as goals get harder, there is some evidence that acceptance falls off (Erez and Zidon, 1984), although this may not result in complete rejection.

Although logically separate, usage of these terms and the methods employed to measure them seem to have been confounded in the literature (Earley and Kanfer, 1985). It seems intuitively more correct to use the term 'commitment,' which has an intrapersonal meaning as well as being applicable to any type of goal. As Salancik (1977) has argued, commitment can be thought of as a binding of the individual to behavioural acts; in a sports context, individual commitment to self-set or participatively set goals may be a more useful concept than the acceptance to goals assigned by the coach, partly because of the generally less autocratic nature of sports coaching and partly, as we have seen, because sports persons seem likely to use covert goal-setting strategies.

It may be postulated that, given two people with similar levels of ability, the person with the higher level of commitment to a difficult goal will perform better, have higher levels of persistence, and so on. However, the predicted commitment–performance relationships have often been difficult to demonstrate in industrial/organizational studies (e.g. Locke *et al.*, 1984; Yukl and Latham, 1978). The problem for experimenters may have been a ceiling effect; commitment to goals is relatively easily achieved, and low variability in (high) levels of commitment means that experiments using correlational techniques to investigate the relationship between goal commitment and performance have often been unsuccessful. Nevertheless, in a number of recent carefully controlled studies, a relationship between commitment and performance has been demonstrated when steps were taken to ensure that variability in the former was adequate (e.g. Earley, 1986; Erez and Arad, 1986; Erez and Zidon, 1984).

Erez and Zidon's (1984) experiment, which involved a letter-cancelling laboratory task, is particularly interesting. Subjects were assigned a different goal before each trial; these varied in difficulty from very easy to very difficult, as determined in earlier pilot work. Goal acceptance was measured at the beginning of each trial and performance was the dependent variable. They found that as task difficulty increased, acceptance decreased but remained positive until subjects were faced with a task on which they had less than a 0.30 probability of success; at this point, many of the subjects began to reject the goal, increasingly so as even more difficult goals were set. The performance data showed that so long as goals were accepted, the usual positive linear relationship between goal difficulty and performance was found. However, as acceptance changed to rejection, this positive relationship changed to a negative one. Overall, therefore, the relationship between goal difficulty and performance was rather like an inverted-U curve; in other words, subjects still tried and succeeded, in spite of feeling less than happy about the situation, right up to the point where they judged that they had a less than one in three chance of success on the task.

This threshold is of very considerable interest; if a manager or coach knows just how far he can push when setting challenging goals, he may be able to maximize output or performance. However, it is important to note two things; first, that Erez and Zidon deliberately manipulated subjects to encourage them to reject fairly hard goals; and secondly, that there were still some individual differences, with some subjects still trying to reach impossible goals long after most others had given up. Clearly, the precise level of the acceptance/rejection threshold is subject to individual differences and the demand characteristics of the situation.

It is worth noting that Garland (1983) pointed out that many laboratory-based studies of goal setting have in fact produced the familiar positive monotonic goal difficulty–performance relationship even for very difficult goals, and, of course some of Erez and Zidon's subjects behaved in this way. On the other hand, virtually no field studies have used extremely difficult goals, which might have been rejected, and thus the generalizability of Erez and Zidon's laboratory results to the real world has not yet been well tested. In addition, it is even more difficult to make clear predictions about what might be expected in sports settings, although Hardy, Maiden and Sherry (1986) were able to show how goal acceptance fell off with the stress of competition.

Somewhat ahead of the evidence, recommendations to coaches and physical educators about presenting performers with difficult, but attainable goals had been made by several writers (e.g. Botterill, 1978, 1980; Gould, 1986; McClements and Botterill, 1979). The key word has been 'realistic', and the assumption is made that goals which are too difficult will result in a diminution in effort, a drop-off in motivation, a deterioration in performance, or even an abandonment of the goal. In effect, these suggestions reject Locke's (1968) contention that performance and goal difficulty are related monotonically and predate Erez and Zidon's (1984) result.

One recent study which challenged the transferability of Erez and Zidon's (1984) result to a sports context was described by Weinberg et al. (1987). They presented groups of subjects who were enrolled in a fitness training class with easy, moderately difficult, very difficult and highly improbable goals in a sit-up task. They found, using a questionnaire method, that virtually all of the subjects in every group accepted these goals, and that goal difficulty level did not affect acceptance. Nor did groups differ in respect of their intention to try to attain these goals, even though each group apparently accurately perceived the level of difficulty of their assigned goal.

However, the performance of the groups was not significantly related to the difficulty of the goal they received; in fact, it seems that each group performed at or near average, since each one reached the easy goal which 75 per cent of subjects had reached in earlier experiments. It is therefore not at all clear either whether laboratory studies will generalize to the field or to sports-related contexts. The whole question of the relationships between commitment, performance and goal difficulty in sports remains open at the present time; although Hardy, Maiden and Sherry (1986) pioneered this area, much work remains to be done.

The problem of individual differences

Much of the research on goal setting, as we have seen, is the stuff of the workplace; there seems to be an exploitative, managerial feel to it. For a coach working with individuals or a small team, each of whom is involved in their sport for its own sake, the problems he or she sees are perhaps less collective than is the case in a factory. In fact, when a sport psychologist is consulted, it is usually about an individual with a very specific problem. More often than not, the coach will claim that the athlete has 'low motivation', or succumbs to stress; what can goal setting do to help individuals, rather than productivity?

In this respect, the early literature on goal setting is less than helpful; Locke et al. (1981) acknowledged that individual differences had received very little attention from researchers. They reviewed the available evidence on two aspects of individual differences which had been explored. The first series of studies concerned themselves with demographic variables, such as age, sex, race, education and job tenure, and produced very inconsistent results. A second group of studies considered personality factors, such as needs for achievement or independence, higher-order need strength (the degree to which a person wants variety, autonomy and feedback in his work) and locus of control. Once again, the evidence showed that personality differences seemed inconsistent in moderating the effects of goal setting. Locke *et al.* concluded that 'the only consistent thing about the studies of individual differences in goal setting is their inconsistency' (p. 142).

This was perhaps a little defeatist; in fact, self-concept variables seemed more promising. There were very few studies available at that time which were concerned with the effects of goal setting on how people thought of themselves but they seemed to show that:

(a) individuals with high self-assurance increase effort when faced with difficult goals; those with low self-assurance work less hard as goal difficulty increases (Caroll and Tosi, 1970);

(b) feedback should be positive for high self-esteem people; it helps them to reach their goals. Low self-esteem people, on the other hand, seem to be more affected by negative feedback than are high self-esteem people, and perform even worse (Dossett, Latham and Mitchell, 1979; Schrauger and Rosenberg, 1970). The message is that positive feedback is good for everyone;

(c) high self-esteem people seem to be able to work harder with fewer practical rewards, appearing to appreciate completion of tasks for their own sake (Yukl and Latham, 1978).

To be fair, Locke *et al.* said these results were 'intriguing', but in the absence of further work could take the matter no further. Since, then, however, considerable interest in individual differences in goal setting has been evident.

One of the most useful advances has been made recently by Hollenbeck and Brief (1987), who reviewed the literature on individual differences and goal setting again. They identified studies in which self-set goals, rather than assigned goals, were used. Relationships between self-concept variables, such as generalized self-esteem, perceived task-specific ability, locus of control, need for achievement, and ability or past performance, and the dependent measure of chosen goal difficulty were all statistically significant. That is, under self-set conditions, individual differences in self-concept seem to determine the level of goal difficulty chosen; in addition, commitment to these goals is uniformly high. Hollenbeck and Brief then suggested that the way that people react to assigned goals, rather than self-selected goals, will depend on the similarity between these and the goals they would have selected for themselves; specifically, that people will react negatively to goals which differ widely from those which they would have set on their own. Because of this, commitment to assigned goals will vary; only individuals high in self-regard will show commitment to, and the ability to reach, difficult assigned goals.

After giving several self-concept tests to a sample of about 100 students, a factor analysis of these data by Hollenbeck and Brief suggested that a two-factor solution accounted for most of the variance. These factors were generalized self-esteem and perceived task-specific ability. In the laboratory anagram-solving task that followed, these factors seemed to have differing effects on goal-related and performance processes, depending on whether goals were self-set or assigned. In a self-set goals condition, subjects with high perceived task-specific ability set higher goals, while generalized self-esteem seemed virtually unrelated to chosen goal difficulty. Goal commitment was higher, and the goal difficulty–performance relationship was stronger for subjects in this condition than for those in the assigned goal condition.

In contrast, when subjects were assigned goals, perceived task-specific ability was related to the expectancy of attaining the assigned goal: that is, people who knew they were competent expected to do well. Generalized self-esteem, on the other hand, was related to assigned goals in a curious way. Subjects with high self-esteem considered that it was more important to reach the goals that had been set for them than subjects with low self-esteem, and the usual positive goal difficulty–performance relationship appeared. Subjects with low self-esteem, on the other hand, showed a negative goal difficulty–performance relationship; they did better with low goals rather than high goals.

This last result is important. It substantiates what many practitioners already know from experience, and confirms earlier work on feedback by Dosset, Latham and Mitchell (1979) and Schrauger and Rosenberg (1970); it also has parallels in the field of test anxiety (e.g. Sarason, 1978). People with low self-esteem are vulnerable to confirmation of their perceived status (e.g. Brockner, 1983), and a method of goal setting which disconfirms these perceptions at an early stage seems to be necessary. The message from this work seems to be that self-set goals (and possibly participatively set goals, depending on the degree of input from the learner) do not expose low self-esteem individuals to the same trauma as assigned, difficult goals.

In a sports setting, self-concept variables may be a much more important consideration than in an industrial/organizational context. Positive self-regard is widely acknowledged to be a crucial variable in sporting success. In particular, perceived task-specific ability, or self-efficacy, has been shown to discriminate between good and excellent performers in a range of sports, such as gymnastics (Mahoney and Avener, 1977), rifle shooting (Doyle, Landers and Feltz, 1980) and wrestling (Highlen and Bennett, 1979; Gould, Weiss and Weinberg, 1981).

Unfortunately, it is not clear from these studies whether athletes feel efficacious because they are skilled performers or whether they can turn in skilled performances because they feel efficacious. The likelihood is that the trade is in both directions; Feltz (1983) showed this to be the case for novice divers. For a non-elite performer for whom the coach sets goals, the expectancy of reaching these goals may well vary with perceived self-efficacy. Whether this is important is, as yet, an open question. However, by involving the learner in choosing and setting his or her own goals, goal commitment is higher than when goals are assigned. It may therefore be useful to work participatively with performers in goal setting in sports; as always, however, such a speculation awaits empirical investigation.

Interpersonal factors

It is hardly surprising that the way that goal setting is approached by the superior/coach can have an effect on its success. A number of parameters have been identified which have a greater or lesser impact on the goal-setting process.

Feedback

Knowledge of results (KR) has long been known to have a facilitative effect on learning and performance, particularly in the motor skill area (e.g. Ammons, 1956; Bilodeau and Bilodeau, 1961; Newell, 1974; Schmidt, 1982). Most coaches and many athletes will be aware of this, at least at a conversational level, and will probably use KR in training.

The effects of KR are usually regarded as twofold. First, it is thought to cue the performer about the nature and size of any errors which he or she is making; he or she is assumed to be capable of making use of this knowledge to improve his or her performance. Secondly, KR is concerned with motivating the recipient to increase his or her effort and/or persistence. Payne and Hauty (1955) called these the directive and incentive functions of KR, respectively. The second of these, however, sounds very much as if it may have similar effects to those of goal setting. And yet goal setting occurs prior to performance and KR is contingent upon it. Any coach wondering whether to use KR or goal setting might at this point be somewhat confused about which theoretical concept to believe and where improvements in performance come from.

This paradox was discussed by Locke, Cartledge and Koeppel (1968), who reviewed studies where both goal setting and KR were manipulated. Their conclusion was unequivocal: KR has no effect unless goals are set, either explicitly by the experimenter or covertly by the subject in response to the feedback. This is not very surprising; it simply means that people 'take on board' the feedback and do something about it; Locke (1968) called this his mediating hypothesis.

Locke *et al.* (1981) confirmed Locke, Cartledge and Koeppel's (1968) analysis that KR without goals has no effect on performance and went on to show that later research had demonstrated the obverse—that goals without KR fail to affect performance. This led Locke to modify his mediating hypothesis. Goals and feedback are, according to Locke *et al.* (1981), reciprocally dependent, and both are necessary for performance to improve. This point had been made before by Bandura (1977) and was amplified by Bandura and Cervone (1983). The results of studies such as that of Anderson *et al.* (1988), who showed that KR interventions improved the performance of a university ice-hockey team, are probably clouded by the likelihood that players set covert goals for themselves (see also the section on competitive anxiety). Anderson *et al.* found that further improvements could be extracted from players by explicit goal setting, confirming that both explicit goal setting and KR are necessary for the maximum improvements in performance to occur.

Surprisingly, a meta-analysis of the literature by Tubbs (1986) found only weak evidence for the effects of KR on goal setting; later, however, Mento, Steel and Karren (1987) were able to clarify this finding. They reported that those studies which used hard, specific goals showed considerable beneficial effects of feedback; overall, however, the literature was equivocal, as reported by Tubbs. To the 'hard-pressed' coach, it must surely sound somewhat self-evident to say that research has shown that giving people specific, challenging goals and letting them know how they are getting on results in improvements in performance. However, there is a message to take away. It is that performance must be measurable if feedback is to be effective. It's no use giving general feedback, like 'Well done', that sort of thing—or is it?

Supportiveness and trust

Most field and laboratory studies on goal setting have used assigned goals, probably because this is the way it happens in the workplace. This implies that the supervisor or experimenter is perceived to have some degree of legitimate authority; compliance with this authority may explain why assigned goal setting works at all (French and Raven, 1959; Oldham, 1975; Orne, 1962). However, some people are better than others at managing, doing experiments, or coaching. In the industrial field, this was acknowledged by Likert (1961), who, in his System 4 management theory, pinpointed supportive relationships, participative decision-making and goal setting as the hallmarks of a successful manager. Because much goal setting research has been applied to organizations, and perhaps because much of the early thinking in the area was almost behaviourist in flavour, such cognitive and social factors have received surprisingly little attention. Many psychologists nowadays would claim to be more interested in these aspects than any other; in transferring goal setting research to other contexts it may not be possible to ignore them.

In an early attempt to come to terms with these problems, Latham and Saari (1979) examined the proposition that goal-directed performance will depend, to some extent, on interpersonal factors such as the 'perceived supportiveness' of the experimenter. Likert (1961) had defined the supportive manager as someone who is perceived by the subordinate as primarily interested in building and maintaining the subordinate's sense of personal worth. He predicted that managerial supportiveness will lead to better performance by the subordinate.

In fact, Latham and Saari (1979) found that this was not the case. They varied the way they spoke to the subjects during the experiment, appearing either to be supportive and caring, or distant and uninterested in the subjects. The results showed that supportiveness *per se* did not affect performance, but that is not the end of the story. They found an interaction between the degree of supportiveness and the way that goals were set. The experimenters approached goal setting in one of three ways: they either assigned goals, an autocratic approach; set 'do-your-best' goals, a *laissez-faire* approach; or they participated with subjects in setting goals, a democratic approach. (They also arranged for the assigned and participatory goals to be of identical level.) They found that when they were being supportive, and goals were being set participatively, it gave 'subordinates and supervisors the confidence to set high goals, which in turn led to high levels of performance' (p. 154). This is one of the few experiments where participation in goal setting proved to be markedly more effective than assigning goals.

Trust in authority has also been shown to be an important factor in goal setting. Oldham (1975) found that perceptions of trustworthiness were related to an intent to work hard for a goal which had been assigned by a supervisor with legitimate authority; subordinates often reject messages (which could be about goals) from untrustworthy supervisors (Baird, 1974). Similarly, Earley (1986) showed that a US sample of workers who were given information which could help them attain assigned goals accepted this information from either supervisors or union shop stewards. The effect of accepting and using the information was to improve both the way they viewed their goal and their performance. In England, however, workers would only accept information from their shop stewards; this information had exactly the same effect as with the American group, whereas information from managers was rejected and goal acceptance and performance were lower. Earley regarded this result as evidence that worker–management relationships in England are based on deep mistrust.

The results of these sorts of studies seem to show that you get more out of people if they feel you are a decent sort of person. Perhaps this comes as no surprise to people involved in sport, but it is revealing to find out that such a commonsensical idea works via goal setting. Whether you are a naturally 'hard' coach or someone who prefers a more participative approach to getting the best from your performers, it seems that goal setting is the underlying mechanism which motivates people. If you want to maximize its effects, this research suggests that the latter approach may have its advantages. However, it is notoriously difficult to change the way you deal with people, and it may be better simply to rely on the technique of goal setting rather than seem to appear insincere. It is equally true that putting pressure on people to achieve goals can improve their performance (Andrews and Farris, 1972; Hall and Lawler, 1971), so long as this pressure is not excessive (Andrews and Farris, 1972; Forward and Zander, 1971).

Participation in goal setting

Latham and Saari's (1979) and Earley's (1986) results suggest that two useful things can happen if a manager or coach is trustworthy, supportive and democratic rather than distant and autocratic in his approach. The first is that support and participation can lead to higher goals being set than might be unilaterally assigned by the manager or coach; in turn, these higher goals lead to better performance. The second is that participatively set goals are accepted more readily, as are goals which are assigned by an apparently trustworthy or supportive superior.

Another reason for the success of participation in Latham and Saari's experiment may be that subjects seemed to have a clearer grasp of what to do when they participated in the goal setting, possibly because they asked questions to clarify what was required of them before deciding what they felt they could realistically achieve. Given that a goal is a representation of future action, participation seems to result in a more clearly focused and richer percept, and that can be no bad thing.

These findings notwithstanding, there is no firm evidence in the bulk of the goal setting literature that participatively set goals are significantly more effective than assigned goals; both Tubbs (1986) and Mento, Steel and Karren (1987), in their meta-analyses of the literature, showed that the difference between assigned and participatively set goals was small and relatively unimportant, although it was slightly in favour of participatively set goals. However, in sharp contrast, Erez and her colleagues (e.g. Erez, Earley and Hulin, 1985; Erez, 1986; Erez and Arad, 1986) found a consistently large difference, with assigned goals being markedly less useful. Thus, it seems that while there is agreement that participatively set goals are effective, there is some confusion with respect to assigned goals. One possibility is that cultural differences are involved; most goal setting work has been done in the USA, while Erez' work has been undertaken in Israel.

Recently, Latham, Erez and Locke (1988) attempted to resolve this confusion. Their results suggest that a subtle difference in goal setting techniques, which may be cultural of course, could explain the differing results. Latham *et al.* found that goals assigned using a 'tell' style were less effective than goals assigned using a 'tell and sell' style (cf. Tannenbaum and Schmidt, 1958); Erez and her Israeli colleagues used the former style, unlike American management and experimenters who characteristically used the latter. They found that these different styles produced different amounts of goal commitment and performance, and thus the apparent differences in the literature were once again attributable to interpersonal factors in goal setting.

These results complement those of Latham and Saari (1979) and Earley (1986); the perceived attributes of the goal setter, and the way he or she goes about setting goals, are probably confounded. A consistent story is thus beginning to take shape, although all the details are not yet clear. It would seem that perceived genuineness and skilfulness in persuasion, rather than autocracy, can result in the acceptance and attainment of goals assigned by a superior. Better still, participation in goal setting with such an authority figure may result in even better performance because the subordinate may set even higher goals than would the superior acting alone.

Contextual factors

Goals are not set in isolation. They are bound up with both the nature of the task itself, which may be either simple or complex, and the context in which it occurs. There are a number of fundamental differences between sport and the workplace which mean that some of the findings of goal-setting research undertaken in the latter context may not easily transfer to a sporting context. For example, in sport, unlike most industrial/organizational tasks, the process of skill learning will often involve performers in a very lengthy period of training to reach their personal best. For them, the 'dream goal' may seem far away. And most importantly, most sports are undertaken in an atmosphere of intense competition, which adds to the stress inherent in performing a possibly dangerous or complex activity. Nevertheless, a number of useful findings and concepts from industry have at least some relevance for sport, and increasingly, work on goal setting is being done within sport itself.

Task difficulty

All tasks, or sports, are not the same. One dimension of difference which has received surprisingly little attention by researchers in industrial/organizational settings is that of difficulty. Generally, difficult tasks are either more complex, demand greater information-processing capabilities, or require higher levels of skill, knowledge or effort to accomplish (see Wood, 1986, for a discussion and the development of a metric of task difficulty). In sports, the differences between track and field events and, say, golf or competitive sailing exemplify this continuum. In the former, performance is often of a very short duration, is affected by a relatively small number of uncontrollable variables, and can be estimated by a simple time or distance measure. In more complex sports, success is dependent on being able to deal with several unpredictable things like the wind, the texture of the grass on the green, and so on, and may be of a protracted nature. In practice, finding a suitable measure for such a performance is extremely difficult and complicates the job of goal setting.

Locke *et al.* (1981) had little to say about goal setting with tasks of varying difficulty or complexity beyond speculating that hard goals might lead to the development of more effective strategies, and thus better performance. In fact, they pointed out that 'If the requisite strategies are not developed, then increased motivation provided by goals will be negated' (p. 133). Recently, Wood, Mento and Locke (1987) reviewed the growing literature on task difficulty and goal setting and performed a meta-analysis on the data. They found that the usual goal difficulty–performance relationship and the goal specificity–performance relationship were both affected by task complexity. Generally, as the tasks became more complex and difficult, both these relationships became weaker, although this was more pronounced for the goal difficulty–performance relationship. Wood *et al.* attributed these results to the strategy development effect of goal setting, as Locke *et al.* had proposed.

These findings may seem to suggest that when the task itself is tricky, goal setting may be less effective. However, there is a further twist to the tale. Based on as yet unpublished results from their laboratory, Wood *et al.* suggested that in complex tasks specific, challenging goals operate with a time lag. That is, while the benefits of goal setting may not be immediately obvious, the development of strategies seems to result in performance improvements later on. This makes a certain amount of sense. Goals are representations of to-be-performed actions, and it would not be unreasonable to expect that strategies might be developed covertly during mental rehearsal as people try to puzzle out how best to achieve their goals. We might expect such a process to occur when the task, or sport, is complex; one view of the function of consciousness is that it enables us to do just this.

However, there is a further explanation for the effects which Wood, Mento and Locke (1987) reported. All sports, and many tasks, have a motor component, and it may be that these cognitive processes have an indirect impact on the performance of motor skills. If strategy selection is going on during skilled performance, rather than before, it may be that the attentional demands of this cognitive activity will result in suboptimal control of motor activities. The result will be an apparent decrease in the level of performance, although for a quite different reason than the arousal or strategy selection hypotheses would suggest.

One way in which goal setting theory and practice has attempted to deal with difficult goals is by introducing the concept of proximal and distal goals. Locke *et al.* (1981) could say only that this aspect of goal setting had not yet received much attention. One might speculate that this reflects the context in which most goal setting occurs, where there is an interest in maximizing individual output of subtasks as a way of improving overall productivity in an industrial/organizational setting. This is very different from contexts in which individuals are trying to master a difficult and complex task, perhaps over a time-scale of months or years. Such a situation occurs in education, and in clinical psychology, and it will come as no surprise that the explanations for the success of goal setting in these contexts are very different from those offered by workers in the industrial/organizational field. Most sports are perhaps better viewed from this perspective too.

The idea of breaking a distant, 'dream' goal into apparently achievable subgoals describes a third property of goals (other than difficulty and specificity) which has shown to be at least comparable in importance to these two. Goal proximity affects both performance and attainment motivation (e.g. Bandura, 1977; Bandura and Simon, 1977; Bandura and Schunk, 1981). That is, people respond better when their goals are apparently closer to hand than when they are distant, future goals, or when they have no goals. This approach has been used in classrooms with some success (e.g. Bandura and Schunk, 1981; Schunk, 1983).

Locke and Latham (1985) suggested that in sport, setting subgoals may be an important technique for athletes and coaches to use. They quote the apocryphal tale of John Naber, the 1976 Olmpic 400-metre backstroke gold medallist, who, quite spontaneously, adopted a goal-setting programme based on this approach. In 1972, he became aware that he had four years to improve his best time by four seconds if he was to stand a chance of winning his medal, and calculated that he could achieve this if he could improve his times by about four milliseconds for every hour of training. This represents only a fifth of the time it takes to blink, and he felt that this was an achievable proximal goal. He does not report if he used feedback in his training, but it is virtually certain that he must have; there is ample evidence to predict that he would have been unsuccessful if he had not (Locke et al., 1981).

Of course, this is another anecdotal account, and although there are a number of studies which suggest that proximal goal setting works well in other fields, the research evidence in sport is very limited. McClements and Laverty (1979) presented a mathematical model of performance improvement, based on the law of diminishing returns. Because there must be an absolute limit to an individual's performance, the approach to this is likely to be asymptotic; it follows that more and more effort is needed to make smaller and smaller advances. This learning curve can be used to generate subgoals which will not be separated by equal intervals, as in John Naber's account, but will represent realistic increments in performance given steady commitment to training over an extended time. As McClements and Botterill (1979) pointed out, goal setting is an exercise in predicting the future; determining the shape of this learning curve for an individual so that distal and proximal goals may be identified may be easier said than done.

GOAL SETTING AND COMPETITIVE STATE ANXIETY

Competition in relation to goal setting can mean very different things, depending on whether the context is a laboratory or organizational/industrial one or whether we are concerned with competitive sport. In the former context, competition has often been seen as a confounding factor in goal setting research, which has tended to contaminate experimental results (e.g. Latham and Baldes, 1975; Komacki, Barwick and Scott, 1978). Not surprisingly, attempts have been made to reach an understanding of how goal setting and competition (or more strictly, competitiveness) interact in the work context.

Locke (1968) suggested that competitiveness may result in the spontaneous setting of higher goals than might otherwise be set, and that it may lead to greater goal commitment. Forward and Zander (1971) and White, Mitchell and Bell (1977) showed that higher goals are often set in competitive situations; Mueller (1983) confirmed that more difficult goals are set, but that greater goal commitment does not necessarily occur when competition is encouraged. However, it is important to note that this work on informal competitiveness may have very little relevance for competitive sport, where the competition is formalized and the motivation for reaching goals is very different from that found in the workplace. In this very different context, goal setting is beginning to be used in a quite different way—not to improve productivity, but to help athletes deal more effectively with the stress of competition.

There are a number of factors which need to be considered in any discussion of the use of goal setting in a sport context. For instance, it is vitally important to draw the distinction, as Locke and Latham did, between training and competition. Of course, the essential difference between training and competition is stress; there is no doubt that competition is more stressful than training (e.g. Passer, 1981). There are a number of reasons for this. As Locke and Latham (1984) described, a stressful situation arises when three requirements are fulfilled. These can occur in training but are unavoidable in competition. First, an important outcome or value must be threatened. This is commonly the case in competition, where the most valuable (and most uncertain) outcome is winning. However, it may also be the case that success can seem elusive where the athlete in training is seeking only to improve his or her performance. Secondly, there must be a possibility of performing so as to attempt to reach some criterion, for example by running faster than before—or anyone else. Thirdly, there must be a fundamental uncertainty about the success of the attempt to reach the criterion. Nobody can expect to perform at their optimum all the time, and in competition the performances of others add to the uncertainty. It also seems likely that a certain amount of anxiety is generated because of the evaluative element in competition (cf. Simon and Martens, 1979). In addition, many sports have an element of risk associated with them—diving, gymnastics or rock-climbing, for example— where tiny mistakes or unforeseen factors can have dramatic consequences, and where anxiety is more than legitimate.

Two contrasting approaches have been taken to help athletes deal with the problems caused by competitive stress, based on the taxonomy of coping suggested by Cohen and Lazarus (1979). They described intrapsychic, or emotion-focused coping, which is primarily aimed at dealing with anxiety and other unpleasant emotions, and action-oriented, or task-centred coping, which is aimed at removing the causes of the unwanted emotions. Emotion-focused methods commonly used in sport include relaxation techniques, attention management strategies which involve focusing attention on a neutral stimulus such as the navel, and self-talk. Many athletes also find that social support to help them 'talk out' their emotions can be a helpful technique, while others may use alcohol or other substances to change either their emotions or their perceptions of the situation.

In contrast to these mental skill and other emotion-focused approaches to managing anxiety, goal setting offers a task-centred way of tackling some of the underlying causes of anxiety. It has been argued that goal setting can be used in this way both in training and in competition itself. Unfortunately, however, goal setting is a 'double-edged sword'. As Locke and Latham (1985) pointed out, formal competition and goal setting have a lot in common, in that they both involve criterion-referenced performance. In formal competition, however, the criterion is a personalized, external event, the winning competitor's performance, rather than the impersonal performance standard more commonly found in work settings. In addition, the criteria in competitive sport are continuously moving as performance standards improve, not to mention what happens during, say, a middle-distance race. The similarity between goals and competition is thus quite striking, so it should come as no surprise that, as Huber (1985) pointed out, goals themselves can be thought of as stressors. This is because they satisfy all Locke and Latham's (1984) criteria for generating stress—they are important, require action, and may not always be reached. The parameters of goal setting which research has shown to be crucial—difficulty, specificity and proximity—can be seen as the inevitable consequences of this paradox, and reflect the need to balance the positive and negative aspects of goal setting. Difficult, challenging goals must inevitably generate anxiety; on the other hand, goals which are specific avoid the trap of ambiguity, which is itself a source of anxiety (Locke and Latham, 1984). In a similar way, a succession of proximal goals reduces the anxiety which might be generated by a distal, extremely difficult goal, simply because it is perceived as more likely that they may be reached.

In training, goals, especially proximal goals, can be used to improve an athletes's self-confidence, strength, stamina and skills. This makes him or her less likely to be affected by competitive stress. The stress caused by these training goals themselves can be discounted—in fact, it may even, as Locke and Latham suggested, help the athlete improve his or her anxiety management skills. However, goals to be set during competition, if they are to be effective in containing some of the stress of competing, must follow the basic rule that additional stress caused by goal setting itself should be minimized. Two main approaches to this tricky problem have emerged. The first has focused attention on the relative difficulty of goals used in competition and those used in training; the second has considered the nature of the goals themselves.

Recently, Cale and Jones (1989), in a laboratory task, measured cognitive and somatic anxiety with the CSAI-2, the Competitive State Anxiety Inventory-2 (Martens *et al.*, 1990), goal acceptance and performance when very easy, challenging, and very difficult goals were set. Rather like Erez and Zidon (1984), they found that very easy goals were universally accepted, acceptance of the challenging goals was variable, and the very difficult goals were rejected. More importantly, however, they also found that cognitive anxiety rose and self-confidence fell just before the attempted performance of the challenging and very difficult goals; somatic anxiety was not affected by goal difficulty. This confirms that difficult goals themselves are sources of cognitive anxiety and underlines the importance of identifying just how much anxiety is generated by goals of varying difficulty.

Hardy, Maiden and Sherry (1986) threw a little light on this still murky area with a study which may be of some practical help to the coach or athlete trying to set goals for competition which do not themselves generate too much additional anxiety. They also used the CSAI-2 with a collegiate soccer team, and showed that cognitive and somatic anxiety were very high just before an important match, but much lower on the days before and after. Each team member was asked to perform a ball control task, with various levels of goal difficulty, at these times. The highest goal difficulty level was that which had been attained earlier in training. Significantly, both goal acceptance and goal attainment scores fell off as anxiety levels rose as the competition approached. Goals which may have been accepted and attained in training may therefore be rejected in competition, and this work has considerable practical value for coaches who would wish at least to try to give their athletes a set of performance goals for competition. However, what represents an appropriate reduction in goal difficulty is an as yet incompletely answered empirical question, and there is an urgent need for more research on this important aspect of goal setting.

It is also becoming clear that it is important to choose the right type of goal for competition. Roberts (1986) suggested that where a performer's personal goal is the attainment of a successful outcome in competition, he is most likely to suffer from competition-related stress; Burton and Martens (1986) found that wrestlers who gave up the sport were more likely to focus on winning or losing as a measure of their competence, a result confirmed by Ewing (1981) and Whitehead (1986) for children in sporting situations. As Roberts (1986) stressed, goals which help the athlete to avoid this stress trap are those which focus on performance rather than outcome. This seems to be a common theme in research in this area, particularly when a developmental perspective is assumed. Maehr and Nicholls (1980), for example, discussed how goals in sport change with age. They found that children begin by having mastery goals, where they are concerned only to improve their skills and performance; develop competence goals, where the outcome (winning or losing) becomes important; and may come to embrace social approval goals, where the social rewards from significant others for winning or avoiding losing are most salient.

A similar point was made recently by Elliot and Dweck (1988) in the context of children's academic performance. They differentiated between what they called learning goals, which they regarded as promoting mastery and challenge-seeking behaviour, and what they called 'performance' goals, where the real goal is to appear to others as competent. It is unfortunate from our point of view that they chose this name for the latter, which appears to confound Maehr and Nicholl's outcome and social approval goals; perhaps this is because of the very different contexts in which these ideas were developed. They found that these different sorts of goal had quite profound consequences, which in turn depended on the self-concept of the subjects. In a problem-solving experiment, both high and low perceived ability children were given these different types of goal. Elliot and Dweck found that low perceived ability children who were given 'performance' goals evidenced negative affect, avoidance and learned helplessness; although high perceived ability children persisted better, and appeared to be less upset by performance goals, they claimed not to like failing in public. In contrast, learning goals resulted in both high and low perceived ability children being unconcerned about failure *per se*, and both groups were more persistent and came up with more problem-solving strategies. The message seems to be that mastery or learning goals help all children to avoid negative feelings such as anxiety.

For all these reasons, it is often suggested that in competition, outcome or 'win' goals should never be used. Instead, it is proposed that performance or mastery goals should be used. These may act as a way to encourage a winning performance, while at the same time keeping the althlete's attention away from thoughts of winning (and evaluation). The implicit hope, therefore, is that in competition, appropriate goal setting may act as a stress management device. Locke and Latham (1985), for example, suggested an elaborate points system which emphasizes effective subskill performances within American football, although no doubt a similar strategy could be devised for most sports. Unfortunately, many performers will have their own, covert goals and familial goals, both of which may well be of the 'win' type. The enigma of this approach is that it seems to argue that in an ideal world, sports performers should go into competition with nothing but a set of performance goals at the front of their mind so that competition anxiety does not arise. Unfortunately, many would claim that this removes the very essence of competition, along with its adrenalin and the kudos of winning.

GOAL SETTING THEORIES

Three major theories of the effects of goal setting need to be described. These include Locke's (1968) original goal setting theory, and attempts by others, often working in disparate areas, to apply their own insights to the robust findings from the world of industry. In addition, it is worth mentioning that a very early theoretical analysis from an educational pioneer may have considerable merit, and relevance, for sports coaching. As yet, however, none of these models has emerged as the clear victor, and models which have been developed purely for a sports context have yet to be produced.

Goal setting theories, of whatever colour, are based on the premise that some internal, cognitive processes are involved. For most theories, both representational and comparative processes are implicated, where some sense of the difficulty, effort and benefits involved in reaching a goal is computed. Several recent attempts have been made to integrate expectancy theory and other situational and personal variables, such as self-efficacy and commitment (e.g. Locke, Motowidlo and Bobko, 1986; Hollenbeck and Klein, 1987), but the complexity of the moderating influences on goal setting can make such models either oversimple or unwieldy. An integration will no doubt be forthcoming in the not too distant future, one which hopefully will incorporate the findings from sport which are sometimes not in complete agreement with those from the industrial/organizational field. In spite of these drawbacks, however, considerable insight can be gained from the application of existing models to sport, and a number of tests of their predictions for sporting performance have been made.

Vygotsky's theory

Although most of Vygotsky's work was published in English some 25 years ago, his original research and writings date back to the early part of the century. His primary concern was to model the development of cognitive functioning from a Marxist perspective, thus 'swimming against the tide' of individualism which was—and still is—running in western psychology. He stressed that learning and development cannot be divorced from their cultural social context, and was extremely critical of contemporary Piagetian ideas (Vygotsky, 1962). These, of course, assume that cognitive processes simply unfold in a more or less orderly way; the influence of the mother or later teachers on development is largely ignored.

In contrast, Vygotsky believed that learning and knowledge are cultural, and acquired from more knowledgeable and skilful others through our social interactions with them. He focused on the rather curious fact that when children attempt tasks with adults or more competent peers around, they can often achieve success which would elude them if they tried to tackle the same task alone. These two ability or performance levels he called, respectively, the 'level of potential development' and the 'actual development level'.

His great contribution was to recognize that these mark the boundaries of the learner's 'zone of proximal development'. This 'zone' includes those cognitive functions which are incomplete but in the process of developing. In his view, the role of the instructor is to ensure that learning experience occurs in this zone, 'rousing to life those functions which are in a stage of maturing' (Vygotsky, 1956; p. 278; translated from the Russian, and cited in Wertsch and Rogoff, 1984, p.3). Thus, the primary task of the instructor is to segment the task into subtasks which the learner can successfully accomplish under instruction at each stage of the learning process.

Recent advances in educational psychology have drawn on these ideas. The concept of the teacher as a supporter of learning was described by Wood, Bruner and Ross (1976). Their 'scaffold' metaphor represents the way that the trainer or teacher adjusts the amount of support or help given as the learner's abilities develop; later work by Wood, Wood and Middleton (1978) showed how the best teachers vary the help they give as children succeed or fail, contingent upon learning outcomes. In effect, they adjust subgoals on a moment-to-moment basis and effective teaching (and learning) occurs. In an almost identical way, Williams, Dooseman and Kleifield (1984) and Williams, Turner and Peer (1985) showed that the clinical technique of guided mastery was significantly more effective than the usual methods of desensitization or flooding. In guided mastery, the therapist is much more interventionist than in classical behavioural techniques, ensuring that the patient successfully copes with his graded problem hierarchy on a moment-to-moment basis. This method results in measurable changes in patients' perceived ability to deal with previously noxious situations, and a more or less permanent improvement in coping.

What has all this to do with goal setting in sport? It confirms that three things we already know about from the goal setting literature seem to be fairly general phenomena: first, that learning (or performance) takes place best when goals are somewhat, but not too far, ahead of current ability; secondly, that the sensitive support of a competent other, who can judge and set subgoals, may be vital; and thirdly, that growing confidence results from continuing success in learning, or performance, through achieving a succession of subgoals.

Vygotsky's work predates contemporary theories of goal setting by nearly half a century, but perhaps because it existed in obscure Russian sources until relatively recently, its contribution has largely gone unrecognized in the goal setting literature. It has a great deal to offer people whose job it is to encourage others to improve their performances, and can be seen as a theory of moment-to-moment goal setting. It probably has more to say about the microstructure of how coaches should approach their task, but the parallels with the more macroscopic topic of goal setting are remarkable. Clearly, an underlying principle may be at work.

Goal-setting theory

Given that Locke and Latham in their many publications virtually singlehand-edly developed the principles of goal-setting for industry and organizational settings, it should come as no surprise to discover that they also had something to say about the reasons why the techniques worked. Locke (1968) was very clear that a goal should be seen as a mental representation of an action, and not simply as a stimulus which in some way controls behaviour. In this, goal setting theory broke away from earlier conceptualizations of a goal as something external to the person and made a firm statement that conscious goals are the most immediate and direct regulators of human action. Goals are said to differ from other cognitions, such as needs, values or attitudes, which are regarded as forming a backdrop to action (Locke and Henne, 1986).

The theory asserts that the difficulty–performance and specificity–perform-ance effects of goal setting operate primarily through motivational mechanisms. The four mechanisms which have been identified by Locke and Latham are: (1) the mobilization and exertion of effort; (2) the direction of attention and action; (3) an increase in persistence; and (4) the development of alternative strategies to reach the goal (Locke and Latham, 1984). In one sense, this theory is a halfway house, being partly cognitive and partly motivational; in another sense, it is almost tautological. While it offers the goal setter clear guidelines about the principles of goal setting, it fails to open up the processes by which the practice works in the way that more cognitively orientated theories do.

Together with its corollaries, it has been espoused by some writers in the sports field, such as Fuoss and Troppmann (1981). Incidentally, their acronym SCRAM, standing for specific, challenging, realistic, acceptable and measure-able, describing the properties of effective goals which should lead to improved performance, is difficult to beat. The key to successful goal setting in sport lies in the identification of appropriate values for most of these parameters, and being aware that they are likely to change under the stress of competition. Perhaps that is the biggest task for research in the future.

Expectancy theory

Expectancy theory, sometimes referred to as valence–instrumentality–expectancy (VIE) theory, was first developed by Vroom (1964). The theory proposes that three variables affect an individual's level of motivation to attain a goal. The first is performance expectancy, which Vroom conceptualized as the subjective probability that an act would be followed by an outcome. Campbell *et al.* (1970) modified this concept by proposing that it consisted of two logically separate components: Expectancy I is the subjective probability of reaching a goal and Expectancy II is the subjective probability that the goal will have an outcome, such as a reward. The first of these has been generally referred to as 'effort–performance expectancy', and is very similar to Bandura's self-efficacy construct. Self-efficacy, however, is somewhat wider in scope and includes factors related to the situation and to the performer himself. The second is very similar to the construct of locus of control (Rotter, 1966) and is generally referred to as instrumentality.

Performance valence represents the extent to which performance and/or its outcome is personally valued. Monetary or social rewards are the usual outcomes which people seek from their attainment of a goal in an industrial/organizational context and, of course, these may also be important in certain high-level sports situations. Task mastery, however, may be a more general personally rewarding consequence of goal attainment in recreational sport.

Recently, Garland (1985) proposed a causal model of performance which included these three factors, together with task ability and goal difficulty. His model is an attempt to arrive at an understanding of the cognitive mechanisms which underlie the goal difficulty–performance relationship. In a laboratory task of creativity, Garland found that the model accounted for 63 per cent of the variance of performance, and in a path analysis he was able to show that the hypothesized causal relationships between variables were consistent with his model. Whether the model will generalize to field situations, and sport in particular, remains to be seen.

Social learning theory

Bandura's social learning theory (Bandura, 1977, 1982) is concerned with the judgements a person makes about his or her ability to meet the demands of a given situation competently. Its focus is the internal, cognitive processes by which individuals gauge the likelihood of success and failure in their future endeavours, and the external and internal factors which influence these processes. The central tenet of Bandura's theory is called 'self-efficacy'.

When a person judges that he is perfectly capable of producing the behaviour which will meet an environmental demand he will feel confident, to use the lay term. He will know whether he can act effectively from his experience in previous similar situations, although as Bandura (1977) stated, this judgement will not simply reflect past performance. Other factors, such as situational differences, and personal variables, such as the ability to function under stress, ingenuity and adaptability will be taken into account in a complex appraisal of the new situation and his current level of competence. In Bandura's terms, a confident person has a high level of perceived self-efficacy.

The usefulness of the theory is partly conceptual because it unpacks at least two lay terms, confidence and motivation. Confidence is something which all coaches and athletes strive for, and research has shown how, even at an elite level, a sense of confidence in one's self characterizes successful competitors (Mahoney and Avener, 1977; Highlen and Bennett, 1979). Confidence and self-efficacy, however, are not the same thing. Self-efficacy is largely situationally specific, whereas confidence is a much more global (and wooly) term; it is perfectly possible, for example, to be a supremely confident middle-distance runner whose perceived self-efficacy to run 100 metres in less than 10 seconds is very low indeed.

Bandura also proposed that perceived self-efficacy was the cognitive mediator which underlies a number of familiar, related behaviours: what people choose to do, how much effort they are prepared to expend while they are doing it, and how long they persist in the face of real or apparent difficulties. These are all said to be influenced by beliefs about one's ability to produce a required piece of behaviour; in other words, motivation is related to self-efficacy.

Bandura (1977, 1982) identified four principal sources of information which influence self-efficacy judgements. These are, in order of their effectiveness: performance accomplishments; vicarious experiences, that is, modelling another's actions; verbal persuasion; and attention to emotional arousal. The first of these has the most direct relevance to goal setting, but the last is of considerable interest in relation to the effects of stress. Attending to somatic arousal stimuli, and interpreting them negatively, can lead to a reduction in perceived self-efficacy; it may convince the person that there really is something to worry about. This, in turn, may lead to further anxiety, until the person reaches the conclusion that not only can they not perform adequately, but that the situation they find themselves in is completely untenable. This may result in a dramatic change in their ability to continue, and they may 'seize up' or 'blow out'. Catastrophe theory, described by Hardy in Chapter 4 of this book, is a way of modelling this unfortunate experience.

Early tests of the theory often relied on the conservative, and striking, technique of manipulating self-efficacy indirectly—by verbal suggestion, for example. Bandura and his associates showed that perceived self-efficacy is strongly related to performance (Bandura and Adams, 1977: Bandura, Adams and Beyer, 1977; Bandura et al., 1980). In sport, Weinberg, Gould and Jackson (1979) and Weinberg et al. (1981) showed that endurance on a muscular endurance task was affected by the level of perceived self-efficacy, apparently independently of past performance levels.

However, the situation is not as simple as this study might imply. Later work by Feltz (1982, 1983), using female students attempting somewhat difficult reverse dives for the first time, found that self-efficacy seemed, indeed, to determine their performance. Later in the series of dives, however, the relationship was reversed and performance seemed to affect perceived self-efficacy. This reciprocal relationship between self-efficacy and performance was confirmed in an important study by Locke et al. (1984), who examined a number of variables associated with performance of a simple, open-ended cognitive task. Using path analysis, they confirmed that perceived self-efficacy directly affected current performance. Self-efficacy itself, however, was more strongly influenced by past performances. Locke et al also found that perceived self-efficacy had an indirect effect on performance, but only for subjects who set their own goals, as opposed to having them assigned. These subjects had increased levels of perceived self-efficacy associated with an increase in goal commitment; no such effect was found for subjects who had goals assigned to them by the experimenter. The beneficial effects of sports performers learning to set their own goals, rather than having them imposed by a coach, are as yet poorly documented (e.g. Burton, 1983). However, there would seem to be a strong possibility that Locke et al's (1984) result would generalize to a sport context, especially if a self-learning package (e.g. Hardy and Fazey, 1990) were used.

The common technique of using proximal goal setting may operate via improvements in self-efficacy (Bandura and Schunk, 1981). In their view, proximal goals provide markers of increasing competence as distal goals are approached, and it is this increase in perceived competence which leads to an increase in self-efficacy. Bandura and Cervone (1983) expanded the debate to include both self-efficacy and self-evaluation. They proposed that goals could have an effect on both; self-evaluation, the comparison of actual performance with an internal, idealized standard, has much in common with explanations of self-esteem (e.g. Coopersmith, 1967). Bandura and Cervone, however, regarded the self-dissatisfaction experienced when performances are sub-standard as a motivational factor, and suggested that people will want to reduce the self-dissatisfaction by performing better. In this way, goal setting has the potential both to build self-efficacy and to increase self-dissatisfaction, or motivate performance.

THE FUTURE FOR GOAL SETTING IN SPORT

Goal setting, which has had an impressive pedigree in the industrial/organizational field, is beginning to be used very differently in a sport context. Until now, much of what has been achieved in sport has been at an intuitive level, without the benefit of either theory or empirical research findings to underpin it. This will need to change before the technique gains respectability in its new role. The reasons for its success in business are quite well understood, although there are growing theoretical ideas which may be able to explain its application to competitive stress in sport. The work of Bandura on self-efficacy immediately springs to mind, but there is little doubt that further advances in the theory of goal setting will grow from its employment in sport. However, before that happens, research will need to examine a number of areas where knowledge about the effects or the practice of goal setting is exceedingly sparse. When we consider that the use of goal setting in industry has been going on for nearly 80 years, while in sport it has been around for only 10 years or so, this is hardly surprising.

In attempting to build a coherent model of goal setting in the sport context, both the motivational aspect of goals and their stress management benefits will need to be included in a testable form. Unlike most models of goal setting in industry, such a model will need to focus on the individual, because the looked-for changes to be brought about by effective goal setting are not at the level of plant productivity but in the functioning of the individual athlete. Virtually all of the research already conducted on goal setting has ignored the person for whom the goals are being set; athletes are not 'units of production', and very different approaches to theory and practice are needed. Clearly, any new theory will have to incorporate ideas on multidimensional anxiety, and the first task of researchers will be to gain some very firm purchase on the way that goal setting can affect athletes' responses to competitive stress. A start has been made in this area, but much remains to be done. Because participation in sport is a very personal event, self-concept variables, such as self-efficacy and self-esteem, have important effects on performance. These personality variables will also need to figure prominently in such a theory. Unfortunately, we will know nothing like enough about how these variables interact with goal setting to even begin to model the process.

At a more practical level, coaches will want to know more about how to personalize goals, to match goals to personalities and to match assigned goals to athletes' covert goals, hopefully thus to maximize acceptance and commitment. One technique which may sidestep any problems in this difficult area may be to rely on training athletes to set goals for themselves. Much of previous goal setting has used assigned goals; in sport, learning to self-set goals may turn out to be a very important skill. We need to know a lot more about how athletes do this, and what are its benefits and drawbacks. Most elite athletes use mental rehearsal in their preparation for competition; we also need to find out how mental rehearsal and goal setting might operate together to change both self-concept and goal achievement strategies.

One of the most useful areas of future research will extend the pioneering work on the quantification of goals. The acceptance/rejection threshold for challenging goals immediately springs to mind; more broadly, an appropriate metric, and value, for challenging goals needs to be sought. Being able to set proximal goal difficulty on some series of optimum values may help to accelerate the athlete up the learning curve, boost his or her self-confidence, and protect him or her from competitive stress in the most effective and efficient way. As yet, we know little about how this can be achieved other than a reliance on intuition. Again, the choice of goal difficulties in training and in competition has important implications for the athlete's ability to cope with competitive stress; we urgently need to know about the relative difficulties of training and competition goals in different sports. And talking of different sports, there is a dearth of useful published ideas about how goal-setting programmes can be constructed in complex sports.

This may seem like a catalogue of unanswered questions, and there is no doubt that many others could be posed. The reason is that, at the moment, we are at the beginning of an interesting and exciting new era in goal-setting theory and research. Goal setting is a potentially very valuable tool for both coach and athlete to use to help overcome the stress of competition, but so much remains unclear. It is to be hoped that when a review of research in goal setting in sport is written in the years to come, it will be able to report as fulsomely in its benefits to coaches and athletes in search of new and better ways of protecting against competitive stress as earlier reviews were able to in respect of employee motivation.

REFERENCES

Ahrens, A. H. (1987). Theories of depression: the role of goals and the self-evaluation process, *Cognitive Therapy and Research*, **11**, 665–680.

Ammons, R. B. (1956). Effects of knowledge of performance: a survey and tentative theoretical formulation, *Journal of General Psychology*, **54**, 279–299.

Anderson, D. C., Crowell, C. R., Doman,, M. and Howard, G. S. (1988). Performance posting, goal setting, and activity-contingent praise as applied to a university hockey team, *Journal of Applied Psychology*, **73**, 87–95.

Andrews, F. M. and Farris, G. F. (1972). Time pressure and performance of scientists and engineers: a five-year panel study, *Organizational Behavior and Human Performance*, **8**, 185–200

Baird, J. W. (1974). An analytic field study of 'open communication' as perceived by supervisors, subordinates and peers, *Dissertation Abstracts International*, **35**, 562B.

Bandura, A. (1977). Self-efficacy: toward a unifying theory of behavioural change, *Psychological Review*, **84**, 191–215.

Bandura, A. (1982). Self-efficacy mechanism in human agency, *American Psychologist*, **377**, 122–147.

Bandura, A. and Adams, N. E. (1977). Analysis of self-efficacy theory of behavioral change, *Cognitive Therapy and Research*, **1**, 287–310.

Bandura, A., Adams, N. E. and Beyer, J. (1977). Cognitive processes mediating behavioral change. *Journal of Personality and Social Psychology*, **35**, 129–139.

Bandura, A., Adams, N. E., Hardy, A. B. and Howells, G. N. (1980). Tests of the generality of self-efficacy theory, *Cognitive Therapy and Research*, **4**, 39–66.

Bandura, A. and Cervone, D. (1983). Self-evaluative and self-efficacy mechanisms governing the motivational effects of goal systems, *Journal of Personality and Social Psychology*, **45**, 1017–1028.

Bandura, A. and Schunk, D. H. (1981). Cultivating competence, self-efficacy and intrinsic interest through proximal self-motivation, *Journal of Personality and Social Psychology*, **41**, 546–598.

Bandura, A. and Simon, K. M. (1977). The role of proximal intentions in self-regulation of refractory behavior, *Cognitive Therapy and Research*, **1**, 177–193.

Barnett, M. L. (1977). Effects of two methods of goal setting on learning a gross motor task, *Research Quarterly*, **48**, 19–23.

Barnett, M. L. and Stanicek, J. A. (1979). Effects of goal setting on achievement in archery, *Research Quarterly*, **50**, 328–332.

Bilodeau, E. A. and Bilodeau, I. McD. (1961). Motor skills learning, *American Review of Psychology*, **12**, 243–280.

Botterill, C. (1977). Goalsetting and performance on an endurance task. Paper presented at the Canadian Psychomotor Learning and Sport Psychology Conference, Banff, Alberta.

Botterill, C. (1978). The psychology of coaching, *Coaching Review*, **1**, 1–8.

Botterill, C. (1980). Psychology of coaching, in R. M. Suinn (ed.). *Psychology in Sports: Methods and Applications*. Minneapolis: Burgess.

Brockner, J. (1983). Low self-esteem and behavioral plasticity, in L. M. Wheeler and R. P. Shaver (eds). *Review of Personality and Social Psychology: 4*. Beverly Hills, California: Sage.

Burton, D. (1983). Evaluation of goalsetting training on selected cognitions and performance of collegiate swimmers. Unpublished doctoral dissertation, University of Illinois.

Burton, D. and Martens, R. (1986). Pinned by their own goals: an exploratory investigation into why kids drop out of wrestling, *Journal of Sport Psychology*, **8**, 183–197.

Cale, A. and Jones, J. G. (1989). Relationships between expectations of success, multidimensional anxiety and perceptuo-motor performance. Paper presented at the Annual Conference of the North American Society for the Psychology of Sport and Physical Activity, Kent State University, Ohio, USA.

Campbell, J. P., Dunnette, M. D., Lawler, E. E. III and Weick, K. E. (1970). *Managerial Behavior, Performance and Effectiveness*. New York: McGraw-Hill.

Carroll, S. J. and Tosi, H. L. (1970). Goal characteristics and personality factors in a management-by-objectives program, *Administrative Science Quarterly*, **15**, 295–305.

Cohen, F. and Lazarus, R. S. (1979). Coping with serious illness, in G. C. Stone, F. Cohen and N. E. Adler (eds). *Health Psychology*. San Francisco: Jossey-Bass.

Coopersmith,, S. (1967). *The Antecedents of Self-Esteem*. San Francisco: Freeman.

Danish, S. J. (1983). Learning life's lessons by setting goals in sports, *New York Times*, September 25.

Dossett, D. L., Latham, G. P. and Mitchell, T. R. (1979). Effects of assigned versus participatively set goals, knowledge of results, and individual differences on employee behavior when goal difficulty is held constant, *Journal of Applied Psychology*, **64**, 291–298.

Doyle, L. A., Landers, D. M. and Feltz, D. L. (1980). Psychological skills in elite and subelite shooters. Paper presented at the Annual Conference of the North American Society for the Psychology of Sport and Physical Activity, Boulder, Colorado, USA.

Earley, P. C. (1986). Supervisors and shop stewards as sources of contextual information in goalsetting: a comparison of the US with England, *Journal of Applied Psychology*, **71**, 111–117.

Earley, P. C. and Kanfer, R. (1985). The influence of component participation and role models on goal acceptance, goal satisfaction and performance, *Organizational Behavior and Human Decision Processes*, **36**, 378–390.

Elliot, E. S. and Dweck, C. S. (1988). Goals: an approach to motivation and achievement, *Journal of Personality and Social Psychology*, **54**, 5–12.

Erez, M. (1986). The congruence of goalsetting strategies with socio-cultural values, and its effect on performance, *Journal of Management*, **12**, 83–90.

Erez, M. and Arad, R. (1986). Participative goalsetting: social, motivational and cognitive factors, *Journal of Applied Psychology*, **71**, 591–597.

Erez, M. and Earley, P. C. (1987). Comparative analysis of goalsetting strategies across cultures, *Journal of Applied Psychology*, **72**, 658–665.

Erez, M., Earley, P. C. and Hulin, C. L. (1985). The impact of participation on goal acceptance and performance: a two-step model, *Academy of Management Journal*, **28**, 50–66.

Erez, M. and Zidon, I. (1984). Effects of goal acceptance on the relationship of goal difficulty to performance, *Journal of Applied Psychology*, **69**, 69–78.

Ewing, M. (1981). Achievement orientations and sport behaviors of males and females. Unpublished doctoral dissertation, University of Illinois.

Feltz, D. C. (1982). Path analysis of the causal elements in Bandura's theory of self-efficacy and an anxiety-based model of avoidance behavior, *Journal of Personality and Social Psychology*, **42**, 764–781.

Feltz, D. C. (1983). Gender differences in the causal elements of Bandura's theory of self-efficacy on a high-avoidance motor task. Paper presented at the Annual Conference of the North American Society for the Psychology of Sport and Physical Activity, East Lansing, MI, USA.

Forward, J. and Zander, A. (1971). Choice of unattainable group goals and effects on performance, *Organizational Behavior and Human Performance*, **6**, 184–199.

French, J. and Raven, B. H. (1959). The bases of social power, in D. Cartwright (ed.). *Studies in Social Power*. Ann Arbor, MI: Institute for Social Research.

Fuoss, D. E. and Troppman, R. J. (1981). *Effective Coaching: A Psychological Approach*. New York: Wiley.

Garland, H. (1983). Influence of ability, assigned goals and normative information on personal goals: a challenge to the goal attainability assumption, *Journal of Applied Psychology*, **68**, 20–30.

Garland, H. (1985). A cognitive mediation theory of task goals and human performance, *Motivation and Emotion*, **9**, 345–367.

Gould, D. (1986). Goalsetting for peak performance, in J. M. Williams (ed.). *Applied Sport Psychology: Personal Growth to Peak Performance*, Palo Alto, California: Mayfield.

Gould, D., Weiss, M. R. and Weinberg, R. (1981). Psychological characteristics of successful and non-successful Big-Ten wrestlers, *Journal of Sport Psychology*, **3**, 69–81.

Hall, D. T. and Lawler, E. E. (1971). Job pressures and research performance, *American Scientist*, **59**, 64–73.

Hall, H. K., Weinberg, R. S. and Jackson, A. (1983). The effects of goalsetting on the performance of a circuit training task. Paper presented at TAHPERD Conference, Corpus Christi, Texas, USA.

Hall, H. K., Weinberg, R. S. and Jackson, A. (1987). Effects of goal specificity, goal difficulty, and information feedback on endurance performance, *Journal of Sport Psychology*, **9**, 43–54.

Hardy, L. and Fazey, J. A. (1990). *Mental Training*. Leeds: National Coaching Foundation.

Hardy, L. Maiden, D. S. and Sherry, K. (1986). Goalsetting and performance anxiety, *Journal of Sports Sciences*, **4**, 233–234.

Highlen, P. S. and Bennett, B. B. (1979). Psychological characteristics of successful and nonsuccessful elite wrestlers: an exploratory study, *Journal of Sport Psychology*, **1**, 123–137.

Hollenbeck, J. R. and Brief, A. P. (1987). The effects of individual differences and goal origin on goalsetting and performance, *Organizational Behavior and Human Decision Processes*, **40**, 392–414.

Hollenbeck, J. R. and Klein, H. J. (1987). Goal commitment and the goalsetting process: problems, prospects, and proposals for future research, *Journal of Applied Psychology*, **72**, 212–220.

Hollingworth, B. (1975). Effects of performance goals and anxiety on learning a gross motor task, *Research Quarterly*, **46**, 162–168.

Huber, V. L. (1985). Effects of task difficulty, goal setting, and strategy on performance of a heuristic task, *Journal of Applied Psychology*, **70**, 492–504.

Komacki, J., Barwick, K. D. and Scott, L. R. (1978). A behavioral approach to occupational safety: pinpointing and reinforcing safe performance in a food manufacturing plant, *Journal of Applied Psychology*, **64**, 434–445.

Larsen, D. W. (1983). Coach inspires more than winning, *Seattle Times*, February 14.

Latham, G. P. and Baldes, J. J. (1975). The practical significance of Locke's theory of goalsetting, *Journal of Applied Psychology*, **60**, 122–124.

Latham, G. P. Erez, M. and Locke, E. A. (1988). Resolving scientific disputes by the joint design of crucial experiments by the antagonists: application to the Erez–Latham dispute regarding participation in goal setting, *Journal of Applied Psychology*, **73**, 753–772.

Latham, G. P. and Lee, T. W. (1985). Goal setting, in E. A. Locke (ed.). *Generalising from Laboratory to Field Settings*, Lexington, MA: Lexington Books.

Latham, G. P. and Locke, E. A. (1975). Increasing productivity with decreasing time limits: a field replication of Parkinson's law, *Journal of Applied Psychology*, **60**, 524–526.

Latham, G. P. and Saari, L. M. (1979). Importance of supportive relationships in goal setting, *Journal of Applied Psychology*, **64**, 151–156.

Lewin, K. (1921). Das Problem der Willensmessung und der Grundgesetz der Association; I, *Psychologisches Forschung*, **1**, 191–302.

Lewin, K. (1922). Das Problem der Willensmessung und der Grundgesetz der Association: II, *Psychologisches Forschung*, **2**, 65–140.

Likert, R. (1961). *New Patterns of Management*. New York: McGraw-Hill.

Locke, E. A. (1966). The relationship of intentions to level of performance, *Journal of Applied Psychology*, **50**, 60–66.

Locke, E. A. (1968). Toward a theory of task motivation and incentives, *Organizational Behavior and Human Performance*, **3**, 157–189.

Locke, E. A. and Bryan, J. F. (1966). Cognitive aspects of psychomotor performance: the effects of performance goals on level of performance, *Journal of Applied Psychology*, **50**, 286–291.

Locke, E. A. and Bryan, J. F. (1969). The directing function of goals in task performance, *Organizational Behavior and Human Performance*, **4**, 35–42.

Locke, E. A., Cartledge, N. and Koeppel, J. (1968). Motivational effects of knowledge of results: a goal setting phenomenon? *Psychological Bulletin*, **70**, 474–485.

Locke, E. A., Frederick, E., Lee, C. and Bobko, P. (1984). Effect of self-efficacy, goals, and task strategies on task performance, *Journal of Applied Psychology*, **69**, 241–251.

Locke, E. A. and Henne, D. (1986). Work motivation theories, in C. L. Copper and I. Robertson (eds), *Review of Industrial and Organizational Psychology*, Chichester, England: Wiley.

Locke E. A. and Latham, G. P. (1984). *Goal setting: A Motivational Technique that Works!* Englewood Cliffs, NJ: Prentice-Hall.

Locke, E. A. and Latham, G. P. (1985). The application of goal setting to sports, *Journal of Sport Psychology*, **7**, 205–222.

Locke, E. A., Motowidlo, S. J. and Bobko, P. (1986). Using self-efficacy theory to resolve the conflict between goal setting theory and expectancy theory in organizational behavior and industrial/organizational psychology, *Journal of Social and Clinical Psychology*, **4**, 328–338.

Locke, E. A., Shaw, K. N., Saari, L. M. and Latham, G. P. (1981). Goal setting and task performance: 1969–1980, *Psychological Bulletin*, **90**, 125–152.

Maehr, M. L. and Nicholls, J. C. (1980). Culture and achievement motivation: a second look, in N. Warren (ed.). *Studies in Cross-Cultural Psychology*, New York: Academic Press.

Mahoney, M. J. and Avener, M. (1977). Psychology of the elite athlete: an exploratory study, *Cognitive Therapy and Research*, **1**, 135–141.

Martens, R., Burton, D., Vealey, R. S., Bump, L. A. and Smith, D. E. (1990). Competitive State Anxiety Inventory-2, in R. Martens, R. Vealey and D. Burton (eds). *Competitive Anxiety in Sport*. Champaign, Illinois: Human Kinetics.

Matsui, T., Imaizumi, T., Onglatko, M. C. and Kakuyama, T. (1985). Effects of individual versus group goals and feedback on task performance. Unpublished manuscript: cited in Erez and Earley (1987).

McClements, J. D. and Botterill, C. B. (1979). Goalsetting in shaping the future performance of athletes, in P. Klavora and J. Daniels (eds) *Coach, Athlete and the Sports Psychologist*, Toronto: University of Toronto.

McClements, J. D. and Laverty, W. H. (1979). A mathematical model of speedskating performance improvement for goal setting and program evaluation, *Canadian Journal of Applied Sports Science*, **4**, 116–122.

Mento, A. J., Steel, R. P. and Karren, R. J. (1987). A meta-analytic study of the effects of goal setting on task performance: 1966–1984, *Organizational Behavior and Human Decision Processes*, **39**, 52–83.

Miller, G. A., Galanter, E. and Pribram, K. H. (1960). *Plans and the Structure of Behavior*, New York: Holt.

Mueller, M. E. (1983). The effects of goal setting and competition on performance: a laboratory study. Unpublished master's thesis, University of Minnesota.

Newell, K. M. (1974). Knowledge of results and motor learning, *Journal of Motor Behavior*, **6**, 235–244.

Odiorne, G. S. (1978). MBO: a backward glance, *Business Horizons*, **21**, 14–24.

Oldham, G. R. (1975). The impact of supervisory characteristics on goal acceptance, *Academy of Management Journal*, **18**, 461–475.

Orne, M. T. (1962). On the social psychology of the psychological experiment with particular reference to demand characteristics, *American Psychologist*, **17**, 776–783.

Passer, M. W. (1981). Children in sport: participation motives and psychological stress, *Quest*, **33**, 231–244.

Payne, R. B. and Hauty, G. T. (1955). Effect of psychological feedback on work decrement, *Journal of Experimental Psychology*, **50**, 343–351.

Roberts, G. C. (1986). The growing child and the perception of competitive stress in sport, in G. Gleeson (ed.) *The Growing Child in Competitive Sport*, London: Hodder and Stoughton.

Rotter, J. B. (1966). Generalized expectancies for internal versus external control of reinforcement, *Psychological Monographs*, **80**, (1, whole no. 609).

Ryan, T. A. (1970). *Intentional Behavior: An Approach to Human Motivation*, New York: Ronald Press.

Salancik, G. (1977). Commitment and the control of organizational behavior and belief, in B. M. Straw and G. R. Salancik (eds). *New Directions in Organizational Behavior*, Chicago: St Claire Press.

Sarason, I. G. (1978). The test anxiety scale: concepts and research, in C. D. Spielberger and I. G. Sarason (eds). *Stress and Anxiety*, Washington, DC: Hemisphere.

Schmidt, R. (1982). *Motor Control and Learning: A Behavioral Emphasis*, Champaign, Illinois: Human Kinetics.

Schrauger, J. S. and Rosenberg, S. F. (1970). Self esteem and the effects of success and failure feedback on performance, *Journal of Personality*, **38**, 404–417.

Schunk, D. (1983). Developing children's self-efficacy and skills: the roles of social comparative information and goalsetting, *Contemporary Educational Psychology*, **8**, 76–86.

Shotter, J. (1980). Action, joint action, and intentionality, in M. Brenner (ed.) *The Structure of Action*, Oxford: Blackwell.

Shotter, J. (1984). *Social Accountability and Selfhood*, Oxford: Blackwell.

Simon, J. A. and Martens, R. (1979). Children's anxiety in sport and nonsport evaluative activities, *Journal of Sport Psychology*, **1**, 160–169.

Tannenbaum, R. and Schmidt, E. (1958). How to choose a leadership pattern, *Harvard Business Review*, **36**, 95–101.

Taylor, F. W. (1911/1967). *The Principles of Scientific Management*. New York: Norton.

Tolman, E. C. (1932). *Purposive Behavior in Animals and Men*. New York: Century.

Tubbs, M. E. (1986). Goal setting: a meta-analytic examination of the empirical evidence, *Journal of Applied Psychology*, **71**, 474–483.

Vroom, V. H. (1964). *Work and Motivation*. New York: Wiley.

Vygotsky, L. S. (1956). Cited in Wertsch, J. V. and Rogoff, B. (1984). Editors' notes. In B. Rogoff and J. V. Wertsch (eds). *Children's Learning in the 'Zone of Proximal Development'*. San Francisco: Jossey-Bass.

Vygotsky, L. S. (1962). *Thought and Language*. New York: Wiley.

Ward, C. H. and Eisler, R. M. (1987). Type A achievement striving and failure to achieve personal goals, *Cognitive Therapy and Research*, **11**, 463–471.

Weinberg, R. S., Bruya, L. D. and Jackson, A. (1985). The effects of goal proximity and goal specificity on endurance performance, *Journal of Sport Psychology*, 7, 296–305.

Weinberg, R., Bruya, L. Jackson, A. and Garland, H. (1987). Goal difficulty and endurance performance: a challenge to the goal attainability assumption, *Journal of Sport Behavior*, 10, 82–92.

Weinberg, R., Gould, D. and Jackson, A. (1979). Expectations and performance: an empirical test of Bandura's self-efficacy theory. *Journal of Sport Psychology*, 1, 320–331.

Weinberg, R. S., Gould, D., Yukelson, D. and Jackson, A. (1981). The effect of preexisting and manipulated self-efficacy on a competitive muscular endurance task, *Journal of Sport Psychology*, 4, 345–354.

White, S. E., Mitchell, T. R. and Bell, C. H. (1977). Goal setting, evaluation apprehension, and social cues as determinants of job performance and job satisfaction in a simulated organization, *Journal of Applied Psychology*, 62, 665–673.

Whitehead, J. (1986). Achievement goals and drop-out in youth sports, in G. Gleeson (ed.). *The Growing Child in Competitive Sport*. London: Hodder and Stoughton.

Williams, S. L., Dooseman, G. and Kleifield, E. (1984). Comparative effectiveness of guided mastery and exposure treatments for intractable phobias, *Journal of Consulting and Clinical Psychology*, 52, 505–518.

Williams, S. L., Turner, S. M. and Peer, D. F. (1985). Guided mastery and performance desensitization treatments for severe acrophobia, *Journal of Consulting and Clinical Psychology*, 53, 237–247.

Wood, D. J., Bruner, J. S. and Ross, G. (1976). The role of tutoring in problem solving, *Journal of Child Psychology and Psychiatry*, 17, 89–100.

Wood, D. J., Wood, H. A. and Middleton, D. J. (1978). An experimental evaluation of four face-to-face teaching strategies, *International Journal of Behaviour Development*, 1, 131–147.

Wood, R. E. (1986). Task complexity: definition of the construct, *Organizational Behavior and Human Decision Processes*, 37, 60–82.

Wood, R. E., Mento, A. J. and Locke, E. A. (1987). Task complexity as a moderator of goal effects: a meta-analysis, *Journal of Applied Psychology*, 72, 416–425.

Yukl, G. A. and Latham, G. P. (1978). Interrelationships among employee participation, individual differences, goal difficulty, goal acceptance, goal instrumentality, and performance, *Personnel Psychology*, 31, 305–323.

Chapter 7

Multimodal stress management in sport: current status and future directions

Damon Burton
University of Idaho

I learned early on in my work as an educational sport psychologist that stress management is a topic that is easier to theorize about than to apply effectively. Probably my most frustrating stress management case study occurred during my tenure as sport psychologist for the US Ski Jumping Team and involved an athlete I'll call Tom. Tom had all the classic symptoms of an athlete who 'chokes' under pressure. Tom and his coaches readily acknowledged that he performed better (a) in practice than in competition; (b) in less important competitions than more important ones; (c) when expectations were low rather than high; (d) when his chances of winning were low rather than high; and (e) on his first rather than his second jump.

When I first met Tom, he was beginning his third year on the team. He had initially surprised everyone by jumping his way on to the team and subsequently making the Olympic team, but the longer he was on the national team, the more stress seemed to impair his competitive performance. In competition, Tom tantalized his coaches by training well and often jumping well on the first of his two jumps, but he consistently failed to jump well in situations where it counted. In discussing this problem with Tom, he was very open about his problems and his desire to develop his stress management skills to overcome them. As we began to delve into Tom's stress problems, I discovered that he was an engineering major in college and approached ski jumping very analytically. This approach seemed to help him develop technically in practice but often prompted him to think too much or have negative thoughts in competition.

Stress and Performance in Sport. Edited by J. Graham Jones and Lew Hardy.
©1990 John Wiley & Sons Ltd.

Initially, I decided that the best approach to help Tom to learn to manage stress and perform up to his potential was to teach him a multimodal stress management technique that would help him learn to manage both excessive emotional arousal and negative or unproductive thoughts. A competitive modification of Meichenbaum's (1975) stress inoculation training was chosen, and after explaining the rationale of the program to Tom, we began to develop the requisite physical relaxation (Martens, 1987), self-talk (Burton, 1985) and imagery (Martens, 1987) skills. Tom mastered the individual psychological skills quite well, and imagery and simulated-sport practice of competitive stress inoculation training (CSIT) worked very effectively. However, performance did not improve. Tom's evaluation of competition, particularly his thoughts and feelings prior to and during each jump, produced several interesting insights.

First, he reported that sometimes when he employed CSIT prior to competition to control stress, the procedure left him feeling lethargic and mentally 'flat', a performance state quite different from the one in which he performed his best. Secondly, although he reported being able to counter negative or unproductive pre-competitive thoughts quite effectively, he had difficulty finding a positive 'competitive focus' while jumping that would prevent intruding negative thoughts yet still allow him to perform optimally. Finally, if Tom failed to manage stress effectively and let arousal get too high and/or self-talk become too negative or unproductive, he would reach a point where he felt overwhelmed, making it almost impossible to use stress management techniques effectively.

Regrettably, Tom was one of my biggest failures. None of the modifications or alternative stress management strategies I subsequently tried with Tom were any more effective than CSIT in helping him manage competitive stress effectively enough to perform up to his performance potential. Perhaps the most important implication of this case study for me was the realization that stress management is an extremely complex area. Over time, as I have had a chance to work with other athletes and try other stress management strategies, I have become convinced that increasingly sophisticated stress models are needed to understand this complex process. Thus, conceptual advancements in stress theorization such as Lazarus and Launier's (1978) transactional model of stress and Lazarus and Folkman's (1984) revised stress model, which emphasizes the role of cognitive appraisal and coping processes in stress reduction, offer great promise for helping practitioners gain a better understanding of how to most effectively treat stress disorders.

The purposes of this chapter are therefore fivefold. First, a multimodal stress management model will be introduced that specifies the multiple types of anxiety problems confronted by athletes in sport. Secondly, support for this multimodal stress management model will be provided, including empirical evidence from several lines of research including anxiety, appraisal, and coping. Thirdly, two common multimodal stress management strategies will be described, including examples of how different stress management modalities are combined to achieve an integrated coping response. Fourthly, the effectiveness of multimodal stress management strategies will be evaluated, including empirical findings from both the general psychological and sport literatures. Criticisms of the efficacy of multimodal stress management treatments for enhancing sport performance will also be discussed. Finally, future directions for multimodal stress management research will be addressed, emphasizing the need for more and better evaluation research with athletes as well as the necessity for further refinement in performance and anxiety measurement.

A MULTIMODAL STRESS MANAGEMENT MODEL

Although clinicians such as Meichenbaum (1975) pioneered the development and use of multimodal stress management strategies and documented their effectiveness, the first major theoretical support for a multimodal stress management model came from Davidson and Schwartz's (1976) psychophysiological relaxation model (see Figure 7.1). In examining relaxation intervention studies, Davidson and Schwartz (1976) discovered that different types of anxiety problems demonstrated differential response rates to particular stress management techniques, and that certain types of stress management techniques seemed to work better for specific types of anxiety. They concluded that the mixed results evident in the anxiety intervention literature were probably due to the differences in the degree of compatibility between the type of anxiety being experienced by the client and the ability of the treatment of choice to alleviate that form of anxiety. Thus, these two psychophysiologists set out to develop a relaxation model that would explain the major categories of anxiety typically experienced as well as to provide a conceptual rationale to help clients with specific presenting problems select the most appropriate stress management techniques.

In developing their model, Davidson and Schwartz (1976) incorporated empirical research on the psychophysiology of cognitive and somatic components of relaxation (e.g. Goleman, 1971) with the hemispheric specialization literature indicating differential hemispheric mediation of cognitive and somatic behavior (e.g. Bogen, 1969; Kimura, 1973; White, 1969). Their comprehensive relaxation model not only categorizes four distinct types of anxiety, but it also specifies the relaxation techniques predicted to be most effective in alleviating each anxiety type. In order to facilitate understanding of this multimodal stress management model, a brief description of differences between (a) left and right hemisphere functioning and (b) cognitive and somatic anxiety is provided below.

	LEFT HEMISPHERE		RIGHT HEMISPHERE	
	ANXIETY PROBLEM	INTERVENTION STRATEGY	ANXIETY PROBLEM	INTERVENTION STRATEGY
COGNITIVE ANXIETY	Sequential activation of verbal or analytical behaviors e.g., over-analysis or specific neg-ative thoughts	Transcendental meditation Goal Setting Self Talk * "cue" words * counterarguments Hypnosis - suggestion component	Parallel activation of multiple imagery/spatial behaviors e.g., automated images of disaster	Hypnosis-imagery/ suggestion component Cognitive restructuring techniques that focus on changing self-images
SOMATIC ANXIETY	Sequential activation of specific somatic behavior e.g., tension in specific muscles	Physical relaxation techniques EMG Biofeedback Hypnosis - relaxation component Exercise/stretching	Parallel activation of global somatic behaviors e.g., butterflies in the stomach or cold, clammy hands	Zen meditation Hatha yoga breathing component Autogenic training Biofeedback * skin temperature * skin conductance

Figure 7.1. Multimodal stress management model (adapted from Davidson and Schwartz, 1976).

Differences in hemispheric functioning

For most individuals who are right-handed or mixed dominant, the left hemisphere becomes specialized for sequential processing and is guided predominantly by specific thoughts or verbal self-statements (e.g. Davidson and Schwartz, 1976; Blakeslee, 1980). When athletes are thinking rationally, employing logic and reasoning skills, or using computation or problem-solving strategies, they are predominantly using left hemisphere processing. Thus, the processes of learning new skills, modifying previously learned skills or developing competitive strategies are left hemisphere functions. Conversely, the right hemisphere normally becomes specialized for parallel processing and uses visual/spatial guidance processes to simultaneously integrate many diverse types of inputs (e.g. Davidson and Schwartz, 1976; Blakeslee, 1980). Intuition and creativity, orientation in time and space, emotions, and performance execution are all right hemisphere functions. Thus, once athletes learn how to perform skills correctly, they rely on their right hemisphere to execute these skills automatically.

Cognitive versus somatic anxiety

The distinction between cognitive and somatic anxiety has become quite common in both the psychophysiology of relaxation (e.g. Davidson and Schwartz, 1976; Schwartz, Davidson and Goleman, 1978) and anxiety (e.g.

Liebert and Morris, 1967; Martens *et al.*, 1990; Morris, Davis and Hutchings, 1981; Smith, Smoll and Schutz, 1990) literatures. Cognitive anxiety is the mental component of anxiety caused by negative expectations of success, negative self-evaluation, or diversion of attentional focus, whereas somatic anxiety is the physiological or affective component of anxiety that is directly related to autonomic arousal. Cognitive anxiety is characterized by worry, negative self-talk, attentional distraction, and unpleasant visual imagery, whereas somatic anxiety is reflected in such physiological responses as rapid heart rate, shortness of breath, clammy hands, butterflies in the stomach, and tense muscles.

Four types of anxiety

Davidson and Schwartz (1976) have combined these differences in left and right hemispheric functioning with the unique characteristics of cognitive and somatic anxiety to form the comprehensive multimodal stress management model described below (see Figure 7.1).

Left hemisphere–somatic anxiety (LH—SA)

This type of anxiety is elicited by sequential activation of specific somatic behaviors such as experiencing tension in a hamstring muscle prior to an important 100-meter dash (see Figure 7.1). The model hypothesizes that the sprinter with a tight hamstring could effectively cope with this tension problem by using one or more of the stress management techniques designed to achieve LH–SA relaxation. As illustrated in Figure 7.1, these LH—SA interventions include: any one of a number of physical relaxation techniques (e.g. progressive muscle relaxation), EMG biofeedback training, the relaxation component of hypnosis, or physical exercise, particularly stretching.

Left hemisphere—cognitive anxiety (LH—CA)

This category of anxiety problems is engendered by sequential activation of specific verbal or analytical behaviors (see Figure 7.1). Because the left hemisphere is verbally mediated, athletes with this type of anxiety would have difficulty relaxing because they think too much, are overly analytical, or cannot get specific negative thoughts out of their mind. Davidson and Schwartz's (1976) model predicts that athletes who overanalyze or are plagued with specific negative thoughts could effectively cope with this anxiety problem by selecting one or more LH—CA stress management techniques, including: transcendental meditation, goal setting (i.e. lower goals to keep them realistic), self-talk, both self-instructional 'cue words' and positive affirmations, cognitive restructuring (e.g. counterarguments), and the suggestion component of hypnosis (see Figure 7.1).

Right hemisphere—somatic anxiety (RH—SA)

This type of anxiety is elicited by parallel activation of a number of global somatic behaviors (see Figure 7.1). Because RH—SA involves diffuse body tension and global somatic stress related to the activation of the autonomic nervous system, athletes often experience this class of anxiety through such symptoms as butterflies in the stomach or cold clammy hands. The multimodal stress management model predicts that a volleyball player who typically experiences pre-competitive anxiety in the form of butterflies and clammy hands could effectively reduce her anxiety by using one or more of the stress management techniques designed to achieve RH—SA relaxation, including: Zen meditation, autogenic training, skin temperature and skin conductance biofeedback, the breathing component of Hatha yoga, and vigorous exercise (see Figure 7.1).

Right hemisphere—cognitive anxiety (RH—CA)

This category of anxiety problems is engendered by unwanted cognitions of a visual/spatial, rather than a verbal, nature such as images of poor performance (see Figure 7.1). The images of competitive disaster are often more anxiety-provoking because of the great realism offered by the right hemisphere's parallel processing capabilities that allow integration of simultaneous input from various sensory modalities, so athletes see, hear, touch, smell and taste every aspect of their imagined failure. Davidson and Schwartz's (1976) model predicts that athletes who experience relatively automatic images of competitive disaster can effectively cope with this type of anxiety by selecting one or more RH—CA stress management techniques, including: the imagery/suggestion component of hypnosis, and cognitive restructuring techniques that focus on changing self-images (see Figure 7.1).

Compatibility between anxiety type and treatment modality

Although Davidson and Schwartz (1976) emphasized that stress management strategies will be most effective in reducing compatible types of anxiety, they did not discount possible 'crossover' effects in which the technique also alleviates less compatible types of anxiety. Thus, progressive muscle relaxation will be most effective in reducing specific muscular tension such as a tight hamstring (LH—SA), but it may also provide some benefit in reducing butterflies (RH—SA), eliminating specific negative thoughts of failure (LH—CA), or interrupting images of competitive disaster (RH—CA).

Subsequent empirical investigation by Schwartz, Davidson and Goleman (1978) found that subjects regularly employing a cognitively based stress management technique (i.e. transcendental meditation (TM)) demonstrated lower cognitive anxiety scores than subjects who used a somatically based exercise treatment. Conversely, exercisers demonstrated significantly lower somatic anxiety scores than did subjects who practiced TM. Interestingly, for subjects using TM, cognitive and somatic anxiety were very similar, suggesting that TM was either effective or ineffective at reducing both.

Although evidence from many different lines of research supports Davidson and Schwartz's (1976) multimodal stress management model, much of the subsequent research on anxiety (e.g. Martens et al., 1990; Morris, Davis and Hutchings, 1981) and stress (e.g. Lazarus and Folkman, 1984; Burchfield, Stein and Hamilton, 1985) also suggests that, in practice, the different types of anxiety are difficult to separate and that situational cues that stimulate one type of anxiety will often provoke other types of anxiety as well.

EMPIRICAL SUPPORT FOR A MULTIMODAL STRESS MANAGEMENT MODEL

Despite somewhat limited direct support for the Davidson and Schwartz (1976) model, research with multidimensional anxiety and appraisal and coping lends support to the validity of the cognitive–somatic distinction and the model.

Multidimensional anxiety literature

Recent multidimensional anxiety research both in test anxiety (e.g. Deffenbacher, 1980; Liebert and Morris, 1967; Morris, Davis and Hutchings, 1981; Schwartz, Davidson and Goleman, 1978) and in sport (e.g. Burton, 1988; Martens et al., 1990; Smith, Smoll and Schutz, in press) has supported a multidimensional conceptualization of anxiety comprising distinct cognitive and somatic components (see Chapter 3 by Parfitt, Jones and Hardy in this book for further details). Interestingly, Martens and his colleagues (1990) reported moderate relationships between cognitive and somatic anxiety ranging from 0.30 to 0.76 across 18 studies. Such relationships suggest the conceptual independence of cognitive and somatic anxiety, but they also indicate that many situations probably elicit both types of anxiety. Moreover, empirical findings have generally supported the 'anxiety–performance' hypothesis that cognitive anxiety is more consistently and more strongly related to perform-ance than somatic anxiety in both academic (e.g. Deffenbacher, 1980; Morris, Davis and Hutchings, 1981) and sport (e.g., Burton, 1988) domains. However, some recent studies examining the relationship between multidimensional anxiety and subcomponents of performance (see Chapter 3 by Parfitt, Jones and Hardy in this book) have demonstrated that somatic anxiety is also an important predictor of performance (Jones and Cale, 1989; Jones, Cale and Kerwin, 1988; Parfitt, 1988; Parfitt and Hardy, 1987).

Morris, Davis and Hutchings (1981) noted that cognitive and somatic anxiety are likely to covary in stressful situations because these situations contain elements related to the arousal of each. Borkovec (1976) concurred, although for a somewhat different reason. He suggested that each component of anxiety may serve a conditioned or discriminative function for the other component. For example, if powerful somatic behaviors have been conditioned to a particular stimulus, the responses may be interpreted by the athlete as reason to worry. Athletes may acquire conditioned somatic responses to precompetitive stimuli such as locker room preparation, an audience in the stands, or pre-contest warm-up routines that may trigger them to begin worrying about those somatic symptoms. Conversely, negative thoughts or images of competitive ·disaster may trigger a specific pattern of somatic responses such as clammy hands, butterflies in the stomach, frequent urination, and tension in particular muscles.

The test anxiety treatment literature generally supports the compatibility notion while reinforcing the need to treat both cognitive and somatic anxiety simultaneously. In their review of the test anxiety intervention literature, Morris, Davis and Hutchings (1981) found that when differential effectiveness was demonstrated, compatible treatments were typically more effective. However, it must be noted that in a number of studies, incompatible treatments proved equally effective to compatible ones. Of particular interest, Morris and his colleagues concluded that improvement in actual test performance normally occurred only when there were concomitant reductions in both cognitive and somatic anxiety. Previous research (e.g. Martens *et al.*, 1990; Morris, Davis and Hutchings, 1981; Wine, 1980) has suggested that cognitive anxiety reduction enhances performance in several ways, including: (a) creating positive expectations of success; (b) eliminating distracting negative thoughts and self-rumination; and (c) preventing excessive analysis and evaluation that inhibit flow. Several explanations may indicate why lowering somatic anxiety may also be necessary. First, high somatic anxiety may normally be appraised negatively, prompting cognitive anxiety. Moreover, it may be difficult to reduce cognitive anxiety until somatic anxiety has been lowered to a level where cognitive stress management strategies can be implemented. Another possibility is that somatic anxiety reduction techniques may occupy cognitive processes with productive activities, thus making worry less likely (e.g. Carter, Johnson and Borkovec, 1986).

Thus, contemporary anxiety research not only documents the need to conceptualize cognitive and somatic anxiety as separate constructs, but it also recognizes that treatment may require simultaneous reduction in both types of anxiety.

Stress, appraisal and coping literature

Lazarus and Folkman's (1984) research on stress, appraisal and coping also provides support for this multimodal stress management model. Lazarus and Folkman (1984) emphasized that stress is the product of two types of cognitive appraisal. Primary appraisal assesses the amount of threat an individual perceives in a particular situation, whereas secondary appraisal involves the assessment of one's potential coping resources to combat the threat. Primary appraisal is assumed to be predominantly a cognitive process that nevertheless can be substantially influenced by emotional arousal. Thus, Lazarus and Folkman predicted that minimal stress may be inferred either because (a) no threat is perceived or (b) coping resources are perceived sufficient to deal with the perceived threat. Similarly, high stress can only occur if threat is perceived high and/or coping resources low.

Lazarus and Folkman (1984) distinguished between two categories of coping behaviors: emotion-focused coping (EFC) and problem-focused coping (PFC). PFC strategies are employed when the individual perceives that he/she can do something to remove the threat and include a number of active problem-solving skills. EFC strategies are utilized in situations when it is perceived that little can be done to remove the threat. Thus, these coping strategies are invoked to help the person feel better emotionally while tolerating the threat.

Although their model is primarily a cognitive one, Lazarus and Folkman (1984) have still maintained the worry (i.e. cognitive anxiety) and emotionality (i.e. somatic anxiety) distinctions in the appraisal and coping processes. Preliminary results (Folkman and Lazarus, 1980, 1985) assessing the stress experienced by middle-aged adults and college students suggest that (a) most individuals normally use both EFC and PFC strategies and (b) the types of coping strategies used vary depending on the situational constraints. For example, Folkman and Lazarus (1985) found that PFC was most prominent during preparation for a mid-term exam, whereas the EFC strategy of distancing was more prominent following the exam while waiting for grades to be posted.

Whether cognitive or somatic stress management techniques are EFC or PFC strategies probably depends on the compatibility between the coping strategy and situationally-specific types of threats. For example, if physical tension in the hamstring muscle presents a major threat to a sprinter with an upcoming race, a compatible stress management strategy such as progressive muscle relaxation probably would be a PFC strategy because it could do something directly to reduce the threat. However, if a wrestler is worried about an upcoming match against a vastly superior opponent, progressive muscle relaxation is not highly compatible with this type of cognitive anxiety, thus limiting it to the role of an EFC strategy that will help the wrestler feel better even though prospects for success have not changed. Recently, our own pilot research (Burton and Williams-Rice, 1989) found that female collegiate basketball players used a combination of EFC and PFC strategies to deal with such diverse types of appraised threats as losing, playing poorly, not playing, conflict with the coach or a team-mate, and receiving a technical foul. Moreover, a significant negative relationship was evident between players' scores on PFC and cognitive anxiety whereas only weak relationships were found between EFC and either cognitive or somatic anxiety.

Thus, the limited research on coping strategies in sport and non-sport domains suggests that multiple types of coping strategies are commonly employed to combat stress, and effective coping may require the appropriate use of both PFC and EFC strategies.

MULTIMODAL STRESS MANAGEMENT STRATEGIES

Davidson and Schwartz's (1976) multimodal stress management model seemingly has significant implications for the design and implementation of stress intervention programs. This model clearly suggests that any one stress management strategy (e.g. progressive muscle relaxation) will do a good job at alleviating compatible types of anxiety (e.g. LH—SA) but will be less effective in combating other types of anxiety. However, empirical research clearly demonstrates the strong relationship between cognitive and somatic anxiety (e.g. Martens et al. 1990; Morris, Davis and Hutchings, 1981), and laboratory studies that have tried to manipulate environmental conditions to elicit one type of anxiety without also eliciting the other have found this task very difficult (e.g. Morris, Davis and Hutchings, 1981). Indeed, test anxiety intervention research has documented that subjects almost always had to lower both cognitive and somatic anxiety before they actually improved their test performance. Similarly, coping research suggests that individuals use both EFC and PFC strategies to deal with stress. Therefore, conceptual arguments and empirical data argue convincingly that the best intervention programs should employ multimodal stress management techniques that would attack multiple types of anxiety simultaneously.

Several multimodal stress management intervention packages have been developed over the last two decades that have been applied to sport. However, only two multimodal strategies fulfil the major requirements of this model that techniques should (a) alleviate both cognitive and somatic anxiety, preferably in both the left and right hemispheres, and (b) provide systematic strategies for rehearsal of coping procedures under simulated stressful conditions. These multimodal stress management techniques are Meichenbaum's (1977) stress inoculation training and Smith's (1980) cognitive–affective stress management training. The conceptual model and rationale for each technique will be described in the following sections (see also Chapter 8 by Mace in this book).

Stress inoculation training (SIT)

Meichenbaum's (1975) development of stress inoculation training (SIT) was a direct response to clinicians' frustration with the generalizability of behavioral treatments. For example, with multiphobic clients, the therapeutic benefit of systematic desensitization designed to eliminate one type of phobia often failed to generalize to the client's other phobias. Meichenbaum (1977, 1985) and others who pioneered similar cognitive-behavioral treatments felt that a self-control/skills approach to clinical treatment would overcome these problems because treatment generalization depended on the development of a common set of coping responses that could be used across situations.

Meichenbaum (1977) identified seven treatment components that underlie different types of coping/skills programs such as SIT, including: (1) teaching clients how their self-talk influences their emotional and behavioral problems: (2) training clients to observe their thoughts and images and discriminate how these cognitive events influence maladaptive behaviors; (3) training in basic problem-solving skills; (4) modeling of desirable types of self-talk and imagery; (5) modeling, rehearsal, and encouragement of positive self-evaluation, coping, and attentional-focusing skills; (6) use of behavioral techniques such as relaxation training, coping imagery training, and behavioral rehearsal; and (7) 'in vivo' homework assignments that expose clients to graduated levels of manageable stress.

In fact, it is this graduated coping rehearsal that spawned the name 'stress inoculation'. The concept of medical inoculation against disease involves giving patients a small dose of the disease and then letting their immune system develop natural antibodies to combat it. Through a process of graduated exposure and natural accommodation, the body eventually develops defenses to successfully combat the strongest concentration of the disease. Similarly, stress inoculation attempts to use imagery rehearsal to expose individuals to challenging but manageable levels of stress. As their coping skills improve, individuals are exposed to larger doses of stress until they have developed their coping skills to effectively deal with the most stressful possible situations.

Stress inoculation training comprises three treatment phases: (a) education, (b) rehearsal, and (c) application. During the educational phase, clients are provided with an in-depth explanation of the treatment rationale, including a review of their thoughts and feelings during stress experiences, emphasis on conceptualizing stress as comprising both physiological arousal and stress-inducing self-statements, and help in learning to break stress encounters into phases in order to make the experience easier to deal with. The rehearsal phase involves teaching clients three important types of coping skills: planning and problem-solving, physical relaxation, and self-talk/cognitive restructuring. Finally, the application phase involves providing the client with opportunities during training to test out and practise coping skills under other types of stressful conditions. Imaginary stress is the most common rehearsal strategy, but other types of stress (e.g. electric shock, cold pressor test, and stress-inducing films) as well as realistic failure and embarrassment situations are also employed. Each rehearsal technique is carefully graduated to only expose clients to levels of stress that they are capable of successfully handling, often using stress hierarchies similar to the type employed in systematic desensitization.

Cognitive–affective stress management training (SMT)

Cognitive–affective stress management training (SMT), developed by Smith and his colleagues (Smith, 1980; Smith and Ascough, 1985; Smith and Rohsenow, 1987), is a multimodal stress management program that has a number of conceptual similarities with SIT. As depicted in Figure 7.2, SMT is based on an appraisal/coping model that is derived largely from Lazarus' (1975) work on stress. The model emphasizes the primary premise of cognitive psychology: that emotion and behavior are determined not by the situation itself but by the individual's interpretation of that situation. SMT postulates that cognitive interpretations are a composite of perceptions of physiological arousal and primary (i.e. perceived personal threat), secondary (i.e. perceptions of one's ability to successfully cope with the threat), and tertiary appraisal (i.e. the consequences of those coping efforts) processes. SMT is developed through a five-phase process that is quite similar to SIT, including: (a) pre-training assessment; (b) training rationale; (c) skill acquisition; (d) skills rehearsal; and (e) post-training evaluation (see Figure 7.2).

Both SIT and SMT emphasize that in order for coping skills to be maximally effective, they must be rehearsed and practised under simulated conditions that are as similar as possible to the real-life situations where they will actually be employed. The major difference between the two techniques is the rehearsal procedures used to practice coping skills. Instead of attempting to maintain relatively low levels of stress that are compatible with coping skills, SMT employs 'induced affect' (Sipprelle, 1967; Smith and Ascough, 1985) to allow rehearsal of coping responses under high emotional arousal. The athlete is asked to imagine a stressful competitive situation and then focus on the feeling that the event elicits. Suggestions are provided that the feelings are growing stronger and more intense, and verbal reinforcement is given for indications of increased arousal in order to shape a strong affective response (Smith and

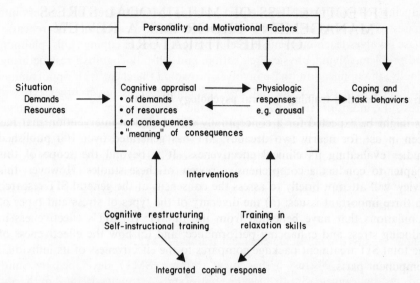

Figure 7.2. Mediational model of stress underlying the cognitive–affective stress management program together with the major intervention techniques used in the development of the integrated coping response (reprinted by permission of Ronald E. Smith from *Social and Behavioral Sciences Documents*).

Ascough, 1985). Once clients become highly aroused, they are instructed to 'turn it off' with their coping responses.

SMT emphasizes the development of functional forms of physical relaxation and self-instructional skills that can be automated for effective use within a several-second timeframe. Initially, coping is accomplished using physical relaxation alone and then through self-instructional skills alone. Finally, both stress management techniques are combined to develop an 'integrated coping response' routine that allows elicitation of both cognitive and somatic relaxation in a one-breath sequence. The integrated coping response combines an adaptive self-statement (e.g. 'I may not like this, but I can definitely stand it!') with the transition phrase 'so' during inhalation and then repetition of the conditioned physical relaxation cue word 'relax' on exhalation.

Because non-specific emotional cues are probably common to a host of different emotional responses across a wide variety of situations, this type of practice should maximize the generalizability of coping skills to a wide variety of stressful situations as well as increase clients' appraisal of their coping resources (Lazarus and Folkman, 1984) and enhance self-efficacy expectations (Bandura, 1986), thus increasing SMT's practical effectiveness.

EFFECTIVENESS OF MULTIMODAL STRESS MANAGEMENT PROGRAMS: A REVIEW OF THE LITERATURE

Stress inoculation training: general psychology literature

As might be expected for a conceptually sound clinical intervention that has been in use for nearly two decades, SIT has generated over 100 published studies evaluating its clinical effectiveness. It is beyond the scope of this chapter to conduct a comprehensive review of these studies. However, this review will attempt briefly to assess the consensus of the general SIT research on three important issues: (a) the diversity of the types of stress and types of populations that have benefited from use of SIT; (b) SIT's effectiveness in reducing stress and enhancing performance; and (c) how the effectiveness of the total SIT treatment package compares to the effectiveness of its individual component parts.

Diversity in application of SIT

A review of the diversity of types of settings and populations to which SIT has been applied needs to focus on whether SIT is used primarily for problem- or emotion-focused coping. Problem-focused SIT treatments are designed to alleviate stress as a strategy to allow individuals to actively do something to remove the source of threat and perform better. The populations and settings that would most benefit from problem-focused coping through SIT include: (a) individuals in very stressful professions, such as registered nurses, school psychologists, teachers, police officers, social workers, probation officers, military recruits, and athletes; (b) individuals suffering performance debilitation due to anxiety problems such as test anxiety, public speaking anxiety, interpersonal or dating anxiety, performance anxiety, and anxiety about confronting significant transitions in life (e.g. re-entering college later in life); and (c) clinical patients who have difficulty coping with daily life due to circumscribed fears and general stress reactions such as animal phobias, fear of flying, neurotic patients in an acute treatment facility, type A individuals, and clients at a community mental health facility.

SIT treatments that are emotion-focused in nature are designed primarily to alleviate stress in order to help the person feel better, even though little can be done to remove the source of threat. The populations and settings that would most benefit from use of SIT for emotion-focused coping include: (a) individuals coping with the stress of upcoming medical procedures such as open-heart surgery, cardiac catheterization, general surgery, and dental procedures; (b) individuals coping with the stress of ongoing health problems such as general pain, cancer, rheumatoid arthritis, chronic tension headaches, burn victims, essential hypertension, dysmenorrhea, and dental pain: and (c) individuals coping with the stress of being victims of rape or terrorist attacks.

Effectiveness in reducing stress and enhancing performance

Careful review of the SIT literature failed to uncover a comprehensive review article assessing the effectiveness of this multimodal technique in reducing stress and enhancing performance. Therefore, to provide a better idea of SIT's effectiveness, a mini-review was conducted of 24 randomly selected SIT outcome studies, 12 each from problem- and emotion-focused coping categories. Of the 12 PFC studies, 10 (i.e. 83 per cent) found SIT to reduce stress and/or anxiety significantly more effectively than did a no-treatment control group, and four of the nine studies (i.e. 44 per cent) that assessed performance improvement demonstrated significantly greater performance increments for the SIT compared to control groups. Thus, although these results suggest that SIT is quite effective in reducing stress, they indicate that SIT is somewhat less efficacious in enhancing subsequent performance.

   None of the 12 EFC studies was concerned with any type of performance measure, but seven of nine studies (i.e. 78 per cent) that included a control group revealed that the SIT group was significantly less stressed than were control subjects. Although this mini-review is a totally unscientific sampling of SIT outcome studies, these results seem to be reasonably representative of the overall literature evaluating this multimodal treatment.

Effectiveness of total SIT package versus component parts

Burchfield, Stein and Hamilton (1985) have conducted an extensive review of 21 test anxiety studies that have compared SIT-related multimodal stress management treatment packages to treatments comprised of their component parts. For both self-reports of test anxiety and behavioral indicators of improved test-taking behaviors, their findings indicated that 24 per cent of the studies found that the cognitive component of the treatment was most effective, 19 per cent reported the somatic component was most effective, 5 per cent indicated that the overall treatment package was superior, and 48 per cent reported no difference in effectiveness between any of the test anxiety treatments. Burchfield and her colleagues noted that because none of these studies measured physiological arousal pre- and post-treatment, it is unclear whether somatic treatments were effective because they modified physiological arousal or because they somehow interfered with cognitive processing. It must be concluded from these data that the exact contribution of the various treatment components to overall SIT effectiveness is uncertain at this time.

Therefore, this review of SIT in the general psychology literature suggests that this multimodal treatment package has been used extensively with a wide variety of populations and a diverse number of settings. Moreover, a non-random mini-review of SIT outcome studies suggests that the technique is effective in reducing stress and anxiety but somewhat less effective in enhancing performance. Finally, the relative contribution of the various components of SIT to treatment effectiveness is unknown at this point.

Cognitive–affective stress management training: general psychology literature

Although SMT is a relatively new stress management program, initial empirical results from three studies testing the efficacy of this treatment have been positive. SMT has been successfully employed with populations of medical students (Holtzworth-Munroe, Munroe and Smith, 1985), problem drinkers (Rohsenow, Smith and Johnson, 1985), and test-anxious college students (Smith and Nye, 1989).

Holtzworth-Munroe, Munroe and Smith (1985) assessed the effects of SMT on stress experienced by first- and second-year medical students. Forty volunteers were assigned to either SMT or control groups, and self-report measures of stress, general anxiety, test anxiety, depression and self-esteem were assessed pre- and post-treatment and at a 10-week follow-up. Group differences at post-treatment were non-significant, but by follow-up, SMT students reported less test anxiety than did control subjects. SMT students also reported greater awareness of tension and greater ability to cope with anxiety than did control subjects. These results clearly suggest that treatment effects may continue to increase over time.

Rohsenow, Smith and Johnson (1985) employed SMT to reduce the dependency on alcohol for stress reduction among college students who were heavy social drinkers. Students reporting excessive drinking were assigned to SMT or control groups, although the SMT group was not told that the focus of the program was to reduce drinking. Results from the six-month investigation revealed that SMT students demonstrated a significant post-treatment reduction in daily anxiety ratings, although these changes were not maintained at 2.5 and 5.5 month follow-ups. The men in the treatment group also showed a significant decrease in self-reported daily drinking rates at post-treatment and the 2.5 month follow-up, although drinking rates returned to near baseline by the 5.5 month follow-up.

SMT students not only developed a significantly more internal locus of control, but they also demonstrated significant improvement on four of 10 irrational beliefs, frustration tolerance, problem avoidance, perfectionism, and personal history. Positive changes in irrational beliefs were strongly correlated with positive mood changes, and reduction in drinking was negatively related with subjects' perceived amount of social support. Finally, subjects who reported drinking to control negative emotions exhibited the largest and most consistent reductions in daily anxiety and anger ratings.

Finally, Smith and Nye (1989) studied test-anxious college students in order to directly compare the effectiveness of covert rehearsal (CR) (i.e. imagined stress) and induced affect (IA) rehearsal techniques. Results revealed that both CR and IA rehearsal groups exhibited significantly greater decreases in trait test anxiety over the course of the treatment than did control subjects, and IA subjects revealed a significantly greater reduction in trait test anxiety than did CR subjects. However, for general trait anxiety, the only significant group difference was between the CR and control groups, with CR subjects demonstrating a greater reduction in trait anxiety than did controls. Locus of control and self-efficacy measures were also employed as dependent measures to test for expectancy generalization. For both measures, each rehearsal group demonstrated significant improvement compared to the control group over the course of the treatment but did not differ from each other.

Finally, significant differences in academic performance were evident between the IA and control groups. Although the academic performance of the CR group did not change over the semester, control subjects actually got poorer grades as the semester progressed, whereas IA subjects improved their grades over the same period. These results not only suggest that SMT is an effective multimodal stress management technique, but they also indicate that IA rehearsal may be superior to the CR techniques typically used in stress inoculation training for rehearsing coping skills.

Stress inoculation trainings: sport literature

Six empirical investigations (Dewitt, 1980; Hamilton and Fremouw, 1985; Mace and Carroll, 1985; Meyers and Schleser, 1980; Meyers, Schleser and Okwumabua, 1982; Ziegler, Klinzing and Williamson, 1982; see also Mace. Chapter 8 in this book) employing stress inoculation-type procedures to enhance sport performance were reviewed for this chapter. Interestingly, four of these six studies used collegiate basketball players as subjects.

Meyers and Schleser (1980) used SIT to help a male collegiate basketball player alleviate 'concentration' problems and improve his performance. In their multiple baseline design, the player significantly improved his performance in four targeted areas: points per game, field goal percentage, field goals made per game, and percentage of total team scoring.

In another study with male collegiate basketball players, DeWitt (1980) randomly assigned six players each to a waiting list control group and a multimodal stress management program that included many SIT components, although he employed EMG biofeedback to develop physical relaxation. The treatment group went through an 11-session program to develop biofeedback and cognitive restructuring skills and then used imagery to rehearse coping skills under varying types of simulated competitive conditions. Details on this investigation are somewhat sketchy, but results indicated that the SIT players received significantly higher performance ratings than did players in the control group.

Hamilton and Fremouw (1985) used a multiple baseline design to evaluate the effectiveness of a SIT program on the cognitions and free throw perform-ance of three male collegiate basketball players. Free throw performance improved significantly for all players, including 88 per cent for player 1, 79 per cent for player 2, and 50 per cent for player 3. Similarly, self-statements for the three players went from 86 per cent negative prior to training to 71 per cent positive following training.

Meyers, Schleser and Okwumabua (1982) used SIT with two female colle-giate basketball players, one a center who experienced concentration and anxiety problems associated with her free throw shooting performance and the other a forward who had similar problems with her field goal shooting performance. Their data demonstrated significant performance increases in the targeted behavior (i.e. free throw shooting for the center/field goal shooting for the forward) but little change on non-targeted behaviors (i.e. field goal shooting for the center/free throw shooting for the forward). Moreover, they employed a return-to-baseline design with the center, and her field goal percentage actually dropped below baseline levels during this period.

Mace and Carroll (1985) employed SIT as a technique to help combat the stress experienced by subjects making their first abseil descent from the roof of a 70-foot building (see also Mace, Chapter 8 in this book). Forty subjects were assigned to one of four groups: SIT (i.e. self-instruction training and simulated practice from a lower height), self-instruction training alone, simulated practice alone, and a control group. Results comparing the four groups on three measures of stress demonstrated that the SIT group had lower scores than the control group on all three stress measures and was less anxious than the simulated practice group on two stress measures.

Finally, Ziegler Klinzing, and Williamson (1982) assessed the impact of SIT on the heart rates and oxygen consumption levels of eight male cross-country runners. Runners received SIT twice weekly for 5.5 weeks, and the results of a 20-minute submaximal run at a constant workload equivalent to 50 per cent of each subject's maximal oxygen consumption revealed that SIT runners demonstrated significantly better cardiorespiratory efficiency than did control subjects.

Cognitive–affective stress management training: sport literature

Early research evaluating the effectiveness of SMT was limited to individual or group case studies with athletes from such diverse sports as football (Smith and Smoll, 1978) and figure skating (Smith, 1980). However, Ziegler, Klinzing and Williamson's (1982) research comparing the efficacy of SIT and SMT on the heart rates and oxygen consumption levels of eight male cross-country runners was the first major empirical test of SMT. Just as with the SIT results reported above, SMT runners demonstrated significantly greater cardiovascular efficiency than did control runners. Interestingly, Ziegler and her colleagues' study was the only one to directly compare the efficacy of SIT and SMT. However, their results demonstrated no differences between the effectiveness of these two multimodal stress management programs.

More recently, Crocker, Alderman and Smith (1988) evaluated the effectiveness of SMT in reducing stress and enhancing the performance of male and female elite junior volleyball players. Members of Alberta's Canada Games men's and women's under-19 volleyball teams were assigned to SMT and waiting list control groups. The treatment group was administered a modified version of SMT in eight modules, presented approximately once a week. Although the two groups did not demonstrate any significant differences on trait or state competitive anxiety, the results indicated that the SMT group emitted significantly fewer negative thoughts in response to videotaped simulations of stressful game situations and had better service reception performance in a controlled practice situation than did the control group. Morever, Crocker (1989) demonstrated that these performance differences were maintained at a subsequent six-month follow-up, although significant gender differences emerged on several other measures. Specifically, women maintained or improved on initial treatment effects in modifying inner dialogue and reducing anxiety compared to men. These gender results parallel findings by Burton (1989), who found that female swimmers utilized goal-setting training more, practiced more on their own, and subsequently benefited more in enhancing competitive cognitions and performance than did their male counterparts.

It can be concluded that although the number of studies testing either of these multimodal stress management strategies in sport is limited, their relative effectiveness appears promising and seemingly warrants additional research.

CRITICISMS OF MULTIMODAL STRESS MANAGEMENT PROGRAMS

Multimodal stress management strategies such as SMT and SIT are probably most effective with athletes who are high in trait anxiety and may not be as effective with athletes with less anxious predispositions. Extensive practical experience in applying first SIT and more recently SMT with athletes has led to some personal frustration. Although I have had some unqualified successes, I have had enough partial successes or outright failures to know that other factors, some theoretical, some personality, and some situational, have a significant influence on overall treatment effectiveness. In this section, I will speculate on why multimodal stress management programs may not be effective in enhancing performance.

Is arousal reduction desirable?

Reversal theory (see Kerr, Chapter 5 in this book), Hardy and Fazey's (1987) catastrophe model of anxiety and performance (see Hardy, Chapter 4 in this book), Martens' (1987) notion of 'psychic energy', empirical research on activation, and my own clinical experience all seemingly question the desirability of arousal reduction for performance enhancement. Instead, they suggest that relatively high levels of arousal are necessary for peak performance, but accompanying cognitions must be positive so that high arousal states can be appraised as facilitative rather than threatening.

Reversal theory

Reversal theory (Apter, 1982) posits that high arousal in a 'telic' or evaluative state will typically be experienced as unpleasant and labeled as 'anxiety', whereas the same high arousal level experienced in a 'paratelic' or non-evaluative state will normally be interpreted positively as 'excitement' (see Kerr, Chapter 5 in this book). Similarly, under evaluative conditions athletes will experience low arousal as 'relaxation', whereas under non-evaluative conditions underarousal is interpreted as 'boredom'. Thus Kerr (1989) suggests that for anxious athletes, rather than decreasing arousal levels to achieve relaxation, most of them simply need to change their interpretation of the situation so that the arousal is experienced as excitement. This change in interpretation should not only allow the athlete to feel better, but it should also maintain the high arousal level that seems necessary in order to perform optimally.

The catastrophe model

Hardy and Fazey's (1987) catastrophe model of anxiety and performance also predicts that at least moderately high levels of physiological arousal are necessary for peak performance to occur (see Hardy, Chapter 4 in this book). According to the model, physiological arousal is only damaging to performance if it is accompanied by high levels of cognitive anxiety reflecting negative appraisal of success in that situation. However, the model also predicts that once such a performance slump has occurred, a considerable change in cognitive appraisal is required before optimal performance can be restored.

Psychic energy

Martens (1987) concurs with both these views regarding the importance of cognitive appraisal. He suggests that positive psychic energy always facilitates performance and athletes cannot have too much of it. Conversely, he proposes that negative psychic energy always hurts performance and any amount of it is too much. Because optimal performance occurs only under high levels of positive and low levels of negative psychic energy, lowering of negative psychic energy levels alone will not guarantee peak performance. Martens argues that in order for coaches to help their athletes perform optimally they must learn techniques that they can teach to their athletes for reducing negative psychic energy while at the same time increasing positive psychic energy.

Empirical research

Theoretical and empirical research on activation by Thayer (1985) and Neiss (1988) has supported the multidimensionality of arousal, suggesting that activation has a qualitative as well as a quantitative dimension. In fact, Neiss (1988) concluded that high levels of arousal alone will not necessarily inhibit performance unless the activation is appraised as debilitative rather than facilitative. Although the research supporting this theoretical point is limited, future researchers need to systematically assess its validity empirically.

Clinical experience

My own experiential knowledge gained through working with hundreds of athletes has recently convinced me that lowering arousal may be undesirable because of the detrimental impact of low arousal levels on performance. In my work with Tom, the case study mentioned at the beginning of the chapter, clinical intervention with a competition version of SIT was largely experienced by Tom as leaving him feeling lethargic and mentally 'flat', suggesting that SIT had lowered arousal too much. However, Tom always seemed to have difficulty reading his body well and being aware of what he was thinking and feeling. In an effort to help alleviate this problem, we decided to use a heart rate monitor to help Tom become more aware of arousal patterns prior to and during jumps.

During this period, the team was in Planica, Yugoslavia for the World Ski Flying Championships. During the week of training, Tom monitored his heart rate on the 90-meter training hill. Interestingly, fairly stable arousal patterns were evident on good jumps, whereas his arousal patterns demonstrated huge variability on poor jumps. Tom continued to wear the heart rate monitor on the first day of the two-day ski flying competition off the 120-meter hill.

Interestingly, Tom's first jump was the best of his life, and the next two were only slightly less successful.

In analyzing the arousal patterns of these three jumps, two interesting facts were evident. First, the arousal patterns during the final minute prior to push-off and through all three jumps were very similar. Secondly, the maximum heart rate during these jump sequences was 35 beats per minute higher than for any jump off the 90-meter hill. Indeed, Tom later reported that he was highly aroused because the risk of falling and injury during ski flying scared him to death. However, his interpretation of these high arousal levels seemed to be quite different from his interpretation of high arousal in other competitions. Instead of labeling his arousal as anxiety, Tom identified his major emotion as fear. This small change in cognitive appraisal of his emotions resulted in a totally different set of coping responses. Fear seemingly prompted him to concentrate totally on what he had to do technically rather than worrying about other competitors or competitive outcome. Although these data were a little difficult to interpret initially, I have since become convinced that fear not only helped Tom develop a cognitive mindset in which he concentrated totally on his performance, but it also helped him to maintain a high arousal level necessary for optimal performance. Unfortunately, on most other occasions, Tom's use of SIT helped achieve positive changes in his cognitive focus only at the expense of reducing his arousal level too much to jump his best.

Last year I began teaching a new course for athletes called Mental Training for Peak Performance. Instead of teaching the athletes in this course specific SIT or SMT stress management techniques, I taught them the component stress management skills but allowed them to personally design their own stress management program around their personal competitive plan (Orlick, 1986). Interestingly, two of the students, one a runner and the other a basketball player, independently developed highly effective stress management programs by combining 'energization' with typical cognitive and somatic relaxation techniques used in SIT or SMT. Both athletes reported that when experiencing stress, physical relaxation was critical in lowering their arousal levels to a point where they could use cognitive restructuring techniques effectively. However, once cognitions were more positive and goals were reestablished, conditioned energization was necessary to raise their arousal level to the point where they could perform optimally. This 'discovery' made immediate sense, and subsequent use of these procedures with other athletes from a variety of sports has been much more successful than use of a multimodal stress management program alone.

This change in procedure for teaching stress management has actually prompted a broadening of program focus. Instead of attempting to 'sell' athletes on the value of stress management, the focus of our psychological skills training (PST) program has shifted to the need to develop a 'flow frame-of-mind' (Csikszentmihalyi, 1977) or an 'optimal performance state' (Orlick, 1986; Unestahl, 1979, 1982). Thus, in order to attain flow, athletes need to develop the ability to quickly and effectively manipulate muscular tension, arousal level, self-talk, competitive images, and goals according to the demands of the situation. That means that athletes must be able to raise as well as lower arousal level, make self-talk more pessimistic as well as optimistic, and lower goals as well as raise them. This change in philosophical approach has actually brought stress management procedures more in line with Martens' (1981) ideal of 'psychological skills training'. Moreover, this new focus has enhanced the receptivity of most athletes to developing stress management skills.

Although stress management skills have long been an important performance enhancement tool in sport (e.g. Suinn, 1976; Nideffer, 1976; Orlick, 1980), they have somewhat of a negative, problem-focused connotation with athletes. The optimal performance state approach emphasizes that most athletes only have to manage stress in certain situations, and stress management is only one tool for helping athletes consistently attain a flow state. When presented within this framework, most athletes have responded much more enthusiastically to the development of stress management skills.

Evaluating arousal reduction: techniques to teach athletes to achieve the flow frame of mind

Although the empirical support for energization is non-existent, researchers who feel that its conceptual logic makes it worth including in a future multimodal stress management outcome study are provided with a brief description of how to develop and implement this strategy. Energization procedures were modified from those that are normally employed to teach athletes physical relaxation. In physical relaxation training (PRT), athletes are taught to physically relax both LH—SA and RH—SA by combining yoga breathing with one of the three PRT strategies described by Martens (1987). Formal PRT practice is done once daily at night for as long as it takes to achieve a level of relaxation of at least '8' on a 1–10 scale. Once this criterion level has been reached, the athletes perform a 'conditioned relaxation' procedure (Bernstein and Borkovec, 1973) designed to develop an association between feelings of relaxation and a 'cue word' such as 'relax'. Each time athletes exhale they say their cue word to themselves while concentrating on feelings of relaxation throughout their bodies. Usually, performing this pairing process for 15–20 breaths per session for several weeks will be sufficient to develop the ability to achieve a conditioned relaxation response in one breath during stressful situations, although continued practice is needed to automate the skill.

Similarly, energization involves combining arousal mobilization techniques with quick, panting, Lamaze-type breathing to mobilize both LH and RH arousal. Formal energization is done once daily in the morning using self-directed (Gauron, 1984) or imagery techniques to energize the person to at least a level of '8' on a 1–10 scale. Once the criterion level has been reached, athletes develop 'conditioned energization' by saying their cue word (i.e. power, push, go-for-it) every third exhalation for approximately 60 breaths. After sufficient pairing, athletes report that energization cue words develop the ability to raise arousal and mobilize energy reserves within 3–5 seconds in practice and competitive situations. Once basic energization skills are developed, athletes are also taught the energization technique of transforming energy. Thus, runners might use the wind, their own anger at themselves, a team-mate or their coach, or even the energy from a runner ahead of them as an energization source.

We have coined the term 'optimal coping response' to describe the strategy we recommend athletes employ to combine energization with the integrated coping response. First, the athlete performs the integrated coping response during a one-breath sequence (e.g. [inhale] 'I may not like this, but I can definitely stand it!'. . . 'so' [exhale]. . . 'relax!'). Then, while changing to a faster breathing pattern, the athlete uses the transition word 'now' and repeats the energizing cue word every third breath (e.g. [breath, breath, breath] . . . 'now' [breath, breath, breath] . . . 'go for it').

FUTURE DIRECTIONS IN MULTIMODAL STRESS MANAGEMENT RESEARCH

Types of research needed

The previous review documents that relatively limited evaluation research has been conducted to assess the efficacy of multimodal stress management programs in sport. Thus, the most critical future need is to increase the amount of evaluation research assessing the effectiveness of multimodal stress management strategies such as SMT and SIT in ecologically valid settings with athletes.

Only a few SIT studies have investigated the effectiveness of the total treatment package compared to its component parts. Although the Davidson and Schwartz (1976) conceptual model strongly argues for inclusion of each of the components of SIT and SMT, empirical verification of the contribution of each of these components to overall program effectiveness is needed. Moreover, research is also needed to assess the impact on treatment effectiveness and performance of (a) varying specific component techniques within the multimodal package (e.g. using progressive muscle relaxation *versus* EMG biofeedback to alleviate LH—SA), and (b) altering the way skills are integrated during performance (e.g. integrated coping response of SMT *versus* a more unstructured integration of component stress management skills).

Future stress management evaluation research needs to take into consideration important personality and situational moderator variables that probably influence multimodal stress management program effectiveness. Although the influence of many of these variables on treatment outcome has not been extensively studied, personality variables that should theoretically moderate stress management effects include: trait anxiety, trait self-confidence, self-talk patterns/styles (i.e. irrational beliefs), coping strategies, and performance/outcome orientation. Similarly, situational variables such as type of sport, skill level of the competitor, level of competition, emphasis on winning, and amount of social support are also likely to moderate treatment effects. Therefore, although these types of evaluation research are difficult and time-consuming to conduct, it seems imperative that such research be performed if our knowledge about stress management is to evolve.

Not only does there appear to be a significant need to increase the quantity of evaluation research on multimodal stress management packages, but the quality of that research must also be improved as well (see also Mace, Chapter 8 in this book). A review of this evaluation literature suggests that two major measurement refinements seem particularly critical if the true impact of multimodal stress management programs on stress and performance are to be reliably and validly measured. First, intraindividual performance measures need to be employed that take differences in skill level into consideration. Secondly, anxiety measures need to be developed that assess frequency, intensity, and valence of symptomatology (Jones, in press; see Parfitt, Jones and Hardy, Chapter 3 in this book).

Refinements in performance measurement

Recently, a number of researchers (e.g. Burton, 1988; Gould *et al.*, 1987; Martens, 1977; Martens *et al.*, 1990; Parfitt, Jones and Hardy, Chapter 3 in this book; Sonstroem and Bernardo, 1982) have called for greater precision in performance measurement in order to more accurately assess relationships between psychological variables (e.g. anxiety) and performance or to evaluate the degree of performance improvement in evaluation research. These researchers have criticized previous investigations that have used either imprecise competitive outcome measures (e.g. win/lose) or performance measures that employed between-subjects (i.e. interindividual) comparisons that failed to control for differences in skill level. They argue that interindividual performance measures make it impossible to determine whether differences in performance scores (e.g. 100-meter dash time) are the result of mediating factors such as anxiety or simply differences in innate skill level.

Burton (1988) recommended using 'intraindividual' performance measures that control for differences in skill level by comparing current performance to average or best previous performance. For example, intraindividual perform-ance measures would compare (a) a golfer's or bowler's score today with his average score for the season (i.e. handicap), (b) a basketball player's free throw accuracy in a particular game with her season's free throw percentage, or (c) a sprinter's 100-meter dash time with his best previous performance (i.e. seasonal or career personal record (PR)).

The ability of intraindividual performance measures to control for differ-ences in skill level provides a greater level of measurement sensitivity that can more accurately tease out (a) the exact influence of psychological variables (e.g. anxiety) on performance or (b) the impact of stress management inter-vention programs on performance. For example, even though the impact of elevated levels of anxiety may not be sufficient to change the outcome of a contest or a competitor's place in a race, it can add several tenths of a second to a 100-meter dash time or several strokes to a golfer's score. Similarly, a stress management treatment may help that golfer chop several strokes from his score or a sprinter to cut several tenths of a second from her 100-meter dash time without necessarily changing the outcome of the contest or place in a race. Without the use of more sensitive intraindividual performance measures, these significant performance improvements may go unnoticed.

Refinements in anxiety measurement

Recently, researchers investigating both anxiety (Lewthwaite, 1988) and activa-tion (Neiss, 1988; Thayer, 1985) have called for needed refinements in how these constructs are measured. The two major concerns with current method-ology are: (a) the need for trait measures to assess both behavioral frequency and intensity and (b) the necessity for both state and trait inventories to assess the degree to which symptoms listed on anxiety inventories are perceived to be helpful or detrimental to performance (Jones, in press; see also Parfitt, Jones and Hardy, Chapter 3 in this book).

Frequency and intensity of anxiety symptoms

Most self-report measures of trait anxiety list a number of 'anxiety-related' symptoms and ask respondents to check how often they experience each. Clearly, this technique emphasizes the quantity rather than the quality of symptoms in determining anxiety level. Such scoring procedures mean that an individual who has a large number of symptoms will be labeled high in trait anxiety, regardless of the intensity of those symptoms, whereas athletes with a few intense symptoms will nevertheless be categorized low in trait anxiety even if the intensity of those symptoms is quite high. Thus, in order to eliminate this potential for incorrect diagnosis, future anxiety instruments need to be constructed to measure both intensity and frequency in order to accurately assess true trait anxiety levels.

Degree to which symptoms are helpful or detrimental

Items on anxiety inventories are assumed to measure anxiety, a negative emotion. However, even though individuals may experience these 'anxiety-related' symptoms, great variability is evident in the degree to which particular individuals may perceive those symptoms to be negative or detrimental to their performance. For example. 'I feel nervous' and 'I am concerned about this competition' are two items from the somatic and cognitive anxiety subscales of the CSAI-2, respectively. Both items represent pre-competitive feelings and cognitions about those feelings that may be perceived as positive and helpful in facilitating mental preparation and performance by some subjects. Thus, if subjects indicate that they are experiencing these symptoms intensely, those responses would be scored as anxiety even though the actual emotion experienced was excitement or appropriate attentional focus. Thus, future anxiety instruments need to employ measurement formats that can allow subjects to categorize whether a particular symptom is negative and detrimental (i.e. anxiety) or a more positive and helpful emotion (i.e. excitement or motivation) that not only is unlikely to impair performance but may actually help it. Currently, Robin Vealey and I are in the process of revising SCAT and the CSAI-2 to better reflect these critical measurement considerations. However, preliminary work suggests that the complexity of such measurement procedures makes this a difficult process.

SUMMARY

This chapter has presented a model of multimodal stress management that identifies four distinct types of anxiety. Although support for this model is somewhat limited, conceptual and empirical evidence does support the development of multimodal stress management techniques that can alleviate both cognitive and somatic anxiety that are left and right hemisphere based. Two contemporary stress management techniques were identified and described that met the requirements of this model, stress inoculation training and cognitive–affective stress management training.

The general psychology and sport literatures assessing the treatment effectiveness of these two multimodal stress management packages were reviewed. Although preliminary evidence on the efficacy of these treatment packages in reducing stress and enhancing performance is promising, concerns remain about whether simply reducing stress will, by itself, ensure performance enhancement. Finally, based on this review of the current status of multimodal stress management programs in sport, future research directions were discussed, including the need for more evaluation research, more research comparing the total treatment package to its component parts, and research that considers the influence of personality and situational moderator variables on treatment impact. Moreover, further refinement in anxiety and performance measurement was also called for in order to ensure that true treatment effectiveness is validly assessed.

ACKNOWLEDGEMENTS

The author would like to thank Barb Jaeger for her help on research for this chapter.

REFERENCES

Apter, M. J. (1982). The experience of motivation, in *The Theory of Psychological Reversals*. London: Academic Press.
Bandura, A. (1986). *Social Foundations of Thought and Action: A Social Cognitive Theory*. Englewood Cliffs, NJ: Prentice-Hall.
Bernstein, D. A. and Borkovec, T. D. (1973). *Progressive Relaxation Training: A Manual for the Helping Professions*. Champaign, Illinois: Research Press.
Blakeslee, T. R. (1980). *The Right Brain*. Garden City, NY: Doubleday.
Bogen, J. E. (1969). The other side of the brain II: an appositional mind, *Bulletin of the Los Angeles Neurological Societies*, **34**, 135–162.
Borkovec, T. D. (1976). Physiological and cognitive processes in the regulation of anxiety, in G. Schwartz and D. Shapiro (eds). *Consciousness and Self-Regulation: Advances in Research*, Vol. 1. New York: Phelem Press.
Burchfield, S. R., Stein, L. J. and Hamilton, K. L. (1985). Test anxiety: a model for studying psychological and physiological interrelationships, in S. R. Burchfield (ed.). *Stress: Psychological and Physiological Interaction*. New York: Hemisphere.
Burton, D. (1985). Psychological skills training manual for the US Ski Jumping Team. Unpublished manuscript, University of Idaho.
Burton, D. (1988). Do anxious swimmers swim slower? Reexamining the elusive anxiety–performance relationship, *Journal of Sport and Exercise Psychology*, **10**, 45–61.
Burton, D. (1989). Winning isn't everything: examining the impact of performance goals on collegiate swimmers' cognitions and performance, *The Sport Psychologist*. **3**, 105–132.
Burton, D. and Williams-Rice, B. T. (1989). Coping with stress: competitive coping strategies and their impact on precompetitive anxiety and basketball performance. Paper presented at the meeting of the Northwest District of the American Alliance for Health, Physical Education, Recreation, and Dance, Boise, ID.

Carter, W. R., Johnson, M. C. and Borkovec, T. D. (1986). Worry: an electrocortical analysis, *Advances in Behavioral Research and Therapy*. **8**, 193–204.

Crocker, P. R. E. (1989). A follow-up of cognitive–affective stress management training, *Journal of Sport and Exercise Psychology*, **11**, 236–242.

Crocker, P. R. E., Alderman, R. B. and Smith, F. M. R. (1988). Cognitive–effective stress management training with high performance youth volleyball players: effects on affect, cognition, and performance. *Journal of Sport and Exercise Psychology*, **10**, 448–460.

Csikszentmihalyi, M. (1977). *Beyond Boredom and Anxiety*. San Francisco: Jossey-Bass.

Davidson, R. J. and Schwartz, G. E. (1976). The psychobiology of relaxation and related states: a multi-process theory, in D. Mostofsky (ed.). *Behavioral Control and Modification of Physiological Activity*. Engelwood Cliffs, NJ: Prentice-Hall.

Deffenbacher, J. L. (1980). Worry and emotionality in test anxiety, in I. G. Sarason (ed.). *Test Anxiety: Theory, Research and Applications*. Hillsdale, NJ: Erlbaum.

DeWitt, D. J. (1980). Cognitive and biofeedback training for stress reduction with university athletes, *Journal of Sport Psychology*, **2**, 288–294.

Folkman, S. and Lazarus, R. S. (1980). An analysis of coping in a middle-aged community sample, *Journal of Health and Social Behavior*, **21**, 219–239.

Folkman, S. and Lazarus, R. S. (1985). If it changes it must be a process: study of emotion and coping during three stages of a college examination, *Journal of Personality and Social Psychology*, **48**, 150–170.

Gauron, E. F. (1984). *Mental Training for Peak Performance*. Lansing, NY: Sport Sciences Associates.

Goleman, D. (1971). Meditation as meta-therapy: hypotheses toward a proposed fifth state of consciousness, *Journal of Transpersonal Psychology*, **3**, 1–25.

Gould, D., Petlichkoff, L., Simons, J. and Vevera, M. (1987). The relationship between Competitive State Anxiety Inventory-2 subscale scores and pistol shooting performance, *Journal of Sport Psychology*, **9**, 33–42.

Hamilton, S. A. and Fremouw, W. J. (1985). Cognitive-behavioral training for college basketball free-throw performance, *Cognitive Therapy and Research*, **9**, 479–483.

Hardy, L. and Fazey, J. (1987). The inverted-U hypothesis: a catastrophe for sport psychology and a statement of a new hypothesis. Paper presented at the meeting of the North American Society for the Psychology of Sport and Physical Activity, Vancouver, BC.

Holtzworth-Munroe, A., Munroe, M. S. and Smith, R. E. (1985). Effects of a stress management training program on first- and second-year medical students, *Journal of Medical Education, 60*, 417–419.

Jones, J. G. (in press). Recent developments and current issues in competitive state anxiety research. *The Psychologist*.

Jones, J. G. and Cale, A. (1989). Relationships between multidimensional competitive state anxiety and cognitive and motor subcomponents of performance, *Journal of Sports Sciences*, **7**, 129–140.

Jones, J. G., Cale, A. and Kerwin, D. G. (1988). Multidimensional competitive state anxiety and psychomotor performance, *Australian Journal of Science and Medicine in Sport*, **20**, 3–7.

Kerr, J. H. (1989). Anxiety, arousal, and sport performance: an application of reversal theory, in D. Hackfort and C. D. Spielberger (eds). *Anxiety in Sports: An International Perspective*. New York: Hemisphere.

Kimura, D. (1973). The asymmetry of the human brain, *Scientific American*. **228**, 70–78.

Lazarus, R. S. (1975). The self-regulation of emotions, in L. Levi (ed.). *Emotions: Their Parameters and Measurement*. New York: Raven.

Lazarus, R. S. and Folkman, S. (1984). *Stress, Appraisal, and Coping*. New York: Springer.

Lazarus, R. S. and Launier, R. (1978). Stress-related transactions between person and environment, in L. A. Pervin and M. Lewis (eds). *Perspectives in Interactional Psychology*. New York: Plenum.

Lewthwaite, R. (1988). Threat perception in competitive trait anxiety: the endangerment of important goals. Manuscript submitted for publication.

Liebert, R. M. and Morris, L. W. (1967). Cognitive and emotional components of test anxiety: a distinction and some initial data, *Psychological Reports*, **20**, 975–978.

Mace, R. D. and Carroll, D. (1985). The control of anxiety in sport: stress inoculation training prior to abseiling, *International Journal of Sport Psychology*, **16**, 165–175.

Martens, R. (1977). *Sport Competition Anxiety Test (SCAT)*. Champaign, Illinois: Human Kinetics.

Martens, R. (1981). Psychological skills for athletes, in J. Seagrave and D. Chu (eds). *Olympism*. Champaign, Illinois: Human Kinetics.

Martens, R. (1987). *Coaches' Guide to Sport Psychology*. Champaign, Illinois: Human Kinetics.

Martens, R., Burton, D., Vealey, R. S., Bump, L. A. and Smith, D. E. (1990). Competitive State Anxiety Inventory-2 (CSAI-2), in R. Martens, R. S. Vealey and D. Burton. *Competitive Anxiety in Sport*. Champaign, Illinois: Human Kinetics.

Meichenbaum, D. (1975). A self-instructional approach to stress management: a proposal for stress inoculation training, in C. D. Spielberger and I. G. Sarason (eds). *Stress and Anxiety*, Vol. 1. Washington, DC: Hemisphere.

Meichenbaum, D. (1977). *Cognitive Behavior Modification*. New York: Plenum.

Meichenbaum. D. (1985). *Stress Inoculation Training*. New York: Pergamon.

Meyers, A. W. and Schleser, R. (1980). A cognitive behavioral intervention for improving basketball performance, *Journal of Sport Psychology*, **2**, 69–73.

Meyers, A. W., Schleser, R. and Okwumabua, T. M. (1982). A cognitive behavioral intervention for improving basketball performance, *Research Quarterly for Exercise and Sport*, **53**, 344–347.

Morris, L. W., Davis, D. and Hutchings, C. (1981). Cognitive and emotional components of anxiety: literature review and revised worry–emotionality scale, *Journal of Educational Psychology*, **73**, 541–555.

Neiss, R. (1988). Reconceptualizing arousal: psychobiological states in motor performance, *Psychological Bulletin*, **103**, 345–366.

Nideffer, R. M. (1976). *The Inner Athlete*. New York: Crowell.

Orlick, T. (1980). *In Pursuit of Excellence*. Champaign, Illinois: Human Kinetics.

Orlick, T. (1986). *Psyching for Sport*. Champaign, Illinois: Human Kinetics.

Parfitt, C. G. (1988). Interactions between models of stress and models of motor control. Unpublished doctoral thesis. University of Wales, Bangor.

Parfitt, C. G. and Hardy, L. (1987). Further evidence for the differential effects of competitive anxiety upon a number of cognitive and motor subsystems, *Journal of Sports Sciences*, **5**, 62–63.

Rohsenow, D. J., Smith, R. E. and Johnson, S. (1985). Stress management training as a prevention program for heavy social drinkers: cognitions, affect, drinking, and individual differences, *Addictive Behaviors*, **10**, 45–54.

Schwartz, G. E., Davidson, R. J. and Goleman, D. J. (1978). Patterning of cognitive and somatic processes in the self-regulation of anxiety: effects of meditation versus exercise, *Psychosomatic Medicine*, **40**, 321–328.

Sipprelle, C. (1967). Induced anxiety, *Psychotherapy: Theory, Research, and Practice*, **4**, 36–40.

Smith, R. E. (1980). A cognitive–affective approach to stress management training for athletes, in C. Nadeau, W. Halliwell, K. Newell and C. C. Roberts (eds). *Psychology of Motor Behavior and Sport—1979*, Champaign, Illinois: Human Kinetics.

Smith, R. E. and Ascough, J. C. (1985). Induced affect in stress management training, in S. R. Burchfield (ed.). *Stress: Psychological and Physiological Interaction*, New York: Hemisphere.

Smith, R. E. and Nye, S. L. (1989). Comparison of induced affect and covert rehearsal in the acquisition of stress management coping skills, *Journal of Counseling Psychology*, **36**, 17–23.

Smith, R. E. and Rohsenow, D. J. (1987). Cognitive–affective stress management training: a treatment and resource manual, *Social and Behavioral Sciences Documents*, **17**, 2.

Smith, R. E. and Smoll, F. L. (1978). Psychological intervention and sports medicine: stress management training and coach effectiveness training, *University of Washington Medicine*, **5**, 20–24.

Smith, R. E., Smoll, F. L. and Schutz, R. W. (in press). Measurement and correlates of sport-specific cognitive and somatic trait anxiety: the sport anxiety scale, *Anxiety Research*.

Sonstroem, R. J. and Bernardo, B. (1982). Intraindividual pregame state anxiety and basketball performance: a re-examination of the inverted-U curve, *Journal of Sport Psychology*, **4**, 235–245.

Suinn, R. M. (1976). Body thinking: psychology for Olympic champs, *Psychology Today*, **10**, 38–43.

Thayer, R. E. (1985). Activation (arousal): the shift from a single to a multidimensional perspective, in J. Strelau, F. H. Farley and A. Gale (eds). *The Biological Bases of Personality and Behavior. Vol. 1: Theories, Measurement Techniques and Development*, Washington, DC: Hemisphere.

Unestahl, L-E. (1979). The Scandinavian practice of sport psychology, in P. Klavora and J. Daniel (eds). *Coach, Athlete, and the Sport Psychologist*, Champaign, Illinois Human Kinetics.

Unestahl, L-E. (1982). Inner mental training for sport, in T. Orlick and J. T. Partington (eds). *Mental Training for Coaches and Athletes*, Ottawa: Coaching Association of Canada.

White, M. (1969). Laterality differences in perception, *Psychological Bulletin*, **72**, 387–405.

Wine, J. D. (1980). Cognitive–attentional theory of test anxiety. In I. G. Sarason (ed.), *Test Anxiety: Theory, Research and Applications*. Hillsdale, N. J.: Erlbaum.

Ziegler, S. G., Klinzing, J. and Williamson, K. (1982). The effects of two stress management training programs on cardiorespiratory efficiency, *Journal of Sport Psychology*, **4**, 280–289.

Chapter 8

Cognitive behavioural interventions in sport

Roger Mace
Newman and Westhill College, University of Birmingham

Research into the multidimensional nature of anxiety and into the validity of the 'inverted-U' hypothesis has raised many questions not only pertaining to how the different expressions of anxiety affect skilled performance but also regarding the actual experience of anxiety itself (see Chapters 2–5 in this book for a review). How, for example, the way in which a person's previous experience, attitude and self-statements mediate the experiential aspect of anxiety has attracted considerable interest. Research by Mahoney and Avener (1977) and Fenz (1975) provided the initial stimulus here. In a study of elite gymnasts, Mahoney and Avener (1977) compared those who made the United States Olympic team with those who were unsuccessful in the qualifying meets. They found that while all the gymnasts were anxious during the competition, there were differences between the two groups at different times. Prior to the competition the successful gymnasts were more anxious than the unsuccessful gymnasts. However, during the crucial moments of actual performance this pattern was reversed. Interviews suggested that the successful gymnasts tended to use their anxiety as a stimulant to better performance. The less successful seemed to arouse themselves into near panic states by self-doubting verbalizations and images of impending tragedies.

The mediating role of cognitions was also recognized by Fenz (1975). Following a series of studies on stress and parachuting, he concluded that the performance of a parachutist is related to the way he has learned to cope with anxiety about his forthcoming jump. Fenz's research indicated that jumpers who were rated as poor performers tended to show increasing levels of anxiety right up to the actual jump, whereas jumpers who were rated as good performers began to reduce their anxiety to a more moderate level prior to the jump.

The research by Mahoney and Avener (1977) and Fenz (1975) suggests that focusing on absolute levels of anxiety may be of less value than an under-

Stress and Performance in Sport. Edited by J. Graham Jones and Lew Hardy.
©1990 John Wiley & Sons Ltd.

standing of patterns of anxiety change and the procedures used by athletes to cope with anxiety. It was research such as this, together with the changing conceptions of anxiety, arousal and stress, that prompted further study of the influence of cognitive factors upon performance during the last decade. At the same time, an important development was taking place in clinical psychology. Following many years of applying behaviour modification techniques, a number of clinical psychologists began to investigate more closely the role of cognitive factors in stress and anxiety research. It can be argued that the subsequent developments acted as both a major stimulus and a guide to the direction and focus of future research in sport psychology.

COGNITIVE BEHAVIOUR MODIFICATION

Many of the psychological techniques used in sport today for skill enhancement and psychological stress management have evolved as a result of the development in mainstream psychology of cognitive behaviour modification. This has variously been referred to as 'cognitive behaviour therapy' or simply 'cognitive therapy'. Before examining the application to sport of the techniques that characterize this approach, it is necessary to look into the underlying principles and concepts.

It can be argued that the development of cognitive behaviour modification within clinical psychology began in the 1970s, which Mahoney (1974) referred to as 'an emerging era of the thinking behaviourist' (p.4). The principles involved are based on a mediational model in which cognitions such as images and self-statements play a vital role in behavioural responses. During the last 25 years a gradual shift in stance towards a more cognitive approach by a number of clinical psychologists formerly adopting behaviour therapy techniques can be detected. A major impetus towards this cognitive direction came from Homme's (1965) work on coverant control. Homme's technique involved the alteration of maladaptive thoughts by reinforcing alternative cognitions. The rationale behind his method was that covert processes follow the same laws of learning that govern overt behaviours. The work of Ellis (1962, 1970) also had a significant impact on the development of cognitive behaviour modification. He developed an approach in clinical psychology called rational emotive therapy. According to Ellis, irrational interpretations of objective reality are the fundamental cause of emotional disorders. He identified 12 irrational beliefs, one or more of which he believed could be discovered at the root of any clinically presenting emotional disorder. Ellis proposed that the task of therapy is to assist the client to recognize self-defeating irrational thoughts and replace them with more constructive rational ones.

A variation of cognitive psychotherapy, that of self-instructional training, was developed by Meichenbaum (1973). This involved training the client to identify and become aware of maladaptive thoughts (self-statements). The therapist modelled appropriate behaviour while verbalizing effective strategies; the client then performed the target behaviour, first by verbalizing aloud the appropriate self-instructions and then by covertly rehearsing them. The overall aim was to replace anxiety-inducing cognitions with constructive problem-solving self-talk.

The approach developed by Beck (1970, 1976) was another important influence. In this approach the ultimate goal is similar to Ellis', that is, the development of rational, adaptive thought patterns. In both Ellis' and Beck's approaches, clients become aware of their thoughts and learn to identify irrational and distorted thoughts, which are replaced by rational, more objective ones. However, Beck does not limit the core irrational beliefs to 12 but emphasizes the idiosyncratic nature of each individual's irrational beliefs. Another difference between their approaches is that Beck invokes the concept of 'automatic thoughts'. These are thoughts that seem to come automatically and involuntarily when the person is thinking negatively. They precede and mediate emotional responses. Beck also suggested that automatic thoughts contain implicit appraisals and that they may be outside awareness. However, he claimed that automatic thoughts can be made accessible to the individual by training him or her to become aware of them.

The work of Lazarus (1966) was also very influential in the development of cognitive behaviour modification. Lazarus proposed an integration of the concepts of threat, appraisal and coping. He differentiated appraisal into two forms, primary appraisal and secondary appraisal. Primary appraisal concerns judgements regarding the degree of relevance of the stimulus event to the individual plus an assessment of the availability of relevant coping skills. Secondary appraisal involves judgements regarding the consequences of implementing the available coping strategies.

A further development occurred as a result of Bandura's (1977) social learning theory. Bandura's ideas went beyond covert conditioning and a major concept is that behaviour modification techniques result in changes in self-efficacy. Expectations of self-efficacy determine coping strategies and are modified by a number of factors, for example performance accomplishments, vicarious information, physiological changes and verbal persuasion. Bandura suggested that the various cognitive behavioural approaches which have been developed all have in common the idea that both behaviour (maladaptive and adaptive) and affective patterns are mediated *via* cognitive processes, for example selective attention and symbolic coding.

It can be argued, therefore, that there were three major factors which led to the development of a cognitive behavioural approach: first, research showing that cognitions are subject to the same laws of learning as overt behaviour; secondly, an acceptance that attitudes, beliefs, expectancies, attributions, etc., are central to producing, predicting and understanding behaviour;

thirdly, a desire among many practitioners to combine cognitive treatment strategies with behaviour contingency management.

Particularly relevant to sport psychology is the recent development in cognitive behaviour therapy of approaches labelled 'coping skills therapies'. Examples include modified systematic desensitization (Goldfried, 1971), anxiety management training (Suinn and Richardson, 1971) and stress inoculation training (Meichenbaum, 1977). In these approaches, clients are taught 'coping skills' such as relaxation techniques combined with imagery and self-statement training. As an integrative approach, coping skills therapy contains elements of many different theories and concepts, such as Homme's covert conditioning, Lazarus' primary and secondary appraisal, Ellis' cognitive restructuring and Bandura's social learning theory.

COGNITIVE BEHAVIOURAL INTERVENTION STRATEGIES IN SPORT

Cognitive behavioural intervention strategies appear to have great potential in the context of sport, particularly with regard to stress management. In addition to relaxation training and mental practice, these techniques emphasize cognitive restructuring. Athletes who are continually exposed to situations which elicit high levels of psychological stress frequently develop maladaptive thoughts and images resulting in poor performance. Negative self-statements regarding their inability to cope and mental images of performing badly often occur. Such self-statements and images are considered by cognitive behavioural therapists to be aspects of covert behaviour which can be modified in much the same way as overt behaviour. Cognitive behavioural techniques used for stress management in sport have relied on the cognitive restructuring techniques developed in clinical psychology which were discussed earlier.

The emergence of cognitive behavioural intervention programmes in sport was preceded by rapid development during the 1970s of the application of a variety of psychological techniques in sport. When Straub (1978) referred to the mind as 'sports sciences' last frontier' (p. 1), a number of sport psychologists responded to the challenge and an increasing number of articles advocating a variety of mental preparation and training techniques appeared in sport psychology and coaching journals. In addition to general articles discussing the application of a variety of techniques (e.g. Feltz and Landers, 1980; Gerson, 1980), others examined the value of specific techniques, for example hypnosis (Frager, 1979; Hatfield and Daniels, 1981; Pulos, 1981), biofeedback (Daniels and Hatfield, 1981) and mental practice (for a review and meta-analysis see Feltz and Landers, 1983; Weinberg, 1982). Many of the programmes developed were specifically related to stress management, and a variety of techniques such as relaxation and visualization skills were advocated.

Many of these techniques arose from the development of cognitive behaviour modification although any particular programme may not have been labelled as such. In an attempt to bring some order to such developments, Wilson and Bird (1982) presented a model which illustrated the use of many self-regulation techniques in sport, and explained the underlying principles so that coaches and athletes could select the techniques which were most appropriate to their needs and interests. Wilson and Bird suggested that techniques could be categorized under four headings: performance enhancement; inner self (how one perceives and values oneself, including self-esteem and self-confidence); stress management; rehabilitation and recovery. Within each category a number of psychological techniques and programmes were recommended, such as mental rehearsal for performance enhancement and thought stopping for stress management. Furthermore, as Wilson and Bird pointed out, it is possible for one technique to be used for more than one purpose.

The emergence of cognitive behaviour modification as a new approach in mainstream psychology also gave direction to developments in the application of psychological techniques in sport. By the early 1980s a cognitive behavioural approach to training psychological skills was clearly identifiable and intervention programmes were developed based on the underlying principle that cognitions mediate anxiety. Since many techniques may be described as cognitive behavioural, it is clearly necessary in a review such as this to be somewhat selective regarding which studies to examine in order to evaluate the 'state of the art'. For example, in this review a distinction is drawn between mental rehearsal which focuses on the development of coping skills as part of an intervention programme and mental rehearsal used on its own with the aim of enhancing performance. Only studies which include mental rehearsal as a 'coping skill' will be included. The aim is to review research employing complete programmes and packages with athletes. Since what constitutes performance enhancement and what constitutes preventing performance disruption is not always clear, no attempt will be made to distinguish between behavioural intervention programmes which aim to enhance performance and those which aim to prevent performance disruption in situations which would normally evoke high levels of anxiety. It can be argued, for example, that an athlete who habitually performs below par in a competition, but following an intervention programme produces a higher level of performance similar to that achieved in practice, has successfully used the techniques to prevent performance disruption. Conversely, it can be argued that if his competition performance is at a consistently higher level than previously, then enhancement has occurred.

COGNITIVE BEHAVIOURAL RESEARCH IN SPORT

A cognitive behavioural approach to stress management has the advantage that many of the coping skills training programmes allow counsellors to emphasize one or more of the various components, for example a specific relaxation technique or cognitive restructuring. This flexibility is an important factor because recent research has revealed that anxiety is extremely complex. In a discussion on the multidimensional nature of anxiety, Hodgson and Rachman (1974) proposed that emotional behaviours are multi-response phenomena comprising verbal–cognitive, motor and physiological systems. Similarly, Lehrer and Woolfolk (1982) suggested that cognitive, somatic and behavioural expressions of anxiety reflect the operation of discrete systems. They pointed out that these systems do not correlate highly. Furthermore, they suggested that in behaviour therapy the various types of anxiety may respond best to different kinds of treatment.

Clearly, this has implications for the use of intervention strategies in sport. Counsellors teaching stress management techniques must carefully consider the possibility of different effects on the different systems. It is possible that the effect of an intervention programme may be specific to the expression of anxiety emphasized in the training sessions (see Burton, Chapter 7 in this book). Biofeedback, for example, may result in lower heart rates but have little effect on cognitive anxiety. Conversely, an intervention programme which only emphasizes cognitions may affect cognitive anxiety but have little impact on physiological arousal. It has been suggested (Lehrer and Woolfolk, 1982) that cognitions have a mediating effect on the other systems. If this is the case, then a cognitive-orientated technique is clearly indicated.

The research discussed below focuses initially on three cognitive behavioural intervention packages, visuo-motor behaviour rehearsal (VMBR), cognitive–affective stress management training (SMT) and stress inoculation training (SIT). All three packages involve a variety of coping skills which counsellors may emphasize according to the needs of the individual and the situation. In addition, studies are discussed that have incorporated training in coping skills which have a cognitive behavioural orientation. It is interesting to note that many of the studies considered show a specificity in training effects.

Visuo-motor behaviour rehearsal

In his work with Olympic skiers, Suinn (1972a, b) developed a programme called visuo-motor behaviour rehearsal (VMBR). Basically, VMBR involves an initial relaxation phase, visualizing performance (imagery) during a specific stressful situation (e.g. competition), and performing the skill during a simulated stressful situation. It appeared that the programme was successful but, as Suinn pointed out, the results were inconclusive due to lack of experimental control. However, his work provided a stimulus for controlled studies aimed at providing experimental support.

Following the early work of Suinn (1972a, b), Lane (1980) reported the findings of a series of VMBR studies with athletes under relatively controlled conditions. In a study with tennis players he found that performance scores for the VMBR group showed a tendency to become better than a relaxation only group. Differences, however, were not statistically significant. Lane also used VMBR to improve the shooting ability of basketball players. He found that experimental subjects improved significantly compared to control subjects. However, the results must be treated with caution as only six subjects, three in each group, participated. In addition, there was a lack of control for attention-placebo effects.

In an unpublished controlled study aimed at enhancing the shooting ability of basketball players, Kolonay (1977) (as reported by Weinberg, Seabourne and Jackson, 1981) compared VMBR with mental imagery alone and relaxation alone. The VMBR group listened to a 10-minute relaxation and free throw audiotape on 15 occasions prior to practice sessions. Other groups listened to either the relaxation tape alone or the imagery tape alone, or engaged in irrelevant activity. Kolonay's results indicated that only the VMBR group showed a significant improvement in shooting accuracy when individual pre- and post-test scores were compared, and concluded that the VMBR training led to an increase in free throw percentage accuracy. However, the statistical analysis did not establish whether the groups differed significantly from each other.

In an attempt to replicate these findings in a different sporting context, Weinberg, Seabourne and Jackson (1981) used VMBR in karate training. They strengthened the design by employing an attention-placebo group. During the initial session, subjects in the VMBR, relaxation, imagery and attention-placebo control groups were given instruction and an audiotape on their particular training strategy. They were then asked to use the audiotape at home each day. Following a six-week period during which each group of subjects met together twice a week for practical training, a variety of performance tests were administered. These were broken down into three categories: skill tests, combinations of skills, and sparring (actual competition). In addition to performance measures, state anxiety was measured using Martens' (1977) Competitive State Anxiety Inventory. The results indicated that VMBR and relaxation groups exhibited lower levels of state anxiety immediately prior to competition than the imagery and attention-control groups. The results regarding performance indicated that there was a significant effect only in the sparring condition, with the VMBR group achieving better performance than all other groups. Weinberg et al. concluded that the results of the investigation provided partial support for the effectiveness of VMBR in enhancing karate performance. While the results should be treated with caution because of the small sample size (eight in each group), it is encouraging that positive results were obtained in possibly the most important situation, that is, competition.

In a follow-up study in karate, Seabourne, Weinberg and Jackson (1984) discussed the equivocal nature of the results of studies employing VMBR and suggested that inconsistent findings might have been due to the nature of administration of the VMBR. They pointed out that many studies have not individualized the technique to the particular needs of individual subjects, and argued that a key factor in the success of any cognitive intervention strategy is the close interaction of counsellor and subject. In their study subjects were assigned to either an individual VMBR group or an attention-placebo control condition. Similar measures to Weinberg, Seabourne and Jackson's (1981) earlier study were taken (state anxiety and three measures of performance). The results indicated that following a 16-week training programme, the VMBR group exhibited significantly greater decreases in state anxiety than the placebo group. Performance results indicated that the VMBR group displayed greater levels of improvement over time than the placebo group on all three measures of karate performance: that is, skill, combinations and sparring. The results of their study support the effectiveness of VMBR. Unlike a number of other studies, Seabourne et al. used a reasonably large sample (26 in the control group and 18 in the VMBR group), and their statistical analysis revealed clear and significant differences between groups. Two important features in their study are, firstly, the length of time of training (16 weeks) and, secondly, the individualized approach. It is possible that for VMBR to be effective there must be a reasonable number of training sessions, which ideally will be modified according to individual needs and progress.

Cognitive–affective stress management training programme

One of the most comprehensive programmes for stress management training in sport was developed by Smith (1980). His cognitive–affective stress manage-ment training programme (SMT) was based on a mediational model of stress which recognized the crucial role of cognitive mediators of emotionality. Smith argued that intervention strategies such as cognitive restructuring, self-instruc-tion training and training in relaxation skills could be employed to modify the cognitive behaviour of athletes so as to develop an 'integrated coping response'. As Smith pointed out, stress responses are not triggered by the situation but by what athletes tell themselves about the situation and their ability to cope with it.

The SMT programme represents an attempt to combine a number of clinical treatment techniques into a comprehensive programme for the self-control of emotion. It begins with a conceptualization phase during which athletes are taught to understand the nature of their stress response. This is followed by a phase of training in relaxation, evaluating self-statements and replacing negative self-statements regarding, for example, failure and disapproval with positive self-statements. These coping skills are then practised and rehearsed under conditions which approximate the 'real-life' situations in which they will eventually be employed. In SMT, a major feature which distinguishes it from other intervention programmes is the use of a psychotherapeutic procedure known as 'induced affect'. This is employed to generate high levels of emotional arousal which are reduced by the subject using the coping responses acquired in the preceding training sessions. The comprehensive nature of SMT means that it appears particularly valuable for stress management training in sport. It is surprising, therefore, that there are few reported studies using this programme. One possible explanation is that SMT should not be employed by those not having formal training in clinical procedures. As Smith (1980) pointed out, the induced affect procedure is a clinical technique capable of eliciting strong affective responses, sometimes of an unpredictable nature and intensity. Accordingly, the use of SMT with athletes demands a high level of skill and experience on the part of the trainer.

One study that did employ SMT in a sports context was conducted by Ziegler, Klinzing and Williamson (1982) with cross-country runners. They examined the effect of two stress management programmes, SMT and stress inoculation training, on cardiorespiratory efficiency. The results indicated that subjects who received either of the stress management programmes used significantly less oxygen during a treadmill run than a no-treatment control group. While this study suggested that either intervention programme might be potentially very valuable, further research is clearly necessary, particularly when one considers that the total sample size was only eight and there was no attention-placebo control group. The control group only met the experimenter for the pre- and post-tests, whereas the treatment groups had two sessions a week over a period of five and a half weeks. It is interesting to note that in a similar study Kenney, Rejeski and Messier (1987) obtained different results. They examined the effects of a multimodal cognitive behavioural distress management programme on novice runners' psychological responses and running efficiency. Their findings indicated that the programme resulted in more positive affect and lower ratings of perceived exertion but had no effect on physiological or biomechanical efficiency.

Stress inoculation training

In a perceptive article, Long (1980) presented a cognitive behavioural model for stress management. She discussed cognitive factors in stress such as appraisals, expectations, attitudes and memories, and suggested that the recently developed coping skills therapies could be applied successfully to sport. Long drew attention, in particular, to stress inoculation training (SIT), an intervention programme which had been developed by Meichenbaum (1977).

SIT (Meichenbaum, 1977, 1985) has been successfully used with people in a variety of situations, including medical patients (e.g. Kendall, 1983), police officers (e.g. Novaco, 1980), teachers (e.g. Forman, 1982) and adults needing help to cope with stress (Long, 1983, 1984, 1985). A major feature of this intervention strategy is the development of positive self-statements, which have been claimed to be powerful mediators of anxiety (see Girodo and Wood, 1979). The conceptual model underlying stress inoculation training is a transactional one. As Meichenbaum (1985) stated, stress is viewed as neither a stimulus nor a response, but rather as the result of a transaction, influenced by both the individual and the environment. From a transactional perspective, stress is defined as a cognitively mediated relational concept. It reflects the relationship between the person and the environment that is appraised by the person as taxing his or her resources and endangering his or her well-being. This view can be related to Lazarus' (1966) concept regarding the integration of threat, appraisal and coping. Lazarus argued that how individuals appraise stressful events (primary appraisal) and how they appraise the expected outcome of implementing their coping skills (secondary appraisal) determines the nature of stress. The SIT programme involves exposing the individual to small, manageable units of stress and incorporates the use of modelling and reinforcing self-statements. Stress inoculation is, therefore, a multidimensional approach to stress management which is based on the principle of immunization. It comprises three phases: the education phase; the rehearsal phase; and the application phase. Meichenbaum (1985) has recently renamed these the conceptualization phase; the skills acquisition and rehearsal phase; and the application and follow-through phase. When applied to athletes, the approach used within each of these phases will obviously differ from the approach used with clinical patients. However, the underlying principles and stages are still applied.

In the education phase the counsellor discusses with subjects the effect of high levels of anxiety on psychological and physiological responses and their subsequent effect on performance in sport. Subjects should be encouraged to discuss their own experiences and a collaborative working relationship should be developed. In establishing a rationale for learning psychological skills to control anxiety, subjects should be encouraged to view the stress reaction as a series of stages rather than one automatic fear response. The stages suggested by Meichenbaum (1977) are:

1. Preparing to face the stressor;
2. Impact and confrontation;
3. Coping with fear;
4. When the fear has been overcome.

When used with subjects who have developed specific problems, such as a maladaptive approach to training or a set of negative images and self-statements which affect performance detrimentally, it may be necessary to employ a variety of means to collect all the relevant information regarding the nature of the subject's stress.

The major objective of the skills acquisition phase is to help subjects develop a variety of coping skills. The training procedures normally include relaxation training followed by imagery and self-instructional training. It may also be necessary to use cognitive restructuring procedures with athletes who have developed specific problems. Whenever possible, the intervention programme should be tailored to suit the needs of the individual. During the skills acquisition stage there is a need to convey to the subjects that the amount of gain is tied to how much one practises.

The final phase of the programme is where subjects practise using the coping skills taught. They are exposed to small manageable units of stress which are gradually increased. The rationale for this procedure is that successfully using the coping skills to overcome small units of stress may have a beneficial effect regarding coping in similar but more stressful situations. This phase can include imagery and behaviour rehearsal, role playing, modelling and graduated *in vivo* practice.

At the time of writing the present review, SIT has received at least preliminary examination in the context of sport. For example, in the study with cross-country runners discussed earlier, Ziegler, Klinzing and Williamson (1982) examined the effect of stress inoculation training on cardiorespiratory efficiency. In an attempt to make a more concerted assessment of the value of SIT in sport, Mace and his colleagues have recently reported a series of investigations using this technique. Their initial study (Mace and Carroll, 1985) examined the effect of SIT on the level of anxiety experienced by subjects just prior to abseiling from the roof of a 70-ft (21.2 m) building. In order to assess the various components of SIT as well as the full intervention programme, 40 volunteer subjects were semi-randomly assigned (to allow for equal numbers of males and females in the various groups) to one of four conditions: SIT (which incorporated self-instructions training and practical training in abseiling from a low height), self-instructions training alone, practical training alone, and no training (control group). On completing the training, subjects made two consecutive test abseils from 70 ft (21.2 m). Three indices of each subject's anxiety level were recorded just before they commenced to abseil: an intensity score derived from the word or phrase chosen by subjects from the Perceived Stress Index (Jacobs and Munz, 1968) which best described their feelings; the intensity score appropriate to the word or phrase chosen by a trained observer from the Perceived Stress Index (PSI) as best suiting the subject's demeanour; and a state anxiety score from the state

version of Spielberger, Gorsuch and Lushene's (1970) State Trait Anxiety
Inventory (STAI). Overall analyses indicated that groups varied significantly
in terms of both self-reported stress and observer-estimated stress. The stress
inoculation group had significantly lower self-reported stress intensity scores
than both the control group and the practical training group. In addition,
they had lower scores than the control group and the practical training group
on observer-estimated stress.

For state anxiety, there was a significant variation among groups, but *post
hoc* tests failed to establish clearly where the difference lay. Inspection of the
group means indicated that the stress inoculation group and the control group
showed the greatest divergence: the former showed the lowest anxiety scores,
the latter the highest. Mace and Carroll concluded that the programme was
effective in attenuating anxiety but, in view of the lack of control for attention-
placebo effects, unequivocal pronouncements of efficacy were unwarranted at
that stage.

Their second study (Mace, Carroll and Eastman, 1986a) examined the effect
of SIT on the level of self-reported stress and anxiety, overt signs of distress
and the psychophysiological impact of abseiling. Twenty volunteer subjects
were randomly assigned to either a no-training control group or a SIT group,
following which both groups of subjects had to complete a test abseil from
the roof of a 70-ft (21.2 m) building. Prior to descent, two self-report measures
and an observer's estimate of stress were recorded (similar to Mace and
Carroll, 1985). In addition, heart rate was monitored just prior to and
throughout the abseil using a telemetry system. The results indicated that the
stress inoculation group showed significantly less self-reported stress on the
PSI than the control group. They also showed significantly less state anxiety.
A similar picture emerged for the observer-rated stress on the PSI. However,
a comparison between the groups on heart rates immediately before, during
and after the test abseil revealed that the impact of the abseil stress was not
attenuated for the stress inoculation subjects. All subjects displayed very large
increases in heart rate just prior to abseiling. The mean scores for the two
groups were 146 (control group) and 141 (stress inoculation group) beats per
minute and two subjects recorded heart rates in excess of 180 beats per minute.
Correlations were computed between heart rates and the various other
measures. The coefficients were extremely low. These results essentially replicated those reported in the earlier study and add further weight to the
contention that SIT may be a powerful means for attenuating self-reported
anxiety. Furthermore, these more recent data give credence to the views of
Hodgson and Rachman (1974) and Lehrer and Woolfolk (1982) discussed
earlier: that is to say, that there are cognitive, somatic and behavioural
expressions of anxiety which may not be synchronous and which may be
differentially affected by different modification strategies.

Since neither of the abseiling studies provided data on the effect of SIT on performance, a further controlled study was carried out in a gymnastics setting which, it was anticipated, would normally evoke high levels of anxiety (Mace and Carroll, 1986a). Eighteen subjects were assigned to either an attention-placebo control group or a SIT group. Following preliminary training, subjects were asked to perform a gymnastics sequence under low and high stress conditions. In addition to self-report, an observer's rating of distress, and a psychophysiological measure of distress, performance of the routine was also judged from a videotape by an internationally qualified judge. The results indicated that the intervention strategy was effective in attenuating self-report and the observer's rating of distress. However, as with the abseiling studies, there was no noticeable effect on heart rate. An important finding was a significant difference between the groups for performance. The results indicated that the intervention programme prevented performance disruption. Unlike subjects in the control group, subjects in the stress inoculation group did not display a significant performance decrement when performance in the high stress condition was compared to performance in the low stress condition. While the small subject numbers and the lack of a reliability check on performance scores advise caution, two aspects of this study are worth emphasizing: first, the attempt at an attention-placebo control, and secondly, the finding of performance effects.

In a small group study, Mace and Carroll (1986b) examined the effect of SIT on squash players. Three players volunteered for the study, having reported that too much anxiety was impairing their game. Three other matched subjects provided a control group. In order to obtain baseline measures of anxiety, all subjects were asked to complete the state version of the STAI immediately before each of five important league and team matches. The experimental subjects were given eight training sessions. Following the initial 'education phase', they received training in relaxation, mental rehearsal and self-instruction. On finishing training, all subjects were asked to complete a further five state anxiety scales prior to matches. While full data were only available for two subjects in each group, experimental subjects showed a significant decrease in anxiety levels. Control subjects, on the other hand, showed little difference between the two sets of anxiety measures.

Following the four studies discussed above which investigated the effectiveness of SIT for controlling anxiety in stressful situations, two further studies were conducted with gymnasts who had developed a maladaptive mental approach to training and competing. In each case the problem was more complex than just increased levels of anxiety and reflected an idiosyncratic set of responses to the difficulties they faced.

The first case study (Mace, Eastman and Carroll, 1986) concerned a young female gymnast of regional squad potential who had ceased to make progress when she resumed training after a series of injuries and underwent SIT to help her regain her form. During preliminary interviews, which were audiotaped, it became clear that when she was about to attempt difficult moves she generated a set of negative self-statements. The subject also experienced images which were not conducive to developing a positive mental approach. She had a recurring mental image of a person over-rotating and landing on her head, and although she tried hard to visualize this person performing the move skilfully, the imagined person kept over-rotating. In order to replace the negative self-statements and images with positive ones, an intervention programme of relaxation, visualization and self-statement training was devised. This comprised eight treatment sessions which covered the education, rehearsal and application phases. After the intervention programme, the subject's comments, which were recorded during a two-hour training session, indicated that SIT had been successful in developing a set of positive self-statements and images. Her performance improved considerably and a few months after the intervention she performed very well to win a silver medal in an interclub competition. A month later she won the club championships to become senior ladies champion.

The second case study concerned a male gymnast who had represented his country in Olympic gymnastics (Mace, Eastman and Carroll, 1987) but had developed a maladaptive mental approach to performing in competition on the pommelled horse. Preliminary interviews revealed that immediately before competing he became very tense, his arms started to shake and he had doubts about being able to complete his routine. In addition, he was unable to use visualization, a technique which he employed for mental preparation before performing on the other five pieces of apparatus in Olympic gymnastics competitions. Further interviews also strongly suggested that the subject had developed a set of negative self-statements of which he was unaware. An intervention programme comprising 10 sessions of training in relaxation, visualization and making positive self-statements was implemented. Recorded interviews and comments made by the subject on completion of the training indicated that the programme had been successful. For many years the subject had experienced problems performing on the pommelled horse and he had frequently suffered falls in competition. Towards the end of the programme his performance began to improve. He also became more confident and he used his stress-coping skills in competition. In the National Championships he was able to relax, visualize his routine and make positive self-statements. Shortly after this competition he successfully completed his routine to a high standard without any falls to win the individual title in the Midlands Regional Championship.

Both of these case studies lend further support to the efficacy of the stress inoculation technique for mental training in sport. However, the shortage of systematic performance data and the lack of extensive follow-up measures remain weaknesses.

In a review of their studies, Mace, Carroll and Eastman (1986b) argued that their research clearly indicated the potential value of SIT both for generally controlling anxiety in sport and for helping individuals who have developed a maladaptive psychological approach to training and competing. A number of important issues have arisen as a result of these studies, but one of particular 'significance is the differing effects of SIT on self-report, behavioural and psychophysiological measures of stress. In the second study on abseiling reported by Mace, Carroll and Eastman (1986a), the training resulted in considerably less self-reported and observer-rated stress. However, the training had little effect on heart rate increase elicited by the abseil stress. This has important implications for the use of stress management intervention programmes in sport. As Lehrer and Woolfolk (1982) pointed out, the various systems of arousal and anxiety expression may respond best to different kinds of treatment; for example, cognitive anxiety may be best treated by cognitive techniques, somatic anxiety by somatic techniques and behavioural anxiety by behavioural techniques. It would appear, therefore, that before using a stress management programme, careful consideration should be given to the different response systems and how elevated levels may influence performance in a particular sport (see Jones and Hardy 1989 and Parfitt, Jones and Hardy; Chapter 3 in this book). Consideration should also be given to which response system is the most important from a self-regulation point of view. Finally, the emphasis on the particular response system within a stress management programme and an individual's idiosyncratic mode of responding needs to be analysed prior to intervention.

Additional studies involving a cognitive behavioural approach

A number of other studies have been conducted into the effect of intervention strategies in sport which are cognitive behavioural in orientation but have not used an established treatment package. In a study with novice scuba divers, Griffiths et al. (1981) randomly assigned subjects to a biofeedback relaxation group, a meditation group or a control group. They found that both forms of relaxation training resulted in significantly lower levels of anxiety, which was measured using the state version of Spielberger, Gorsuch and Lushene's (1970) STAI, immediately before an underwater task. However, there were no significant differences between the groups on heart rate, respiration rate or performance.

In a follow-up study (Griffiths et al., 1985), experimental subjects were given training in relaxation and cognitive rehearsal of an underwater task. They were then given two performance tests. The first, bail-out, required the subjects to don and remove scuba equipment underwater. The second was a deep-water quarry dive. Prior to the tests, bail-out only was cognitively rehearsed.

The results revealed significantly lower levels of state anxiety in the experimental group than in the control group, who were given training in scuba diving but no relaxation or cognitive rehearsal training, immediately before both tests. However, a significant difference between the same two groups for performance was found only for the bail-out task, which had been cognitively rehearsed. The results also showed no difference between the groups on respiration rate. Although these results are interesting, the design of the study raises questions regarding the efficacy of the cognitive and somatic training. First, the control group was trained in a different semester to the experimental group. Secondly, only three training sessions (listening to an audiocassette tape programme designed to reduce diver state anxiety and improve underwater performance) were given to the experimental group.

In an interesting study, Murphy and Woolfolk (1987) investigated the effects of two differing cognitive behavioural intervention programmes on competitive anxiety and performance on a fine motor skill accuracy task. Subjects were randomly assigned to three experimental conditions: (a) a cognitive behavioural relaxation group, (b) a 'psyching up' arousal group and (c) a control group. The cognitive behavioural relaxation group showed significantly greater reductions in anxiety during performance than the other two groups. However, the experiment failed to show that the intervention which resulted in lower anxiety automatically resulted in performance gains on the fine motor task. The design involved a test–retest and both the relaxation group and the control group improved. However, the 'psyching up' group showed no significant improvement. It is possible that this treatment resulted in an overaroused state for performance which prevented the normal test–retest gains. Clearly, this has implications for the type of intervention to be used in a particular sport. It is possible that the wrong strategy could actually do more harm than good (see Chapters 4 and 5 in this book).

A study reported by Hamilton and Fremouw (1985) provided some further support for the use of cognitive behavioural interventions in sport. A single-subject multiple-baseline design was used with three intercollegiate basketball players who consistently displayed a low ratio of game-to-practice free throw percentages, suggesting that competition stress resulted in a considerable performance decrement. Each subject was given an intervention training programme of approximately 10 hours, comprising: deep muscle relaxation; identification of negative self-statements; development of positive self-statements; and *in vivo* rehearsal during team practice. The results obtained indicated significant cognitive changes as measured by having subjects reconstruct their thoughts while watching videotape. Positive statements increased from 14 per cent before training to 71 per cent after training. Negative and 'other' self-statements decreased from 86 per cent before training to 29 per cent after training. All subjects also showed a considerable improvement in shooting performance, the overall mean improvement being 72.5 per cent.

Although Hamilton and Fremouw's study failed to control for placebo effects and involved only a few subjects, the size of the effects was sufficiently impressive to merit attention.

In an article on performance enhancement through cognitive intervention, Silva (1982) reported on three single case studies employing an A–B design. In each case the techniques used were problem indentification, cognitive restructuring and self-instructional imagery. The first study was with a male ice hockey player who consistently lost emotional control and fouled his opponents, resulting in his accumulating an average of 4.72 minutes penalty time each game. Following the intervention programme, the subject's average penalty time was 2.30 minutes per game, a reduction of 57 per cent. The total programme time was three hours per week for six weeks. The second study was with a basketball player who felt that he was overaroused and tried too hard to play well, resulting in playing errors which led to numerous personal fouls. Before the intervention programme he committed an average of 4.3 fouls per game and had been disqualified from nine out of 13 games used for baseline measures. Following the intervention programme, the subject reduced fouling by approximately one foul per game and in the 10 games analysed he was disqualified only once. The intervention programme lasted eight weeks and the average contact time per week was three hours. In a third study, Silva employed a cognitive behavioural programme to help a basketball player who was unable to shoot at the same level in competition as he did in practice. Prior to intervention the player had a competition free throw percentage of 53.86. This percentage increased to 74.9 following the intervention programme, a dramatic increase of 21.05 per cent. The programme which this subject followed lasted 10 weeks with an average contact time of four hours per week.

While the results of these case studies are encouraging, the lack of control again counsels caution. As with the case studies reported earlier by Mace and Carroll (1986b) and Mace, Eastman and Carroll (1986, 1987), it is not possible to attribute the effects unequivocally to the intervention programme. A variety of factors could have contributed to the benefits observed: the athlete receiving special attention, spending more time mentally rehearsing skills, and a general raising of expectancy levels regarding success.

SUMMARY AND FUTURE DIRECTIONS FOR RESEARCH

The results of a number of the controlled studies, and in particular the case studies reviewed in this chapter, suggest that cognitive behavioural intervention programmes are potentially valuable for attenuating anxiety immediately before attempting tasks which elicit high levels of psychological stress. Furthermore, it appears that such training can be effective in preventing performance decrement as a result of an athlete experiencing a high level of anxiety. It can be argued, therefore, that the original theoretical position of intervention strategies based on a mediational model has been upheld. The results of the studies examined in the present review provide support for the view that cognitions mediate anxiety and that these cognitions are themselves open to modification with the result that the associated anxiety is ameliorated. However, this view must be accepted with caution as many of the studies examined have methodological weaknesses in design, control and appropriate assessment of the effects of the intervention programme. These weaknesses will be discussed later in proposing future directions for research in the field.

Although the studies reviewed highlight the complexity of expressions of anxiety, the anxiety–performance relationship and idiosyncratic responses (see Chapters 2–5 in this book), it is possible that the overall effect of cognitive behavioural interventions is derived from promoting a change in self-efficacy (Bandura, 1977). Bandura defined self-efficacy as the strength of one's conviction that one can successfully execute a behaviour required to produce a certain outcome. Bandura also argued that having a serviceable coping skill at one's disposal undoubtedly contributes to one's sense of personal efficacy. He suggested that psychological procedures, whatever their form, alter the level and strength of self-efficacy, which, in turn, influences performance. Bandura argued that expectations of personal mastery affect both initiation and persistence of coping behaviour; they determine how much effort people will expend and how long they will persist in the face of obstacles and aversive experiences. Bandura's analysis of how self-efficacy influences performance does not discount the importance of skill level and motivation. Expectations alone will not produce the desired performance if the physical requirements are lacking. It should also be noted that Bandura stated that self-efficacy cognitions are situation-specific rather than a reflection of a global personality trait.

Research in sport has tended to support Bandura's concept of self-efficacy. Particularly relevant to the present series of studies is an early field study conducted by Mahoney and Avener (1977). They investigated the relationship between feelings of confidence and performance in gymnastics. The results revealed that gymnasts who reported experiencing doubts about performing well tended to perform poorly during competition. However, these results should be treated with caution as a causal relationship could not be inferred. Further research in recent years has provided additional empirical support for Bandura's theory with regard to motor performance (Feltz and Albrecht, 1986; Feltz, Landers and Raeder, 1979; Weinberg, Gould and Jackson, 1979; Weinberg, Seabourne and Jackson, 1981). In an interesting study examining self-efficacy, anxiety reduction and performance in gymnastics, McAuley (1985) used path analytic techniques to test the fit of the data to Bandura's model of self-efficacy and an anxiety reduction model. Whereas self-efficacy was found to be a significant predictor of skill performance, the anxiety–performance path was non-significant. However, as McAuley pointed out, path analysis is not a statistical tool with which to prove or disprove theoretical models. Furthermore, his results must be interpreted with caution because of the small sample which he used.

There are a number of possibilities for future work in this field. Clearly, a programme of research into cognitive behavioural intervention programmes which includes among other things an evaluation of changes in self-efficacy would be particularly valuable in understanding the relationship between coping skills and performance. In one study reported to date, Weinberg (1985) found that the results obtained from an experiment into the relationship between self-efficacy and cognitive strategies in enhancing endurance performance generally supported self-efficacy predictions. Efficacy was manipulated and high self-efficacy subjects performed significantly better than low self-efficacy subjects. However, the efficacy–performance relationship was not mediated by the type of cognitive strategy employed. Regardless of the type of intervention, high efficacy subjects still performed better than low efficacy subjects, suggesting that efficacy expectations have a potent effect. Weinberg also suggested that for a cognitive intervention strategy to influence self-efficacy it may be necessary to tell subjects that a particular intervention strategy will enhance performance, and that belief in the effectiveness of the strategy might be more important than the strategy itself.

Results obtained in a number of the studies reviewed (e.g. Griffiths *et al.*, 1985; Mace Eastman and Carroll, 1986) indicate that it is possible that intervention strategies may have specific effects according to the emphasis on the training programme. Those which emphasize cognitive restructuring, for example, may attenuate self-reported anxiety but have no effect with regard to ameliorating physiological responses to psychological distress.

Given the research evidence indicating a specificity in stress effects in sport (see Jones, Chapter 2 and Parfitt, Jones and Hardy, Chapter 3 in this book), future research could also be directed towards examining the effects of intervention programmes which emphasize different response modalities. If emphasis on specific aspects results in specific effects, then this has important implications for devising programmes for different sports. It may be desirable to devise specific packages which emphasize appropriate aspects for a particular sport, for example respiration control for scuba diving (Griffiths *et al.*, 1987). However, the case studies reported clearly indicate that individuals display idiosyncratic modes of responding to stress and the development of packages should be flexible enough to allow, for example, subjects to use preferred modes of visualization.

In view of the specificity of stress effects and the possibility of devising intervention programmes with a particular emphasis, it could be argued that case studies have an important role to play in future research in cognitive behaviour modification in sport. Although some investigators still hold the view that ideographic study has little place in the confirmatory aspects of scientific activity which looks for laws applying to persons generally, there has been a noticeable shift in stance in recent years regarding the use of single-case experimental designs (see Hersen and Barlow, 1976). The development of such designs stems from an increasing awareness of weaknesses and limitations of traditionally controlled studies which have held a prominent position in psychological research methodology. A weakness of controlled studies, for example, is that while results overall may show no difference between subjects in a control group and subjects in a treatment group, it is possible that the treatment actually worked for some individuals. This is particularly true in investigation into psychotherapeutic procedures such as cognitive behavioural intervention programmes.

> . . . attempts to apply an ill-defined and global treatment such as psycho-
> therapy to a heterogeneous group of clients classified under a vague diagnostic
> category such as neurosis are incapable of answering the more basic question on
> the effectiveness of a specific treatment for a specific individual. (Hersen and
> Barlow, 1976, p. 13)

Although it can be argued that this does not apply to controlled studies using homogeneous groups, the problem of obtaining large numbers of subjects who are homogeneous on relevant characteristics such as skill level and experience in a particular sport is itself a serious limitation of traditionally controlled studies. In recent years, many investigators have realized that tests of global treatments such as cognitive intervention procedures would not be fruitful, and that independent variables must be defined more precisely. More specific questions must be asked; for example, what specific treatment is effective with a specific type of client and under what circumstances?

In additional to obscuring individual outcomes by group averages, the group comparison approach also presents ethical problems, for example deliberately exposing a number of subjects to situations which they may find stressful. It has been argued that an advantage of group studies is that it is possible to generalize findings beyond a specific group. However, if results from group studies do not reflect changes in individual subjects, then the findings are not readily generalizable. It is also difficult to generalize findings at all beyond homogeneous groups, as the demand for homogeneity means that subjects belong to a very specific population. In a number of the group studies reviewed (e.g. Griffiths *et al.*, 1985; Mace and Carroll, 1985), subjects were all novices at a particular sports task. It cannot be assumed with certainty that the results obtained with novices would be similar to results obtained from subjects with some experience. The general efficacy of a particular intervention programme for the stress management of a particular group of performers in a particular sport is, therefore, still problematic.

Weaknesses in the group comparison approach have led many investigators to return to a single case study approach. This development has been given credence by improvements in methodological and statistical procedures. The result has generally been greater precision in defining and manipulating independent variables within a single case such as the systematic alteration of therapeutic approaches in an A–B–A design and the use of the multiple baselines. The development of quasi-experimental designs (for example repeated measures in a period preceding and following a given intervention) by Campbell and Stanley (1963) has also encouraged single case studies. Campbell and Stanley drew particular attention to the limited capacity of this repeated measures design to rule out alternative plausible hypotheses. For example, internal validity could be threatened by specific events occurring between the two measurements. In the context of the present research, winning a major competition (a special event) might significantly enhance the athlete's sense of self-efficacy, thus inflating the post-intervention measures used to evaluate the effect of an intervention programme. They also discussed threats to external validity. For example, validity might be compromised by idiosyncratic preferences with regard to mental training; one person may prefer to rely on self-statements to control pre-competitive anxiety whereas another may prefer to use visualization techniques. Accordingly, it cannot be assumed that if an intervention programme is successful with one athlete an identical programme will be successful with others. In addition to improved methodology, Campbell and Stanley argued that the development of statistical procedures such as correlation-type design using trend analysis has also strengthened the scientific basis of a case study approach.

Although recent developments have led to an increasing use of single case experimental designs, the problem of generality of findings remains a thorny issue. An obvious limitation of studying a single case is that one does not know (a) if the results from this case would be relevant to other cases, (b) if another sport psychologist could use the intervention package and obtain similar results, or (c) if the treatment would work in a different setting.

The direction of future work, as well as its methodology, is also an important consideration. With regard to a single case approach with individuals who have developed a maladaptive mental approach to training and competing, future studies could investigate the role of automatic thoughts. These are defined by Rathjen, Rathjen and Hiniker (1978) as self-statements or images that precede a negative affective state. Rathjen et al. referred to the work of Beck (1976), who has devised four methods of collection: (a) assigning clients 30 minutes each day to think about them and write them down; (b) have clients record thoughts accompanying increased negative affect; (c) collect thoughts in association with negative affect and precipitating environmental events; and (d) collect thoughts during a therapeutic interview. Although these methods were devised for clinical patients, clearly they could be used with sports performers who experience high levels of anxiety. To this list, Rathjen, Rathjen and Hiniker (1978) have added a number of other methods, such as collection during role play or through the use of structured projective techniques such as incomplete sentences or Thematic Apperception Test-like pictures. The aim of these methods is to get the client to recognize the association of affect with negative self-statements or images that the therapist can then correct. Ultimately, the client will learn to reason with or modify cognitions that generate negative affect through the use of related methods.

The present review has examined the use of intervention programmes for modifying cognitions based on a mediational model and it may be a contradiction to talk of modifying automatic thoughts, which may be considered as unconscious cognitions. Cognitions, by definition, refer to what is known and unconscious thoughts are, also by definition, unknown or not in one's awareness. However, the influence of unconscious thoughts on behaviour cannot be ignored. There seems good reason to assume the existence of processes that lie outside awareness. Mahoney (1980), for example, forecast an important role for unconscious thoughts in the future direction of cognitive behaviour therapy. The practical implications are challenging to researchers using intervention programmes with athletes who have a maladaptive mental approach to training and competing. It is possible that automatic thoughts regarding, for example, fear of injury play an important role in terms of performance decrement.

The complexity of human behaviour presents particularly difficult problems for investigators wanting to conduct valid research using a group comparison approach. Nevertheless, this approach is necessary, as there are many questions which cannot be answered by single case experimental designs. For example, a group comparison design is desirable when one wishes to compare two treatment packages such as the relative efficacy of the SMT developed by Smith (1980) and SIT developed by Meichenbaum (1977) (see Ziegler, Klinzing and Williamson, 1982). The single case study with its flexibility can determine individual sources of variability and quickly bring the investigator to the point where he is ready to construct a specific intervention programme for participants in a particular sport. At this point it may be appropriate to test the package in a large group outcome study.

As single case studies become more sophisticated, so the number of questions that can be examined by this approach will increase. However, there are many instances in which single case studies cannot answer applied research questions in sport psychology or, at least, they are inappropriate to the problem in hand. A single case approach may be considered a good way to start an investigation into the general use of cognitive behavioural interventions in sport but may not be the best way to end it.

The present review highlights a number of important issues. One important factor would seem to be the length of time given by researchers to training athletes using cognitive behavioural intervention strategies. It would appear that more positive results have been obtained where considerable time was devoted to training. Seabourne, Weinberg and Jackson (1984) employed VMBR with their subjects over 16 weeks and Mace, Eastman and Carroll (1986, 1987) trained their subjects for a minimum of eight sessions each lasting approximately 45 minutes. The positive results obtained by Silva (1982) may also reflect the considerable time devoted to training each subject.

A second possibly important variable concerns individualized *versus* standardized training. The former would seem to be associated with the more promising results. This possibly reflects the fact that many of the cognitive behavioural techniques used originated in clinical psychology, which focuses on the individual's idiosyncratic problems and expressions of anxiety. Accordingly, the intervention techniques may lose some of their effectiveness when applied uniformly to groups.

Both of these variables, length of time and type of treatment, raise questions which may possibly be best answered by well-designed group studies. However, there are numerous methodological problems which must be resolved for valid research into problems such as these. Unfortunately, many of the group studies reviewed displayed methodological weaknesses, with the result that the overall support claimed for the efficacy of cognitive behavioural interventions in sport must be viewed with caution. Future research should attempt to improve methodological procedures in order to ensure internal validity. Designs must be powerful enough to isolate the independent variable (treatment) as being responsible for any observed experimental effects. In addition, every effort must be made to ensure a high level of external validity in order to generalize findings across relevant domains such as different competitors, different trainers and different sports situations.

In the studies reviewed, a number of weaknesses are evident regarding specific design and control factors. For example, the waiting list control group used in some of the studies (Lane, 1980; Mace and Carroll, 1985; Zeigler, Klinzing and Williamson, 1982) is insufficient to control for attention-placebo effects.

Future research also needs to pay particular attention to task selection. Cognitive behavioural intervention in sport is an applied field of study and as such the experimental tasks should be appropriate to the particular sport under study, thereby maintaining a high level of external validity. In their study of stress inoculation training Mace and Carroll (1985) employed an abseiling task, and although the results indicated that the intervention programme was effective, it cannot be assumed that the programme would be equally effective in other rock-climbing situations. Tasks which retain a close similarity to those actually encountered in a sport would appear to be most appropriate, such as the tasks used by Griffiths *et al.* (1985) in scuba diving,

Mace and Carroll (1986b) in gymnastics and Seabourne, Weinberg and Jackson (1984) in karate.

In many of the controlled studies reviewed, subjects were novices and the groups were generally very small in number. While the use of novices helps to solve the problem of obtaining homogenous groups, it poses a threat to external validity as results obtained with novices may not be obtained with more experienced athletes. Future research, therefore, needs to examine alternative methods of controlling for factors such as ability. For example, greater use may be made of designs employing statistical control, such as analysis of covariance techniques.

The present review of cognitive behavioural interventions in sport has highlighted the need for careful consideration of appropriate assessment procedures in future research in order to maintain methodological rigour. In a number of the studies reviewed there is general support for the view that the various expressions of anxiety—cognitive, somatic and behavioural—are to some extent independent of each other. Future studies, therefore, should be carefully designed to allow assessment at a variety of levels. Self-report, physiological, behavioural and performance measures used in isolation may not provide appropriate or adequate assessment. However, multilevel assessment can provide problems and care must be taken to ensure that exposing subjects to a battery of tests immediately before commencing the experimental task does not pose a threat to both external and internal validity.

Recent research has led to the development of new measures. An increasing awareness, for example, of different expressions of anxiety has led to the development of the Competitive State Anxiety Inventory-2 (Martens *et al.*, 1990), which provides scores for the subcomponents of cognitive anxiety, somatic anxiety and self-confidence (see Chapter 3 in this book). It was also suggested earlier that an examination of the role of unconscious thoughts might be a fruitful area for future study. If this is the case, it will be necessary to develop and validate new tests to investigate this phenomenon in the context of sport.

One overall aim of cognitive behavioural interventions in sport is to enhance performance or, at least, to prevent performance disruption in stressful situations. Accordingly, future research should include performance measures which are reliable and objective. A number of the studies reviewed failed to meet these criteria. In view of the importance of accurate performance assessment, the design of controlled studies should incorporate reliability tests and at least two independent judges, unless objective criteria are available. Reliability tests should not, of course, be restricted to performance assessment. They should be used as widely as possible.

Clearly, appropriate measures are essential for accurate assessment and careful consideration must be given to their selection. Skin conductance, for example may be an appropriate measure of the physiological impact of a stressor in one situation whereas heart rate may be appropriate in another. In addition, some measures may need to be developed and refined through pilot testing. Subsequent item analysis of a self-report questionnaire, for example, may show only certain items to be sensitive. Accordingly, these could be selected for the main study.

To summarize, it is clear that both case studies and group comparison studies have their strengths and weaknesses. However, common to both is a need for methodological rigour. Unfortunately, many of the studies reviewed lack this rigour. Only through improved design, control and accurate assessment can future research clearly establish the efficacy of cognitive behavioural interventions in sport. In a discussion of research procedures, Kendall and Hollon (1979) stated that there can be little doubt that cognitive behavioural theories and interventions have reached a point of youthful maturity. They pointed out that attempts to draw on experimental cognitive psychology are increasing and efforts to integrate cognitive and behavioural theories have become increasingly sophisticated. However, they emphasized that more work is still needed, and in the area of cognitive behavioural assessment the goal remains to increase the breadth and power of explanatory concepts and interventions without sacrificing methodological rigour. That goal also still remains with regard to cognitive behavioural intervention in sport.

REFERENCES

Bandura, A. (1977). Self-efficacy: towards a unifying theory of behavior change, *Psychological Review*, **84**, 191–215.

Beck, A. T. (1970). Cognitive therapy: nature and relation to behaviour therapy, *Behaviour Therapy*, **1**, 184–200.

Beck, A. T. (1976). *Cognitive Therapy and Emotional Disorders*. New York: International Universities Press.

Campbell, D. T. and Stanley, J. C. (1963). *Experimental and Quasi-Experimental Designs for Research*. Chicago: Rand McNally.

Daniels, F. S and Hatfield, B. (1981). Biofeedback, *Motor Skills: Theory into Practice*, **5**, 69–72.

Ellis, A. (1962). *Reason and Emotion in Psychotherapy*. New York: Lye Stuart.

Ellis, A. (1970). *The Essence of Rational Psychotherapy: A Comprehensive Approach to Treatment*. New York: Institute for Rational Living.

Feltz, D. L. and Albrecht, R. R. (1986). The influence of self-efficacy on the approach/ avoidance of a high avoidance motor task, *Psychology & Sociology of Sport: Current Selected Research*, **1**, 3–25.

Feltz, D. L. and Landers, D. M. (1980). Stress management techniques for sport and physical education, *Journal of Physical Education and Recreation*, **51**, 41–43.

Feltz, D. L. and Landers, D. M. (1983). The effects of mental practice on motor skill learning and performance: a meta-analysis, *Journal of Sport Psychology*, **5**, 25–57.

Feltz, D. L., Landers, D. M. and Raeder, U. (1979). Enhancing self-efficacy in high avoidance motor tasks. A comparison of modeling techniques, *Journal of Sport Psychology*, **1**, 112–122.

Fenz, W. D. (1975). Coping mechanisms and performance under stress, in D. M. Landers and R. W. Christina (eds). *Psychology of Sport and Motor Behavior II.* The Pennsylvania State University.

Forman, S. (1982). Stress management for teachers: a cognitive behavioral program, *Journal of School Psychology,* **20**, 180–187.

Frager, S. R. (1979). Hypnosis and behavioral techniques improve swimming performance, *Swimming Technique,* **16**, 77–81.

Gerson, R. F. (1980). A stress, motivation and relaxation training programme, *Athlete Journal,* **60**, (5), 30, 79.

Girodo, M. and Wood, D. (1979). Talking yourself out of pain: the importance of believing that you can, *Cognitive Therapy and Research,* **3**, 23–33.

Goldfried, M. R., (1971). Systematic desensitization as training in self-control, *Journal of Consulting and Clinical Psychology,* **37**, 228–234.

Griffiths, T. J., Steel, D. H., Vaccaro, P., Allen, R. and Karpman, M. (1985). The effects of relaxation and cognitive rehearsal on the anxiety levels and performance of scuba students, *International Journal of Sport Psychology,* **16**, 113–119.

Griffiths, T. J., Steel, D. H., Vaccaro, P. and Karpman, M. B. (1981). The effects of relaxation techniques on anxiety and underwater performance, *International Journal of Sport Psychology,* **12**, 176–182.

Griffiths, T. J., Steel, D. H., Vaccaro, P. and Ostrove, S. M. (1987). Psychological implications for underwater archaeologists, *International Journal of Sport Psychology,* **18**, 1–8.

Hamilton, S. A. and Fremouw, W. J. (1985). Cognitive-behavioral training for college basketball free-throw performance, *Cognitive Therapy and Research,* **9**, 479–483.

Hatfield, B. and Daniels, F. S. (1981). The use of hypnosis as a stress management technique, *Motor Skills: Theory into Practice,* **5** (1), 62–68.

Hersen, N. and Barlow, D. (1976). *Single Case Experimental Designs.* New York: Pergamon.

Hodgson, R. and Rachman, S. (1974). Desynchrony in measures of fear, *Behaviour Research and Therapy,* **12**, 319–326.

Homme, L. E. (1965). Perspectives in psychology: XXIV. Control of coverants, the operants of the mind, *Psychological Record,* **15**, 501–511.

Jacobs, P. D. and Munz, D. C. (1968) An index for measuring perceived stress in a college population, *Journal of Psychology,* **70**, 9–15.

Jones, J. G. and Hardy, L. (1989) Stress and cognitive functioning in sport, *Journal of Sports Sciences,* **7**, 41–63.

Kendall, P. C. (1983). Stressful medical procedures: cognitive-behavioral strategies for stress management and prevention, in D. Meichenbaum and M. Jaremko (eds). *Stress Reduction and Prevention.* New York: Plenum.

Kendall, P. C. and Hollon, S. D. (1979). *Cognitive-Behavioural Interventions.* New York: Academic Press.

Kenney, E. A., Rejeski, W. J. and Messier, S. P. (1987). Managing exercise distress: the effect of broad spectrum intervention on affect, R. P. E. and running efficiency, *Canadian Journal of Sports Sciences,* **2**, 97–105.

Kolonay, B. J. (1977). The effects of visuo-motor behaviour rehearsal on athletic performance. *Unpublished Masters thesis,* Hunter College, The City University of New York.

Lane, J. F. (1980). Improving athletic performance through visuo-motor behavior rehearsal, in R. Suinn (ed.). *Pyschology in Sport: Methods and Applications.* Minneapolis: Burgess.

Lazarus, R. S. (1966). *Psychological Stress and the Coping Process.* New York: McGraw-Hill.

Lehrer, P. M. and Woolfolk, R. L. (1982). Self-report assessment of anxiety: somatic, cognitive and behavioral modalities, *Behavior Assessment*, 4, 167–177.

Long, B. (1980). Stress management for the athlete: a cognitive behavioral model, in C. H. Nadeau, W. R. Halliwell, K. M. Newell and G. C. Roberts (eds). *Psychology of Motor Behavior and Sport.* Champaign, Illinois: Human Kinetics.

Long, B. (1983). Aerobic conditioning and stress reduction: participation or conditioning, *Human Movement Science*, 2, 171–186.

Long, B. (1984). Aerobic conditioning and stress inoculation: a comparison of stress-management interventions, *Cognitive Therapy and Research*, 8, 517–542.

Long, B. (1985). Stress-management interventions: a 15 month follow-up of aerobic conditioning and stress inoculation training, *Cognitive Therapy and Research*, 9, 471–478.

Mace, R. D. and Carroll, D. (1985). The control of anxiety in sport: stress inoculation training prior to abseiling, *International Journal of Sport Psychology*, 16, 165–175.

Mace, R. and Carroll, D. (1986a). Effects of stress inoculation training on self-reported stress, observer's ratings of stress, heart rate and gymnastics performance. Paper presented at the Annual Conference of the British Association of Sport Sciences, Birmingham University, Sept.

Mace, R. and Carroll, D. (1986b). Stress inoculation training to control anxiety in sport: two case studies in squash, *British Journal of Sports Medicine*, 20 (3), 115–117.

Mace, R., Carroll, D. and Eastman, C. (1986a). Effects of stress inoculation training on self-report, behavioural and psychophysiological reactions to abseiling, *Journal of Sports Sciences*, 4, 229–236.

Mace, R., Carroll, D. and Eastman, C. (1986b). Stress inoculation to control anxiety and enhance performance in sport, in J. Watkins, T. Reilly and L. Burwitz (eds). *Sports Science: Proceedings of the VIII Commonwealth and International Conference on Sport, Physical Education, Dance, Recreation and Health.* London: Spon.

Mace, R. Eastman, C. and Carroll, D. (1986). Stress inoculation training to control anxiety in sport: a case study in gymnastics, *British Journal of Sports Medicine*, 10 (3), 139–141.

Mace, R., Eastman, C. and Carroll, D. (1987) The effects of stress inoculation training on gymnastics performance on the pommelled horse: a case study, *Behavioural Psychotherapy*, 15, 272–279.

Mahoney, M. J. (1974). *Cognition and Behavior Modification.* Cambridge, Mass: Ballinger.

Mahoney, M. J. (1980). Psychotherapy and the structure of personal revolutions, in M. J. Mahoney (ed.). *Psychotherapy Process.* New York: Plenum.

Mahoney, M. and Avener, M. (1977). Psychology of the elite athlete: an exploratory study, *Cognitive Therapy and Research*, 1, 135–141.

Martens, R. (1977) *Sport Competition Anxiety Test.* Champaign, Illinois: Human Kinetics.

Martens, R., Burton, D., Vealey, R., Bump, L. and Smith, D. (1990). Competitive State Anxiety Inventory-2, in R. Martens, R. Vealey and D. Burton (eds). *Competitive Anxiety in Sport.* Champaign, Illinois: Human Kinetics.

McAuley, E. (1985). Modeling and self-efficacy: a test of Bandura's model *Journal of Sport Psychology*, 7, 283–295.

Meinchenbaum, D. (1973). Cognitive factors in behavior modifications. Modifying what people say to themselves, in C. M. Franks and G. T. Wilson (eds). *Annual Review of Behavior Therapy: Theory and Practice*, Vol 1. New York: Bruner, Mazel.

Meichenbaum, D. (1977). *Cognitive Behavior Modification: An Integrative Approach.* New York: Plenum.

Meichenbaum, D. (1985). *Stress Inoculation Training.* New York: Pergamon.

Murphy, S. M. and Woolfolk, R. L. (1987). The effects of cognitive interventions on competitive anxiety and performance on a fine motor skill accuracy task, *International Journal of Sport Psychology*, **18**, 152–166.

Novaco, R. N. (1980). Anger and coping with stress: cognitive behavioral interventions, in J. P. Foreyt and D. P. Rathjen (eds.). *Cognitive Behavior Therapy: Research and Application.* New York: Plenum.

Pulos, L. (1981). Self-hypnosis and think training with athletes, *Journal of Psycho-Social Aspects (UK)*, **7**, 1–10.

Rathjen, D. P., Rathjen, E. D. and Hiniker, A. (1978). A cognitive analysis of social performance, in J. P. Foreyt and D. P. Rathjen (eds). *Cognitive Behaviour Therapy: Research and Application.* New York: Plenum.

Seabourne, T., Weinberg, R. and Jackson, A. (1984). Effect of individual practice and training of visuo-motor behavior rehearsal in enhancing karate performance, *Journal of Sport Behavior*, **7**, 58–67.

Silva, J. (1982). Competitive sport environments. Performance enhancement through cognitive intervention, *Behavior Modification*, **6**, 443–463.

Smith, R. E. (1980). A cognitive affective approach to stress management for athletes, in C. A. Nadeau, W. R. Halliwell, K. M. Newell and G. C. Roberts (eds). *Psychology of Motor Behavior and Sport.* Champaign, Illinois: Human Kinetics.

Spielberger, C. D., Gorsuch, R. L. and Lushene, R. E. (1970). *S.T.A.I. Manual for the State Trait Anxiety Inventory.* Palo Alto, California: Consulting Psychologists Press.

Straub, W. F. (1978). *Sport Psychology: An Analysis of Athlete Behavior.* New York: Mouvement Publications.

Suinn, R. (1972a). Behaviour rehearsal training for ski racers: brief report, *Behaviour Therapy*, **3**, 210–212.

Suinn, R. (1972b). Removing emotional obstacles to learning and performance by visuomotor behaviour rehearsal, *Behaviour Therapy*, **3**, 308–310.

Suinn, R. E. and Richardson, F. (1971). Anxiety management training: a non-specific behaviour therapy program for anxiety control, *Behaviour Therapy*, **2**, 498–510.

Weinberg, R. S. (1982). The relationship between mental preparation strategies and motor performance: a review and critique, *Quest*, **33**, 195–213.

Weinberg, R. S. (1985). Relationship between self-efficacy and cognitive strategies in enhancing endurance performance, *International Journal of Sport Psychology*, **17**, 280–292.

Weinberg, R., Gould, D. and Jackson, A. (1979). Expectations and performance: an empirical test of Bandura's self-efficacy theory, *Journal of Sport Psychology*, **1**, 320–331.

Weinberg, R. S., Seabourne, T. G. and Jackson, A. (1981). Effects of visuo-motor behavior rehearsal, relaxation and imagery on Karate performance, *Journal of Sport Psychology*, **3**, 228–238.

Wilson, V. E. and Bird, E. I. (1982). Understanding self-regulation training in sport, *Science Periodical on Research and Technology in Sport*, Oct., B.U.-1.

Ziegler, S. G., Klinzing, J. and Williamson, K. (1982). The effects of two stress management training programs on cardiorespiratory efficiency, *Journal of Sport Psychology*, **4**, 280–289.

Chapter 9

The role of performance routines in sport

Stephen H. Boutcher
University of Virginia

Sport competition can generate considerable anxiety which, in turn, can affect psychological and physiological processes so dramatically that performance can be devastated. Athletes competing in self-paced sports, such as golf, archery, shooting, diving and weightlifting, are especially prone to the deleterious effects of competition, as the opportunities to worry or become distracted are numerous and the demands for continual high-level performance after rest or stoppage are particularly challenging. How do athletes avoid thoughts of failure? How are they able to focus their attention away from cameras and spectators? How do they consistently maintain high standards of performance over many hours of play? One strategy for maintaining performance consistency is the performance routine. It is possible that a systematic, routinized pattern of actions and thoughts can aid athletic performance (Boutcher and Rotella, 1987). Thus, archers and shooters may have a behavioural routine for establishing their stance and shooting position, whereas golfers may waggle the club a set number of times before executing a shot. These athletes may also go through a pre-planned sequence of imagery, arousal setting cues, and other cognitive strategies as part of their complete routine. These routines can be used before or after skill performance or while waiting on the sidelines. Thus, performance routines focus specifically on what the athlete is thinking immediately before, during, after and between skill performance. This chapter focuses on the theoretical and applied aspects of performance routines. In the first section research examining performance routines is described, followed in the second section by possible explanations underlying the effectiveness of these routines. Finally, the third section describes methods for developing performance routines.

Stress and Performance in Sport. Edited by J. Graham Jones and Lew Hardy.
©1990 John Wiley & Sons Ltd.

RESEARCH EXAMINING PERFORMANCE ROUTINES

Empirical support for the existence of performance routines in golf has come from Crews and Boutcher (1987), who used trained observers to record pre-shot routines of female professional golfers in tournament play. They demonstrated that the players' pre-putt and pre-shot behaviours were remarkably consistent over many hours of play. These professional golfers repeatedly took the same amount of time, and the same number of practice swings and glances at the target, before playing each shot. Interestingly, when the pre-shot routine for the full swing and putt were compared, the total time was similar; however, the content and components differed. The majority of golfers did not use a practice swing for the full swing but completed at least one practice swing for the putt. The authors suggested that full shots like the drive and irons require less 'fine-tuning' than the putt. Thus, the greater uncertainty experienced in putting brought about by variables such as undulating greens and variable speeds may require the golfer to spend time 'feeling' and then pre-programming the upcoming putt. In contrast, for Ladies Professional Golf Association players, the full shots may be so well learned and automatic that practice swings are not required.

A second study (Boutcher and Crews, 1987) examined the effects of pre-putt routines on putting performance. Collegiate male and female golfers were assigned to a control or treatment group and underwent a six-week pre-putt routine or putting practice programme. Performance while putting on an actual putting green was recorded before and after the six-week programme. Results indicated that both male and female experimental groups increased the length but decreased variability of their pre-putt routines. Interestingly, the only group to show an increase in performance on the putting task was the experimental female group. The authors suggested that as the males were superior on the putting task the effectiveness of the pre-putt routine may be influenced by putting ability. Thus, poorer putters' performance may benefit more from the consistency and control achieved through learning a pre-putt routine.

The effect of pre-shot routines on novice golfing performance was examined in a third study (Crews and Boutcher, 1986). Male and female students of beginning golf learned and practised a specific routine of actions prior to performing a full swing, whereas men and women controls practised only the swing. Subjective and objective performance measures were completed before and after an eight-week training session. Trained men had higher post-training scores than controls and untrained women, but no significant differences were found between trained women and other groups on either measure. The authors suggested that as trained men had superior skills before and after training, a certain level of skill may have to be established before the pre-shot routine is effective.

Pre-performance routines have also been examined in preliminaries to basketball free throw shooting. Lobmeyer and Wasserman (1986) had varsity and high school basketball players attempt 20 free throws with and without their normal pre-shot routine. Results indicated that free throw accuracy was higher when athletes performed their usual pre-performance pattern. The authors concluded that pre-performance response patterns are behaviourally and psychologically relevant and contribute to the accuracy of the shot.

Similar results have been demonstrated by the examination of pre-performance 'psyching-up' strategies in weightlifting. For instance, Shelton and Mahoney (1978) investigated the influence of cognitive strategies used by competitive weightlifters on hand-dynamometer performance. At an Olympic-style weightlifting meet, subjects were assigned to an experimental or control group. Experimental subjects used their favourite psyching strategy as a means of improving their performance on the strength test, whereas control subjects did not use any pre-lifting strategy. To minimize the effects of unrequested use of the psych-up strategies, control subjects engaged in a distractive cognitive task during the pre-performance interval. Results indicated that subjects using the psych-up strategies showed greater improvement in strength performance than did control subjects. Post-experimental interviews suggested that the most popular pre-lifting strategies were those involving focus of attention. Similar results have been found with a leg-strength task (Caudill and Weinberg, 1982), bench press (Weinberg, Gould and Jackson, 1981) and sprinting (Caudill, Weinberg and Jackson, 1983).

These findings provide preliminary empirical support for the existence of pre-performance routines in a variety of sports, and although methodological weaknesses exist, the overall results suggest that attentional routines can facilitate athletic performance. Unfortunately, none of this research has attempted to identify the mechanisms underlying the pre-performance routine. However, recent investigations in sport psychophysiology have attempted to explore attentional states before and during athletic performance. A number of studies have examined cardiovascular concomitants of attention. For instance, Stern (1976) examined cardiac patterns of sprinters between the 'get set' and 'go' of simulated races. The typical pattern of heart rate (HR) between the 'get set' and the 'go' of the subjects waiting to sprint up a flight of stairs, and to sprint on a bicycle ergometer, was acceleration following 'get set' and deceleration immediately prior to 'go'. This deceleration effect has been found by numerous investigators (e.g. Lacey and Lacey, 1970), demonstrating that before a reaction time task most subjects show HR deceleration while waiting for a stimulus to which they must respond.

Fenz (1975) has also observed cardiac deceleration patterns with skilled and less skilled parachutists. Monitoring HR before an actual parachute jump, Fenz observed that skilled performers demonstrated a progressive increase in HR until they entered the aircraft and then exhibited a decrease in HR while waiting to jump. The lesser skilled jumpers, in contrast, showed a progressive increase in HR right through to the jump.

Cardiac deceleration has also been found with shooters. For example, Landers *et al.* (1980) found HR deceleration with elite rifle marksmen just prior to the trigger pull. Similar deceleration effects were found with archers by Wang and Landers (1990), who demonstrated that HR progressively decelerated seconds before the release of the arrow. Interestingly, both skilled and unskilled archers recorded similar HR deceleration patterns during the aiming period. However, skilled archers demonstrated significantly greater HR deceleration compared to less accomplished archers. The authors suggested that skilled archers may have been more able to control their concentration while performing. Boutcher and Zinsser (1990) found similar deceleration effects with elite and beginning golfers on a putting task. Both groups displayed HR deceleration during the performance of four- and 12-foot putts, although the elite golfers showed significantly greater deceleration. The elite golfers also possessed significantly less variable pre-shot routines. The authors suggested that the greater HR deceleration of the elite golfers may reflect more efficient attentional control.

Attentional states during the pre-performance routine have also been assessed through monitoring EEG activity. For instance, Hatfield, Landers and Ray (1984) examined left- and right-brain EEG activity of elite shooters while shooting and while performing a series of mental tasks. Results indicated that progressive electrocortical lateralization occurred during shooting towards right hemispheric dominance before the trigger pull. Thus, seconds before pulling the trigger shooters exhibited more activity in their right hemisphere compared to their left. The authors suggested that elite marksmen may possess such a high degree of attentional focus that they can effectively reduce conscious mental activities of the left hemisphere, thus reducing cognitions unnecessary to performance of the task.

Research examining the underlying mechanisms of the performance routine is in its infancy and there is much to learn about the interaction of psychological and physiological processes and the resultant effect on athletic performance. However, the continued use of multidimensional research strategies, where observational, questionnaire and psychophysiological techniques are used to examine athletic performance in real-life settings, promises to generate greater understanding in the future.

EXPLANATIONS FOR THE SUCCESS OF PERFORMANCE ROUTINES

Boutcher and Crews (1987) have suggested that at least three explanations exist to account for the effectiveness of pre-performance routines: (1) attentional control, (2) warm-up decrement, and (3) automatic skill execution. Thus, routines may enable athletes to concentrate more efficiently; they may act as a psychological and physiological 'warm-up' prior to skills which are stop–start in nature; and they may also prevent athletes from thinking about the details or mechanics of well-learned skills that are better performed automatically.

Attentional control

Attentional theories attempt to explain the effects of competitive pressure on performance by focusing on disruption of the performer's attentional processes. The rationale here is that performance necessitates focusing attention on task-relevant information while ignoring task-irrelevant cues. Therefore, alterations in attentional processing can result in impaired athletic performance.

Three areas of attentional research have pertinence when the role of attentional control and performance routines is examined: distraction theories, self-awareness theories, and capacity theories. Distraction theories are concerned with loss of attention caused by shifting the focus of attention to task-irrelevant cues, thus ignoring critical task cues. Consequently, concentrating on task-irrelevant cues may lead to the omission of critical task cues, which could deleteriously affect performance. If a golfer focuses solely on thoughts of missing a short putt, it is possible that attention will be disrupted and performance negatively affected. Similarly, if a batsman in cricket does not focus visual attention on the incoming bowler, it is probable that he will not make contact with the ball. Thus, even momentary loss of concentration during the initial flight of the ball may have devastating effects.

An important type of irrelevant information that could disrupt attention is worry or cognitive anxiety (see Parfitt, Jones and Hardy, Chapter 3 and Hardy, Chapter 4 in this book). Sarason (1972) and Wine (1971) have used the distraction capabilities of cognitive anxiety to explain test anxiety effects. According to Sarason and Wine, cognitively anxious individuals typically focus their attention on task-irrelevant thoughts and do not use the appropriate cognitive styles to do well during testing. Thus, individuals who engross themselves in thoughts such as 'I'm not as good as the others, I'm bound to fail' distract themselves and do not give themselves the opportunity to present a true reflection of their ability. The test anxiety situation seems to parallel sport competition, where acute anxiety, in the form of self-debilitating thoughts, has been associated with impaired athletic performance (Kroll, 1982). Task-irrelevant processing can explain performance decrements in a wide range of athletic settings. In pressure settings, for example, performance could be affected by focusing on negative thoughts, whereas in non-stimulating environments irrelevant processing could occur in competitions that take place over hours or days. The ability to offset task-irrelevant processing could be improved with the use of an effective pre-performance routine that consistently directs attention to task-relevant cues.

Another source of distraction information is self-awareness. Carver and Scheier (1981) have suggested that being self-conscious while performing may take away attention from task cues, thus degrading performance. Other authors (Duval and Wicklund, 1972; Scheier, Fenigstein and Buss, 1974) have suggested that it is impossible to attend to oneself and to the environment at the same time. As social facilitation generally tends to increase self-awareness (Carver and Scheier, 1978), the presence of spectators and cameras, which are common at sporting events, has the potential to generate an increased focus on the self, thus distracting the athlete.

The effects of physiological arousal on the ability to selectively allocate attention is another possible influence on attention. Landers (1978, 1981) has applied the work of Easterbrook (1959), concerning narrowing effects on the visual field (see Chapter 2 in this book), to athletic performance. Landers (1978) suggested that this phenomenon has implications for sports performance as many sports require athletes to use their peripheral visual attentional field. For instance, if a scrum half is about to feed the ball to his fly half (scanning the periphery of his attentional field), overarousal may bring about perceptual narrowing. This narrow focus may result in the scrum half failing to detect the position of his fly half in the periphery.

Warm-up decrement

A second possible explanation for the effectiveness of performance routines is warm-up decrement, which is concerned with a loss in motor performance when performance is renewed after a short rest period. If subjects stop and rest during performance of a task, initial performance is typically degraded upon continuation. This phenomenon has been known for decades, and has been found in nearly every motor task studied (Schmidt, 1988). In sport this decrement in performance is of potential importance as many sports are discontinuous and require athletes to perform at high levels immediately after stoppages.

Explanations for warm-up decrement have included forgetting (Adams, 1961), the inhibition hypothesis (Eysenck, 1956) and loss of activation set (Schmidt, 1988). The set hypothesis suggests that performance decrement is caused by a temporary loss of the internal state that underlies the skill to be performed. Thus, rather than forgetting how to perform the skill during the rest period, inactivity dulls psychological and physiological readiness necessary for optimal performance. Support for the activation set hypothesis has been generated in both the motor learning and sport psychology literature. For instance, task force estimation (Schmidt and Nacson, 1971), hand movement speed (Schmidt and Wrisberg, 1971) and linear positioning (Nacson and

Schmidt, 1971) have all demonstrated that resumption of skilled performance following a period of no practice is characterized by lower quality performance. Research examining softball performance (Anshel and Wrisberg, 1988) and handspring vaults (Anshel, 1985) has produced similar results. Furthermore, Jones and Hardy (1988), examining the effects of anxiety on choice reaction and movement time, found that elevated cognitive anxiety was also associated with warm-up decrement. The authors suggested that in anxiety-inducing situations individuals may be slow to develop activation sets so that warm-up decrement can occur early in performance.

All of these studies are consistent in saying that the warm-up decrement effect is caused by a loss of internal adjustment during the rest period. Schmidt (1988) suggested that these findings have considerable relevance for athletic performance which is interrupted. He used the analogy of a race car, suggesting that just as the race car needs to be tuned before maximal performance can be achieved, so too must athletes acquire the optimal state of adjustment for high-level skilled performance. Schmidt (1988) suggested that the ability to establish pschological and physiological 'sets' may be an important determinant of performance in sports such as golf. He proposed that there may be different sets for driving and putting, as well as for the the time between shots, and suggested that the golfer must establish a different set for each situation. Thus, one of the functions of the performance routine may be to 'warm-up' psychological and physiological processes immediately prior to performance by establishing the appropriate set for the following skill.

Automatic functioning

The third area that has relevance for explaining the beneficial effects of performance routines is automatic execution of sport skills. Baumeister (1984) has suggested that competitive pressure generally makes individuals want to do well, so they have a tendency to focus on the process of performance. Under pressure, individuals realize the importance of executing the skill correctly and attempt to ensure success by consciously monitoring the process of performance. Paradoxically, consciousness does not contain the necessary information regarding muscle movement and coordination, and thus degrades performance by trying to control it (Kimble and Perlmuter, 1970). A good example of the inefficiency of conscious control on well-learned skills is provided by Langer and Imber (1979), who showed that attempting to ensure accuracy by consciously monitoring finger movements during typing was detrimental to performance. Also, focusing attention on skills such as piano playing has been found to detract from performance (Keele, 1973). This effect has also been obtained using laboratory tasks by Baumeister (1984), who found that increasing subjects' attention to the process of performing debilitated performance.

This idea of automatic functioning has existed since the turn of the century, having originally been discussed by Bliss (1895) and Boder (1935), and has resulted in what is now called the Bliss–Boder hypothesis. This hypothesis suggests that sport skills should be performed automatically even though the general effect of competition is to induce athletes to consciously monitor performance. One way of avoiding conscious monitoring during performance may be to employ a pre-shot routine. Thus, by focusing thoughts on general task cues it may be possible that athletes can stop themselves from consciously monitoring specific movements that may prevent smooth, coordinated performance.

DEVELOPMENT OF PERFORMANCE ROUTINES

The development of effective performance routines is based on previously acquired psychological skills. Boutcher and Rotella (1987) have outlined a comprehensive performance enhancement programme which provides a structure for performance routine development. The programme consists of four phases which include sport analysis, individual assessment, conceptualization/ motivation, and mental skill development. Given the central role of attention previously discussed, it is important that the athlete has learned to concentrate effectively. Other important psychological skills are imaging, relaxation and coping strategies. The programme will not be described here but it is emphasized that the athlete must progress through a series of stages in order to acquire the mental skills necessary to develop an effective individualized routine.

Individualized performance routines focus specifically on establishing optimal psychological and physiological states immediately before, during, after and between skill performance. The majority of this chapter has focused on the pre-performance routine; however, how athletes think and react after performance of a skill (post-performance routine) and when waiting during competition (between-performance routine) are also important determinants of overall performance. This section outlines possible ways of developing these different routines.

Pre-performance routines

From an applied perspective, the main components of pre-performance routines are attentional control, physiological/psychological control and behavioural consistency. Thus, athletes need to have the ability to focus their thoughts on task-relevant cues, they need to be able to control their psychological and physiological states, and they need to be able to acquire an appropriate routinized set of behavioural actions. The challenge for the athlete is to find the most efficient routine and to repeat this routine before every performance.

Pre-performance routines will vary in content for athletes in the same sport. For instance, in golf there are clear differences regarding the speed of pre-performance routines of the faster, more spontaneous golfers compared to their more methodical, slower counterparts. Similarly, pre-performance routines will vary between sports. Thus, a pitcher's routine when standing on the mound preparing to pitch will have different attentional and behavioural components from those of a springboard diver preparing to dive. Skill level will also influence the type and nature of the routine. If the skill is still being acquired, and not performed automatically, then a less complex, abbreviated routine may be more appropriate.

Pre-performance routines can be divided into either self-paced or reactive categories. An example of a self-paced routine would be penalty-taking in soccer or serving in tennis, whereas an example of a reactive routine would be batting in cricket or wide receiving in American football. During self-paced routines the athlete will initiate movement, whereas in reactive routines the athlete is waiting to react to an environmental cue.

Self-paced pre-performance routines

Self-paced pre-performance routines consist of a series of psychological, psychophysiological and behavioural steps. For instance, in golf a typical routine of professional golfers is as follows:

1. Shot analysis (choice of club);
2. Setting (establishing optimal physiological arousal level);
3. Imagery (visualizing result of shot);
4. Kinesthetic coupling (practising and feeling the upcoming shot);
5. Set-up (the address position);
6. Waggle (small movements of the club);
7. Swing thought (e.g. think 'tempo' or 'rhythm').

Each component of the routine needs to have been developed and refined from previous general mental skills acquired by the athlete. Thus the 'setting' response, which would be at the start of the routine, would have been developed through the acquisition of physiological arousal controlling skills developed previously. For instance, relaxation, imagery and breathing techniques could be used to develop the general skill of relaxation and then specific relaxation cues could be transferred to the routine, so a setting response in a routine could be achieved through the use of a combination of techniques such as a cue word like 'relax' coupled with a breathing technique.

The imaging component of the routine would be developed in a similar manner. Initially, the effectiveness of imaging for each individual athlete would have been assessed. If golfers do favour the use of imagery they could image the flight of the ball or the ball landing on the green or fairway as part of their routine. On the putting green the image may focus on the line of the putt and the ball dropping into the hole. However, if the athlete does not favour imagery this component could be excluded. Imagery may help to avoid focusing on irrelevant task information and provide a way to activate the appropriate set. For instance, research examining the influence of imagery on gymnastics (Ainscoe and Hardy, 1987), tennis (Hardy and Wyatt, 1986) and badminton performance (Hardy and Ringland, 1984) has suggested that imaging immediately before execution may enhance skill performance.

The kinesthetic coupling component is concerned with establishing the feel of the upcoming shot. This component seems to be especially relevant during chipping and putting, as elite golfers tend to rehearse far more when performing these kinds of shots (Crews and Boutcher, 1986). Thus, this component will entail rehearsing the correct action and attempting to repeat this action in actual performance.

The next stage is the set-up. In most accuracy sports, and especially golf, the alignment of the body to the target is of crucial importance. Thus, a ritual which directs attention to the stance, grip, posture, alignment, ball position and so forth is a vital component, and a quick mental checklist supplemented by kinesthetic cues could be performed as part of the routine.

The golfer is now ready to swing the club. Initiation of the swing is often preceded by a 'waggle', which comprises small movements of the hands and club. Waggles usually consist of a forward press of the hands in the address position preceded by a number of small movements of the club away from the ball.

During the swing, which should be automatic and reflexive, a common technique used by golfers is to focus attention on a swing thought such as 'tempo'. Thus, timing the backswing to 'tem' and the downswing to 'po' focuses attention on the overall rhythm and timing of the shot rather than on specifics of the swing.

Clearly, athletes in other sports will require different components in comparison to golfers. The basic principle that applies, however, is that the pre-performance routine establishes a rhythm and a focus of attention that simultaneously prepares the body and mind for the ensuing skill.

The first task for the athlete and sport psychologist attempting to develop an effective pre-performance routine is to establish a sequence of mental steps and behavioural actions similar to those outlined in the golf example. The content and structure will be highly individual and will vary for different sports. The refining and fine-tuning of each component will be a continuous process. Once a routine has been developed, its behavioural consistency can be assessed through videotaping and time analysis (see Crews and Boutcher, 1987). For most sports the preliminary work should occur in practice settings (on the practice range, at the swimming pool), but will eventually be monitored and observed during competition.

Once a routine has been established, distraction strategies can be used to test the consistency and attentional efficiency of the athlete's routine. For instance, loud music could be played during the routine and its resulting effect assessed on video and through discussion with the athlete after performance. Eventually, other irrelevant competition cues such as camera clicks, crowd noises, crowd movement and so forth could substitute for music. Vicarious experimental techniques can also be used to create competition-like environments. Thus, a competitive situation in the Olympics could be created by imaging the feelings of the competition, by structuring the environment to simulate the competitive setting and by playing videotapes of world class athletes-who will be competing in the actual competition. The challenge for athletes in these settings will be the same as in actual competition: to focus attention away from distractive thoughts and concentrate on their own individualized pre-performance routine.

Reactive pre-performance routines

The major difference between self-paced and reactive routines is that in the reactive situation environmental cues will play a more important role. Thus, the separate components may be similar to the self-paced routine but there will be a greater emphasis on focusing attention on vital environmental cues. Vision training (Solomon, Carello and Turvey, 1984) for athletes in sports such as baseball and tennis would seem to be a vital component of the reactive routine.

Post-performance routines

How the athlete reacts and thinks after executing a skill (the post-performance routine) is another area where routines can be utilized. In discontinuous sports there is a tendency for athletes to focus on negative aspects immediately after unsuccessful performance. Thus, a poor shot or a bad pitch can carry over and affect subsequent performance. The post-performance routine attempts to stop this negative transfer. Components of this routine may include affective catharsis, post-performance analysis, kinesthetic rehearsal of the correct skill, coping strategies and mind clearing-techniques. Affective catharsis refers to an emotional release immediately following performance. Some athletes may need to release emotions through verbal or behavioural responses; however, other athletes may not feel the need to release emotion. The analysis component might include a review of the performed skill to monitor any form or technique flaws. Kinesthetic rehearsal might involve performing the correct action to reinforce the feel of the skill. Coping strategies might include a relaxation technique such as the setting cues used at the start of the pre-performance routine. Thus, if the athlete perceives that he/she is overaroused, a quick, efficient coping strategy can be employed to reestablish optimal physiological arousal levels. Finally, mind-clearing techniques to eradicate all thoughts about performance of the last skill can be employed. The athlete may use a technique such as centering (see Nideffer, 1986) to clear the mind and prepare the body for the next skill.

Between-performance routines

The between-performance routine is pertinent for athletes engaged in sports that take many hours to complete and are characterized by periods of inactivity. Thus, football players and basketball players sitting on the bench, golfers waiting for their next shot, and weather delays in tennis will challenge the ability to maintain optimal psychological and physiological readiness. This waiting during performance may induce a warm-up decrement (discussed earlier) and may also give the athlete additional time to worry about losing or performing badly. The between-play routine then is a strategy to use the time between performing effectively. Components of the between-play routine may take the form of attentional distraction techniques and psychological and physiological preparation strategies. Attentional distraction techniques could include imaging personal scenes or successful past performances. For example, the golfer waiting for an upcoming shot could image a private scene such as walking through an Alpine meadow or along a sandy beach. Other distraction strategies could be talking to fellow competitors and spectators, observing the scenery, and listening to music through earphones. Preparation strategies might include a physical warm-up, stretching and use of setting cues as discussed earlier.

CONCLUSION

Research examining the nature of pre-performance cognitions and physiological states has recently gained impetus. As the attentional phenomenon is multifaceted, it appears that a multidimensional assessment of pre-performance attentional states is likely to provide the most fruitful research strategy. Possible measures of attention include questionnaires, interviews, thought-sampling techniques, behavioural analysis, performance, EEG and cardiac activity. Once the mechanisms underlying attention are better understood, strategies to effectively increase athletes' attentional efficiency will more readily be developed.

REFERENCES

Adams, J. A. (1961). The second facet of forgetting: a review of warm-up decrement, *Psychological Bulletin*, **58**, 257–273.

Ainscoe, M. and Hardy, L. (1987). Cognitive warm-up in a cyclical gymnastics skill, *International Journal of Sport Psychology*, **18**, 269–275.

Anshel, M. H. (1985). The effect of arousal on warm-up decrement, *Research Quarterly for Exercise and Sport*, **56**, 1–9.

Anshel, M. H. and Wrisberg, C. A. (1988). The effect of arousal and focused attention on warm-up decrement, *Journal of Sport Behavior*, **11**, 18–31.

Baumeister, R. F. (1984). Choking under pressure: self-consciousness and paradoxical effects of incentives on skilful performance, *Journal of Personality and Social Psychology*, **46**, 610–620.

Bliss, C. B. (1895). Investigations in reaction time and attention, *Studies from the Yale Psychological Laboratory, 1892–1893*, **1**, 1–55.

Boder, D. P. (1935). The influence of concomitant activity and fatigue upon certain forms of reciprocal hand movement and its fundamental components, *Comparative Psychology Monographs*, **11**, No. 4.

Boutcher, S. H. and Crews, D. J. (1987). The effect of a preshot routine on a well-learned skill, *International Journal of Sport Psychology*, **18**, 30–39.

Boutcher, S. H. and Rotella, R. J. (1987). A psychological skills educational program for closed-skill performance enhancement, *The Sport Psychologist*, **1**, 127–137.

Boutcher, S. H. and Zinsser, N. (1990). Cardiac deceleration of elite and beginning golfers during putting, *Journal of Sport and Exercise Psychology.*, **12**, 37–47

Carver, C. S. and Scheier, M. F. (1978). Self-focusing effects of dispositional self-consciousness, mirror presence, and audience presence, *Journal of Personality and Social Psychology*, **36**, 324–332.

Carver, C. S. and Scheier M. F. (1981). *Attention and Self-Regulation*. New York: Springer-Verlag.

Caudill, D. and Weinberg, R. S. (1982). The effects of varying the length of the psych-up interval on motor performance, *Journal of Sport Behavior*, **6**, 86–90.

Caudill, D., Weinberg, R. and Jackson, A. (1983). Psyching-up and track athletes: a preliminary investigation, *Journal of Sport Psychology.* **5**, 231–235.

Crews, D. J. and Boutcher, S. H. (1986). The effects of structured preshot behaviors on beginning golf performance, *Perceptual and Motor Skills*, **62**, 291–294.

Crews, D. J. and Boutcher, S. H. (1987). An observational analysis of professional female golfers during tournament play, *Journal of Sport Behavior*, **9**, 51–58.

Duval, S. and Wicklund, R. A. (1972). *A Theory of Objective Self-Awareness*. New York: Academic Press.

Easterbrook, J. A. (1959). The effect of emotion on cue utilization and the organization of behavior, *Psychological Review*, **66**, 183–201.

Eysenck, H. J. (1956). 'Warm-up' in pursuit rotor learning as a function of the extinction of conditioned inhibition, *Acta Psychologica*, **12**, 349–370.

Fenz, W. D. (1975). Coping mechanisms and performance under stress, in D. M. Landers, D. V. Harris and R. W. Christinia (eds). *Psychology of Sport and Motor Behavior*. Penn State HPER Series: University Park, Pennsylvania.

Hardy, L. and Ringland, A. (1984). Mental training and the inner game, *Human Learning*, **3**, 203–207.

Hardy, L. and Wyatt, S. (1986). Immediate effects of imagery upon skilful motor performance, in D. G. Russell and D. Marks (eds), *Imagery 2: Proceedings of the*

Second International Imagery Conference. Dunedin, New Zealand: Human Performance Associates.

Hatfield, B. D., Landers, D. M. and Ray, W. J. (1984). Cognitive processes during self-paced motor performance: an electroencephalographic profile of skilled marksmen, *Journal of Sport Psychology*, **6**, 42–59.

Jones, J. G. and Hardy, L. (1988). The effects of anxiety upon psychomotor performance, *Journal of Sports Sciences*, **6**, 59–67.

Keele, S. W. (1973). *Attention and Human Performance*. Pacific Palisades, California: Goodyear.

Kimble, G. and Perlmuter, L. (1970). The problem of volition, *Psychological Review*, **77**, 361–384.

Kroll, W. (1982). Competitive athletic stress factors in athletes and coaches, in L. D. Zaichkowsky and W. E. Sime (eds). *Stress Management for Sport*. Reston, Virginia: The American Alliance for Health, Physical Education, Recreation, and Dance.

Lacey, B. B. and Lacey, J. I. (1970). Some autonomic–central nervous system interrelationships, in P. Black (ed.), *Physiological Correlates of Emotion*, New York: Academic Press.

Landers, D. M. (1978). Motivation and performance: The role of arousal and attentional factors, in W. F. Straub (ed.), *Sport Psychology. An Analysis of Athlete Behavior*, New York: Mouvement Publications.

Landers, D. M. (1981). Arousal, attention, and skilled performance: Further considerations, *Quest*, **33**, 271–283.

Landers, D. M., Christina, R., Hatfield, B. D., Daniels, F. S. and Doyle, L. A. (1980). Moving competitive shooting into the scientists' lab, *American Rifleman*, **128**, 36–37, 76–77.

Langer, E. J. and Imber, L. G. (1979). When practice makes imperfect: debilitating effects of overlearning, *Journal of Personality and Social Psychology*, **37**, 2014–2024.

Lobmeyer, D. L. and Wasserman, E. A. (1986). Preliminaries to free throw shooting: superstitious behavior, *Journal of Sport Behavior*, **11**, 70–78.

Nacson, J. and Schmidt, R. A. (1971). The activity-set hypothesis for warm-up decrement. *Journal of Motor Behavior*, **3**, 1–15.

Nideffer, R. M. (1986). Concentration and attention control training, in J. M. Williams (ed.). *Applied Sport Psychology*. Palo Alto, California: Mayfield.

Sarason, I. G. (1972). Experimental approaches to test anxiety: attention and the uses of information, in C. D. Spielberger (ed.). *Anxiety: Current Trends in Theory and Research*, Vol. 2. New York: Academic Press.

Scheier, M. S., Fenigstein, A. and Buss, A. H. (1974). Self-awareness and physical aggression, *Journal of Experimental Social Psychology*, **10**, 264–273.

Schmidt, R. A. (1988). *Motor Control and Learning*. Champaign, Illinois: Human Kinetics.

Schmidt R. A. and Nacson, J. (1971). Further tests of the activity–set hypothesis for warm-up decrement, *Journal of Experimental Psychology*, **90**, 56–64.

Schmidt, R. A. and Wrisberg, C. A. (1971). The activity–set hypothesis for warm-up decrement in a movement-speed task, *Journal of Motor Behavior*, **3**, 318–325.

Shelton, T. O. and Mahoney, M. J. (1978). The content and effect of 'psyching-up' strategies in weight lifters, *Cognitive Therapy and Research*, **2**, 275–284.

Solomon, J., Carello, C. and Turvey, M. T. (1984). Flow fields: the optical support for skilled activities, in W. Straub and J. Williams (eds). *Cognitive Sport Psychology*. New York: Sport Science Associates.

Stern, R. M. (1976). Reaction time and heart rate between the GET SET and GO of simulated races, *Psychophysiology*, **13**, 149–154.

Wang, M. Q. and Landers, D. M. (1990). Cardiac responses and hemispheric differ-
   entiation during archery performance: a psychophysiological investigation of
   attention. Manuscript submitted for publication.
Weinberg, R. S., Gould, D. and Jackson A. (1981). Cognition and motor performance:
   effect of psyching-up strategies on three motor tasks, *Cognitive Therapy and
   Research,* **4**, 239–245.
Wine, J. (1971). Test anxiety and direction of attention, *Psychological Bulletin,* **76**,
   92–104.

Chapter 10

Stress in sport: experiences of some elite performers

J. Graham Jones and Lew Hardy
Loughborough University and University of Wales, Bangor

This chapter describes a series of interviews conducted with elite athletes which enquired about their experiences of stress in sport. The rationale for such a chapter is twofold. First, a criticism which has occasionally been levelled at sport scientists, particularly from the perhaps more practically orientated fraternity, is that they do not always make stringent efforts to apply findings from theoretically driven research. Consequently, in adopting a case study approach, this chapter represents an attempt to investigate the practical application of many of the theoretical issues addressed in the previous chapters. Secondly, both Martens (1987) and Gould and Krane (in press) have commented on the almost over-reliance on quantitative information in the pursuit of an understanding of the competitive state anxiety response and its relationship with sports performance. While recognizing the importance of the quantitative approach in this area, Gould and Krane emphasized the strengths of in-depth interviews with athletes and advocated that anxiety–performance researchers, in particular, should seriously consider such an approach.

Six past or present top-level athletes were interviewed; brief profiles of the athletes are presented below:

Name: Steve Backley
Sport: Javelin
Born: 12 February 1969
   1989 World Cup, Europa Cup and World Student Games Champion
   1989 Grand Prix Event (Javelin) winner—third overall
   1989 British Sports Writers' Athlete of the Year
   1990 Commonwealth Games Gold Medal winner and World Record holder

Stress and Performance in Sport. Edited by J. Graham Jones and Lew Hardy.
©1990 John Wiley & Sons Ltd.

Name: Sue Challis (formerly Shotton)
Sport: Trampolining
Born: 11 August 1965
    British Ladies Champion in 1980, 1981, 1982, 1984, 1985 and 1987
    1983 European Champion
    1984 World Champion
    Second in 1989 European Championships
    Fourth in 1988 World Championships

Name: Alan Edge
Sport: Canoe slalom
Born: 27 April 1954
    Current British Canoe Union National Coach for canoe slalom
    Member of the British team for 10 years
    Placed eighth in the 1975 World Championships (the highest place then
    achieved by a Briton)
    Member of the Great Britain 1979 World Championship winning team

Name: David Hemery
Sport: 400 metre hurdling
Born: 18 July 1944
    Commonwealth Games high hurdles champion in 1966 and 1970
    Olympic Games Gold Medal winner and World Record holder in the 400
    metres hurdles in 1968
    Olympic Games Silver Medal winner in the 4×400 metres hurdles in 1972
    Olympic Games Bronze Medal winner in the 400 metres hurdles in 1972
    Winner of British Superstars in 1973 and 1976 and Past Masters champion
    in 1983

Name: James May
Sport: Gymnastics
Born: 30 January 1968
    Thames television Junior Gymnast of the Year 1983
    British Men's Champion 1989
    Placed fourth in the Individual Apparatus Vault Final at the European
    Championships in 1989
    Placed twenty-seventh in the Men's All-Round Apparatus Championships
    at the World Championships in 1989, highest scorer in the British team
    which was placed thirteenth, the best placing ever achieved by a British
    team
    Gold Medal winner in the Men's Individual Apparatus Vault Final at the
    Commonwealth Games in 1990. Also, Silver Medal winner in the Men's
    Individual Apparatus Rings Final, Bronze Medal winner in the Men's

Individual Apparatus Pommels Final and Bronze Medal winner in the men's All-Round Apparatus Final

Name: Mary Nevill
Sport: Hockey
Born: 12 March 1961
  Captain of Great Britain
  Member of Great Britain Olympic team in 1988
  Member of England team which achieved fifth place in the 1987 World
    Cup, second place in the 1987 European Cup and fourth place in the
    1990 World Cup.

Each interview followed a standardized format in which the athlete responded to identical sequences of questions which were phrased in such a way as to encourage truly open-ended responses. Specific clarification and elaboration probes were also used (cf. Patton, 1980; Scanlan, Ravizza and Stein, 1989; Scanlan, Stein and Ravizza, 1989). The length of the interviews ranged from one and a half to two and a half hours. The content of the interview questions was designed to focus upon the central issues raised in the previous chapters, and related to the general areas of:

—the athletes' perceptions of how big a factor stress was for them in their
  sport;
—the athletes' perceptions and experiences of stress, and its effects, during the
  pre-competition and performance periods;
—the psychological skills and strategies used by the athletes, particularly those
  relating to goal setting, relaxation, imagery and performance routines;
—the athletes' use of concentration and simulation training;
—the athletes' confidence in their ability to perform under the stress of
  competition.

THE ATHLETES' PERCEPTIONS OF HOW BIG A FACTOR STRESS WAS FOR THEM

This section represented a very general enquiry into how large a factor the athletes perceived stress to be in their sport. Evidence discussed by Jones (Chapter 2 in this book) suggested that stress responses are likely to be strongly influenced by a complex interaction between the individual and task by situation demands. Furthermore, other authors also indicated that stress could be either a positive or a negative experience, both in terms of the actual response and its effects upon performance (Parfitt, Jones and Hardy, Chapter 3; Hardy, Chapter 4; and Kerr, Chapter 5 in this book).

Five of the six athletes reported that stress was a large or very large factor in their sport, while Mary Nevill described it as a moderate factor: 'I feel that I can cope with the stress which is imposed on me. Sometimes you get close to the point of not coping, but I feel that as long as I am coping with it I would say it is a moderate factor'. However, Mary did say that there had been instances when she had felt under real pressure and worried about whether she would be able to cope.

Sue Challis reported becoming very anxious and even tearful when feeling under intense pressure. Her perception of stress appeared to be closely linked to her level of confidence, which, to a large extent, she attributed to how well her training was progressing at the time. Sue felt that if training was not going well before a competition then her confidence was reduced and the stress she felt was infinitely bigger, increasing to a point at which she was unsure of her ability to handle it. Conversely, when she was happy with her performance in training, her confidence was high and she felt both physically and mentally prepared: 'When I'm prepared, it (the stress) is positive, and when I'm not prepared it's negative'. She emphasized the fact that, in trampolining, the performer only gets one chance: 'In trampolining you've got to do 10 moves. You do as many straight bounces as you want to start with, and then you do 10 consecutive skills and are judged on those. You can't afford to make a mistake. . . it's about desperately trying to get into 18 seconds the perfection you've been trying to achieve for so many years'.

David Hemery stated that any stress he experienced was self-imposed. Interestingly, he reported feeling under stress both in training and in the competition environment. His experience of stress appeared to be a function of the high expectations he imposed upon himself and of the nature of the event itself. This view was echoed by Sue Challis. Both commented that if one is trying to get the absolute best out of oneself, and at the same time has a very realistic chance of being the best in the world, then the stress is enormous. They were also very conscious of the fact that a considerable amount of effort and hard work over a period of months culminated in a performance of very short duration; an awful lot could go wrong in a matter of a few seconds.

Alan Edge attributed the stress he experienced not only to competitive factors in the environment but also to the uncertainty of the conditions of the river: 'You never know what it is going to be like until within an hour of the competition'. Alan also pointed out several other sources of stress which slalom canoeing possesses. As in skiing, slalom canoeists have to work out how to paddle the course without being able to actually try any of the moves out. The course, therefore, represents a series of complex problems which have to be solved one after the other. Consequently, performers have to resist the temptation to change the way they are going to paddle the course because of other paddlers' results. They can be distracted from their plan if they have to make an unexpected adjustment early on and, during the latter part of the run, they can be distracted into trying to protect their earlier success, or even trying to better it, if the first part of the run has gone 'clean' (i.e. the paddler has not incurred any penalty points for touching gates).

James May identified that 'doing justice to yourself' when performing in front of an audience was a potential source of stress which could be positive or negative. Other sources of negative stress included niggles about minor injuries or physical weaknesses, and moves which he was not quite 100 per cent certain about. He reported that, in team events, the responsibility of being part of a team could also be stressful. Finally, like Alan Edge, James recognized that even if things were going really well, thoughts like 'I could be on to a really good score here if I go through this routine' were potential sources of stress, as were similarly ill-considered comments from coaches or parents (although he had never personally experienced any such comments from his parents).

Steve Backley described stress as a huge but very necessary factor. He viewed it as a very positive factor and estimated that it improved his performance by at least 10 per cent in competition as compared to in training: 'I never think of stress as a negative thing . . . I think that as soon as you admit to stress being a negative factor then it will be'. Steve even described instances in recent events when he had felt that he was not sufficiently stressed and deliberately tried to impose stress upon himself: he associated stress with a high level of physiological arousal which made him feel stronger and more alert.

All of the athletes emphasized the importance of 'being in control'. Steve Backley, for example, needed to feel highly aroused but still in control of himself and the environment. Sue Challis said that when nearing a competition you must have the confidence that you can cope with or control the stress. Similarly, David Hemery commented that his performance 'very much depended on having the stress of competition under control'.

These responses clearly indicate the importance of stress in sport, at least at the highest levels of participation. They also emphasize the importance of self-confidence and the perception of control in mediating the experience of stress (cf. Bandura, 1977: Fisher, 1984). As expected, stress was not necessarily perceived to be a negative phenomenon (see Jones, Chapter 2; Parfitt, Jones and Hardy, Chapter 3; Hardy, Chapter 4; and Kerr, Chapter 5 in this book). On the contrary, several athletes reported that stress could be a very positive factor, for example, Steve Backley and James May. The nature of the particular performance and the environment in which it was performed emerged as important factors in the experience of stress, thus supporting the proposals of earlier chapters (see particularly Jones, Chapter 2 in this book).

THE ATHLETES' PERCEPTIONS AND EXPERIENCES OF STRESS, AND ITS EFFECTS, DURING THE PRE-COMPETITION AND PERFORMANCE PERIODS

Pre-competition

The questions in this section of the interview asked the athletes to relate their experiences of stress during training and the period leading up to competition. Particular emphasis was placed on ascertaining whether stress was perceived positively or negatively (Jones, Chapter, 2; Parfitt, Jones and Hardy, Chapter 3; Hardy, Chapter 4; and Kerr, Chapter 5 in this book), the antecedents of stress (Parfitt, Jones and Hardy, Chapter 3 in this book) and the symptoms experienced (Parfitt, Jones and Hardy, Chapter 3; Hardy, Chapter 4; and Kerr, Chapter 5 in this book).

Steve Backley stated that he always looked forward to the competition and described the pre-competition stress that he experienced as nearly always being positive. It became clear that he needed to be able to impose stress upon himself in order to reach an appropriate state of readiness. Steve actually referred to a couple of major competitions during the past few months prior to which he had not felt sufficiently stressed. His strategy for inducing increased stress is to visualize himself in situations such as lying second in the last round with one throw left to win the competition. As the competition gets closer, 'these short bursts of stress (through visualization) get longer and stronger'. His level of physiological arousal builds up during the days preceding competition and he experiences very strong physiological changes on the competition day which reach a peak within two or three hours of the warm-up: 'I'm off to the toilet every 10 minutes, and I'm very active and chattering away'. However, Steve further reported experiencing 'a kind of release as soon as I start warming up'.

Sue Challis also reported using visualization as a means of simulating the stress of competition during training. This is clearly effective, at least in terms of inducing the stress response, as she reported experiencing nerves and mild panic during some of her training sessions. However, these experiences varied as a function of her progress in training. If her perceptions of her training performance were positive, then 'there's just excitement'; if her perceptions were negative, then her thoughts were that time was running out and that she would not be ready for the competition. Sue described symptoms such as loss of appetite and problems with sleeping during her pre-competition build-up. She also reported being mentally exhausted, largely through worrying about failing. She said that she could start worrying up to three months before a major competition, especially if she perceived that training was not going well. In the context of a less important competition such thoughts did not generally occur until a week to 10 days prior to it, but this varied: 'On a good run-up to a competition, if I suffer (from panic) a week beforehand then I'm alright from then on in—it gets better towards the day; on a bad run-up it might not hit me until the night before, which is obviously the worst thing that can happen. I think, in a way, I bring it on myself to get it over with, to get used to the idea, so I can then just cope with it. You hit rock bottom, then it's just got to go upwards'. Sue's physical symptoms seemed to follow the same pattern as her mental symptoms: 'I think the physical symptoms are a result of the mental worry'.

David Hemery reported that seeing his race opponents just prior to a race was a source of stress. Reading, or being informed, about impressive performances by opponents and then seeing them 'looking good' during warm-up induced feelings of stress in him. David much preferred to focus on himself at this period. In training, he deliberately created stress in himself by visualizing his races so that he felt able to cope with the stress when the time arrived. In fact, his visualization was so vivid that he reported being able to increase both his respiration and his heart rate to near race levels when he visualized races. Physiological symptoms which he experienced included shortness of breath, sweaty fingertips and churning stomach. Interestingly, these physiological symptoms were not always preceded by conscious cognitions about the race. David stated that: 'I would suddenly find that my pulse rate went up and then become conscious that my unconscious had been working on the race . . . there was certainly a prior initiative from a subconscious level, not prompted that I am aware of by any external thing'.

Mary Nevill identified her amateur status as being a source of some pre-competition stress: '. . . Trying to get organized to leave home home for a competition when I've got a job, I've got to do all the other things in life and I've also got to get away for a major international tournament and be well prepared and supposedly rested for it. That is a major factor. There is just not enough time to fit everything in, in terms of preparation for the competition'. Mary saw these factors, together with the attention of the media, as inducing negative stress. She reported being slightly nervous just prior to a match but also excited at the prospect of playing so that any tension which she experienced was relatively pleasant. She reported this as positive stress. Specific symptoms were the common ones of tight stomach and butterflies; however, these were accompanied by feelings of liveliness, sharpness and a readiness to perform. Mary indicated that she does not normally worry about a game. Instead, she concentrates on mentally rehearsing skills, etc., and generally thinking positively. Mary also stated that the bigger and more important the match the more excited and better she feels, and the more she wants to play.

Like Mary Nevill, Alan Edge also identified his amateur status as being important in his experience of stress during the pre-competition period. During the early stages of preparation he found that it was difficult to make time to prepare for events as he would have liked to have done. However, as the competition drew near, Alan used his job to help 'take his mind off the event'. During the period immediately prior to competing he reported that he 'always felt a definite sensation of an easing of stress on the word 'go' . . . Before that . . . in the final five minutes approaching the start I would feel calm and collected and more in control than I did half an hour before. It was always very gratifying . . . and I used to wait for it'.

James May reported that he did experience stress prior to major competitions, but that he generally regarded this as useful since it helped him to get prepared for the competition. However, two situations that he did find had a negative effect on him were losing training time through injury and having problems with a routine during the run-in to competition: 'If you have constructed a routine and it's going badly, even when you have had a day off, then it's going to be a stressful type of activity. You are not going through your routine, and it's getting nearer, and it's almost certainly going to get worse. . . I'm sure it is! My philosophy now is that you have got to be solid in your routines a long time before the competition. If you can't go out and do your 12 routines, you defeat the whole object of going'. The symptoms James reported from this sort of stress were cognitive rather than somatic: 'I don't get any physical reaction, it's more in the mind. If you go to that apparatus and think "I've got to get this move because it's not going well", it's always jumping into your mind. If you have got that sort of move then it makes the whole of the rest of the routine go badly as well'. He attributed the infectious properties of such problem moves to focusing too much attention on the move. James stated that he did experience physiological symptoms nearer to the competition, particularly when he first arrived at the training venue for a competition, or at the arena itself. For a big competition, this could be as much as one week before the actual event. To combat this nervousness, James reported that he usually went through a training session doing only those moves on which he felt completely safe. Sometimes, these moves would not even be from the routines he was going to perform in the competition.

One of the major factors to emerge from this section of the interview was that the athletes perceived pre-competition stress to have both negative and positive potential. All of the athletes indicated that they tried to perceive the stress in a positive way, and at least two of them indicated that they interpreted the felt arousal almost as excitement, thus providing some support for Kerr's (Chapter 5) proposal that interpretation of felt arousal is an important determinant of performance. Another factor to emerge was the athletes' need to simulate the stress of competition before actually encountering it (see Jones, Chapter 2; Burton, Chapter 7; Mace, Chapter 8; and Boutcher, Chapter 9 in this book), mainly through some form of visualization technique. The symptoms of anxiety discussed by Parfitt, Jones and Hardy (Chapter 3 in this book) and Hardy (Chapter 4 in this book) seemed to vary a little between the athletes, although nearly all of them reported a strong increase in their physiological response on the day of competition. The early peaking of anxiety in expert performers reported by Fenz (1975) and Mahoney and Avener (1977) was alluded to by several of the performers, notably Alan Edge, Steve Backley and Sue Challis. The athletes' cognitions about upcoming events suggested that they could experience both intense worry and anticipatory excitement during the weeks or days preceding competition, thus supporting the orthogonality of positive and negative stress states (see Hardy and Whitehead, 1984; Parfitt, Jones and Hardy, Chapter 3 in this book; Thayer, 1978). This would also appear to support Parfitt, Jones and Hardy's (Chapter 3 in this book) and Burton's (Chapter 7 in this book) proposals that the intensity measure of 'anxiety' symptoms (as measured, for example, by Martens et al.'s (1990) Competitive State Anxiety Inventory-2) is rather limited and that performers' perceptions (i.e. direction; see Jones, in press; Parfitt, Jones and Hardy, Chapter 3 in this book) of those symptoms should also be measured.

During performance

This section also enquired about the athletes' experiences of stress, but this time the questions related to during performance rather than prior to performance. Of particular interest were responses to questions which focused upon Jones' (Chapter 2 in this book) and Parfitt, Jones and Hardy's (Chapter 3 in this book) discussion of stress effects upon the different subcomponents of performance.

David Hemery reported that he experienced stress whenever he heard or saw another runner just behind him during a race. He described one such experience during a heat in which he was judging his race so as just to qualify: 'As I cleared the last hurdle with only one man ahead of me and four to go through, looking to my right, a yard behind me were three runners. I almost caught the front bloke up in the last 50 metres, and he was eight yards ahead of me at the time!' Later in the interview, David also described a similar experience during his 1968 Olympic Gold Medal winning run: 'At the eighth hurdle I thought "I don't know if I can maintain this pace". But the instant overthought was "This is the Olympic final, you can't ease down". The next second I heard a step in water to my left. I don't know how far back it was, but I heard it close enough that I believe that I got another shot of adrenaline and I was again running scared'. David finished the race eight yards clear of the second placed runner.

As mentioned earlier, James May commented that being a member of a team was a potential source of stress during a competition. In team events in gymnastics the team's worst score on each piece is discounted, so each team can afford only one mistake per piece if they want to do well. Consequently, 'If the first gymnast gets up on the pommel horse (say) and goes through a clean routine, then it really does set everyone up to do the same. If the first one falls off, then it's tough for the next one because there is far more pressure to produce the team performance'. James interpreted the nervousness he experiences before he performs as positive, provided that he controls it: 'I usually compete slightly better than I have trained'. When asked to describe his nervousness in a little more detail, he replied, 'It comes upon me like a wave through my body and, at that stage, I would be slightly shaky, with a little bit of sweat on my palms and maybe on my feet too. When I go on the floor area you will see me squatting with my hands on the mat so that I can get used to the feel of the mat. It also gets the sweat off my hands and the same with my feet, just to control myself a bit more and make sure it doesn't overtake me. On floor, it usually does help because that bit of tension seems to produce an extra little bit of lift for the tumbles'. James also thought that controlled nervousness could help him achieve more lift, and therefore more time, on vault. However, he did not think that nervousness was always an advantage, particularly if it was not properly controlled. For example, on the pommel horse, 'If you are very nervous, then your body tightens up and pikes. Of course, that brings your feet closer to the horse on every circle, and your hips closer to the handles, and you are off before you know it'.

Steve Backley said that he builds himself for his first throw and 'if the first throw goes well then every time I'll just drop off. I'll just relax and be lethargic. My blinkers come off and I just watch everything around me'. He identified one source of stress as being in a winning position and then someone bettering his throw. He recounted one incident in Budapest in 1989 when he had thrown what he thought would be a winning distance in the third round: 'I took my boots off, put my track suit on and relaxed'. In the final (sixth) round a Russian threw further but Steve reported that this stress was a very positive influence upon him which spurred him to a better, winning final throw. He emphasized the fact that he finds this sort of stress a positive influence which makes him stronger and more alert. He continued by contrasting his performances in training and in competition: 'In a training session, with very low stress and arousal, I can't do a run-up and throw. I can't use my competition run-up because I'm not tall enough or fast enough to hold the positions that I need to do a technically good throw . . . I'll always crash in a low position. In training, because the arousal is not there, my physical and mental abilities are reduced. . . I can't see what I'm supposed to do as clearly because when I am highly stressed I can see things much more clearly'.

Sue Challis stated that there was very little time to think while she was performing her moves on the trampoline. However, if she performed a move which went wrong she could 'feel a tightening up, an electric shock-type feeling from my stomach up towards my head. But I don't lose my head when I'm actually performing. I get that shot of adrenaline but in a way it calms me down to actually try and concentrate harder and really work on one move to recover and to make the rest even better in order to make up for my mistake'. She also reported working herself up into a frenzy just before her first move: 'It gets to a stage where the pressure is so great that you lose the sense of reality and think "oh, well, I'll go", and just do it'. In terms of her performance, Sue felt that intense stress could negatively affect her timing but, on other occasions, 'a burst of adrenaline can actually make you quite a lot stronger'. Interestingly, she commented that 'the worst time is often when a routine is going well. . . say I've done eight moves and nothing has gone wrong, and I'm thinking "I mustn't do anything wrong now, I must hold on". Then I tend to, rather than let loose and do a really good one, tighten up and not dare to quite commit it, in case I commit it wrongly. . . so I tend to back off a bit'.

One of the biggest experiences of stress which Alan Edge could recall was in between the first and second runs during his team's winning performance in the 1979 World Championships. One of the British team, Richard Fox, had already won the individual event with clean runs. Alan was anchor man in the team (the most stressful position), which had recorded the fastest time on the first run but had incurred penalty points for four touches, all of them credited to Alan. After the first run the coach had told them 'if they didn't win the gold they had blown it'. There were two and a half hours to the next run. Alan commented, 'I was thinking "This is it . . . we've never won the team championship. We've always threatened to do it . . . this guy who's coaching us is one of the guys who threatened to but never did it". Foxy was saying "Is God going to give me five clean runs?". . . I remember feeling that it was a big weight to carry'.

Mary Nevill's experiences of stress during performance were mainly in games which were slipping away from her team and without knowing how to prevent it. Characteristic of these situations were 'frustrations that something's going wrong, that we don't seem to be able to put it right. Sometimes, you just can't see what's going wrong, and even if you think you can see what's going wrong, you can't communicate to 11 people at once without getting together, and there's only a limited number of times when you can get together in a team. . . Also, people forget immediately what you say to them in that sort of situation. They've got so many other things to think about'. She identified a succession of penalty corners against her team as also being a source of some stress: 'There is a sort of inevitability about it. If a team has four or five penalty corners in succession then there is a fair chance that they will score off one of them'. Mary stated that positive stress is usually a positive influence on her performance, increasing both her work rate and aggression. She referred to instances when 'everything flows. I suppose everything feels relatively easy; work rate and skills go well and you don't make many mistakes on the ball'. However, she also reported that negative stress, arising largely from trying to combine the pressures of a demanding job with an international hockey career, could negatively affect her performance if she arrived at a competition physically and mentally exhausted.

These responses clearly demonstrate that stress can have specific effects on different subcomponents of performance. Moreover, the proposals of Jones (Chapter 2 in this book) and Parfitt, Jones and Hardy (Chapter 3 in this book) that stress can have both positive and negative effects depending on the precise nature of the performance subcomponent also received support from the athletes' statements. This is perhaps best epitomized by James May's perception of high physiological arousal having a negative effect on some aspects of gymnastics performance (e.g. interfering with the fine movement control required for performance on the pommel horse) and a positive effect on other aspects (e.g. enhanced 'lift' for tumbling and vaulting). The general consensus appeared to be that controlled cognitive anxiety enhanced perform-ance on well-learned tasks and that the increased physiological arousal associated with increased stress enhanced performance on skills requiring speed and strength, but was detrimental to performance in skills requiring fine movements and timing (cf. Jones and Cale, 1989; Parfitt and Hardy, 1987).

PSYCHOLOGICAL SKILLS AND STRATEGIES USED BY THE ATHLETES

Goal setting

Goal setting is viewed as an important technique for the enhancement of both motivation and self-confidence in sport (Beggs, Chapter 6 in this book; Locke and Latham, 1985). The interview questions which related to goal setting specifically asked whether the athletes set goals, why they set them, what types of goals they set and how difficult those goals were.

During his interview, Alan Edge clearly indicated that he used goal setting a great deal during his preparation for races. He reported using a countdown method of structuring his training for World Championships every two years. It was apparent from Alan's interview that his training goals were quite tightly structured and evaluated in terms of period of the year, race experience and the intensity of white water racing (on rapids) required. Alan also reported having a very detailed race plan, with a plan B and even a plan C on occasions, to adjust for mistakes. These plans included very precisely formu-lated process-oriented goals about how he wanted to prepare for and paddle each race. Nevertheless, Alan was quite critical of his evaluation of goal achievement, both in races and in training. In particular, he felt that he did not evaluate the reasons behind his race successes, or the quality of the white water (rapids) on which he trained, as effectively as he might have done. He concluded this section of the interview with: 'We didn't evaluate too well really. We had a rigid format of strength weight training, endurance-based (work) with some quality (work) tied into it, and then a date when you got back in your slalom boat . . . quite crude really. I was (recently) sent a training schedule of goals and performance objectives from a guy who is not even in the Junior (National) Squad, and it made the stuff I was doing when I was in the team look quite poor'.

Mary Neville reported a long-term goal which was to win a medal at the 1992 Olympics. Her shorter-term goals included 'certain imaginary standards of performance which I wish to reach, and I'm not satisfied if I don't make that, and that level might change depending on how I'm playing at the time'. The sorts of goals that she sets for matches include stick-stopping every single penalty corner: 'I would allow myself the leeway of missing one but I'd be very dissatisfied if I missed more than one'. Mary also gets herself goals in terms of maintaining certain work rates during games. She saw goal setting as an important means of enhancing motivation ('Having a long-term goal keeps you going through the difficult times') and confidence ('If you do things well in the game which you planned to do it definitely improves your confidence'). She emphasized the importance of the goals which she sets for herself being difficult but obtainable. Mary also set goals in training: 'If we're practising penalty corners I would want to be stopping nine out of ten. Also, working as a team, we have a full defence and full attack working on penalty corners. Our attack sets targets of how many we will get on target and how many goals we'll score, while the defence also sets targets'.

James May said that he set goals in both training and competition. However, he explained that it is difficult to set objective goals, such as a certain score, for competitions because of the variability in judging standard: 'So normally I would say I can't expect to do better than my average performance in training. So that is the sort of thing I would set, and if it happens that two or three of the performances are better than this because of the competition, then that is a plus'. In training, James structured his goals in conjunction with his coaches. These were directed towards the next Olympic Games in 1992, which was two and a half years away at the time of the interview. Although James' training goals were quite specific and detailed, an important feature of them was that they also allowed him some flexibility: 'I know that a programme for myself would need to be flexible, because you just don't feel like it some days. There is nothing worse than really feeling like not doing something and the coach saying "Well, this is **the** programme, you've got to do it!" '. It became clear during the interview that this flexibility also extended to competition goals, but only to the extent that he would adjust routines which were not going particularly well during the lead-up so that he could retain the competition goal of performing them 'clean'.

Goal setting was a very important part of David Hemery's preparation for life in general rather than just for his races. He reported using outcome goals, performance improvement goals and process-oriented goals from a very early age. For races and training these were very carefully structured and precisely formulated in conjunction with his coach, Billy Smith: 'He actually thought I knew what was right. I knew that what he said was right! Every touchdown time and every hurdle was known by me, and if he said 'I want you to run this time', I could run within a tenth of a second or even spot on, every time. I knew that the touchdown for the first hurdle had to be 6.1 or 6.2 (seconds), the second hurdle would be 10.2, and so on through the whole thing. In the early season I couldn't run the whole race at the 48 second pace, but I could get to hurdle seven at the pace I wanted to run the race at by the end of the year. So I would be aiming for 30.7 at the seventh hurdle, and the workout would be to run twice to get to there as close as I could to 30.7. Then we would stride a 600 metres for the over-distance work. So it was very, very structured'. Later on in the interview David described his training diaries: 'Every day I would have the temperature, the time, the session and what I did in it. I would star it if it was the next step up, averaging the times if there were multiple repetitions to see if there was a progression, always to see if there was a progression. So my own evaluation was extremely important to me in that the progression was towards an ultimate self-improvement'. During races the goal was to execute the race plan, which was structured in exactly the same amount of detail as the training goals, with paces specified for each section of the race. It is an interesting testimony to how well rehearsed all these goals were that David could still quote them 20 years after the event.

Steve Backley reported setting very short-term goals but not in any structured way. In fact, he said that goal setting was not something which he felt he particularly focused on during the pre-competition or competition periods: 'I think very, very short term . . . just to win. The goals that I set are to throw well tomorrow, that's as far as I think. Tomorrow's (training) session would be the immediate goal.' When asked about his goals for a training session, he replied that he had a process-oriented goal of 'just trying to be technically proficient in the throw. It would always be something technical . . . I might want to feel a driving across the ground as I'm throwing rather than block and throw . . . I want to throw technically proficiently, and I want my coach to say "You look sharp" to make me feel as if I'm improving'. Rather surprisingly, Steve was quite definite that long-term goals did not figure strongly in his preparation: 'I could say that I want to win the Gold Medal at the (1992) Olympics in Barcelona, but it doesn't really hold for me in that it's not a very strong sort of feeling that I really desire. . . I do want to be Olympic Champion, but I'll never use that as a goal psychologically . . . I would never use it as a goal to improve my performance, only something technical'.

Sue Challis said that she did not set goals for herself before 1982 'and I think it was a mistake'. She has used goal setting since then in both training and competition. She plans her training goals from day to day and 'sometimes writes them down'. These goals are process-oriented in that she will work on specific aspects of moves. Sue's goals during competition may change according to how her close rivals are performing: 'If a close rival has done a good routine before me then my goal may alter in that rather than just trying to go and do a steady routine to the best of my ability, I might be thinking "I've got to go and jump out of my skin now" '. She does not set herself targets in terms of points as 'that would be silly because you've got five judges and you don't know how they're going to mark'. Like Mary Nevill, Sue believed in setting goals which were difficult but realistic.

Goal setting was, therefore, clearly an important aspect of the athletes' preparation, although the nature of the goal setting varied. For example, David Hemery's goal-setting programme was very structured and detailed while James May's was very flexible. The athletes generally set themselves both process- and product-oriented goals, although it would be fair to say that goals for competition were generally process-oriented. All of them agreed that any goals that they set should be difficult but realistic (cf. Beggs, Chapter 6 in this book; Locke and Latham, 1985).

Relaxation

Research has shown that one of the important factors which distinguishes elite performers from less skilful performers is their ability to control their anxiety at crucial moments (Fenz, 1975; Mahoney and Avener, 1977). This finding was reinforced by the present interviews, reports from which have already indicated the great significance that the athletes attached to being able to control any stress that they experienced. This section of the interview focused on the anxiety control techniques used by the athletes and the particular circumstances in which they used them (see Burton, Chapter 7 and Mace, Chapter 8 in this book).

James May stated that he used relaxation to compose himself if his nervousness started to get out of control: 'The relaxation technique that I have adopted over the past year is a mantra-type. I count down from three to zero and when I get to zero I can produce a calmer approach. I use that (say) if I have got to stand there and wait around for the judges and I feel a rush of nervousness that's too much'. James reported that he chose this technique because it seemed right for him. He indicated that he did not practise it as a separate part of his training, but did practise it whenever opportunities arose naturally during training. For example, he explained that earlier in the year, when he first started working his high bar routine away from the pitted gym and above a hard floor, he had a 'certain amount of anxiety due to the fact that if you miss (the bar) it's not a controlled landing. I always know I can cope with falling off, but there was still a bit of anxiety there and when I went to jump up I always seemed to feel nervous about that fact. So I certainly used it (relaxation) then, and it just lowered me down that little bit to where I could attack the routine without being over the top'.

Steve Backley said that he uses relaxation but not as a means of coping with stress. He uses it mainly as a means of 'clearing and preparing' his mind for visualization and uses it before important training sessions. He described the process as follows: 'Basically, breathing techniques for relaxation over 5–10 minutes. It's about trying to clear your mind rather than put stuff into it. Then it's the 'control room' which for me would be the Loughborough track. I actually watch myself walk out of my room, walk down to the track, see everyone, walk into the pavilion, be in control, carry my javelins and boots, walk out on to the track, stretch and go through my warm-up drills. I'm there. I'm relaxed and in control. Then I'm on to the run-up and I go through what I would do during a throwing session, purely from the point of view of becoming more proficient technically'. Steve uses his breathing technique during the competition: '. . . say up to 30 seconds before I throw, but only if I feel I need it. It's not a ritual; two deep breaths and I'm clear of everything. My mind's clear and I'm ready for the throw. That's about as far as it goes during performance and competition'. Interestingly, however, 'it would usually be because I was underaroused, if I needed perking up. So it's not really a relaxation technique'. Clearly, Steve saw the breathing technique as about quieting the mind or about achieving an appropriate mental state.

David Hemery also used breathing as a means of slowing his pulse rate down just prior to a race: 'The intention was not to waste energy and I managed to do that under what was great stress (just prior to the start of the Olympic final in 1968), with about eight people in a little (waiting) room and a bench in the middle. I lay on the bench and the others started jogging around, while I just stayed there, because that was what my plan was, trying to bring my pulse rate down'. He added 'At will, I tend to be able to relax the whole body without going through the progressive bits. If I just think about that goal I can let all the muscles go . . . I don't really know where I got it from. It was intuitively the right thing to do pre-competition'. David went on to indicate that he practised this relaxation strategy as a natural part of his mental rehearsal of a race plan (see later section on visualization) rather than as a separate part of his training. David also reported using an imagery-based dissociation strategy to control his anxiety when the presence of another runner impinged upon his preparation: 'I was on the practice track watching Jeff Vanderstock who was the expected winner of the (1968 Olympic) Games. He did a start out of the blocks and I felt my throat constrict and recognized that my mind was on him, and I knew that I could not control how fast he ran and that I had to come back inside myself. I left my shoes and spikes on the side and used the in-field to simulate going back to my very early training days where I had been in the situation of running on very firm sand at the low water's edge. I just ran down the field imagining the feeling that I had at that stage, with the sun on my back, feeling the warmth, the power, the strength, the fluidity of flow, and recalling this one day when I had run on the beach. I had no idea how far it was . . . I just kept running and running, lifting up faster and faster, and there didn't seem to be any fatigue. It was just an unbelievable flowing feeling that went on and on and on over hundreds of yards. Eventually I slowed down and jogged back. It was enough to come back into my senses, of what it felt like to be strong and flowing . . . it took my awareness back inside. By the time I had done that I was back inside me and Jeff Vanderstock could do his own thing'.

Sue Challis stated that she uses relaxation techniques 'all the time' during the pre-competition period, but that 'it's not a deliberate "now I'm going to sit down and relax for 10 minutes". It's much more innate. When I went to university I discovered that I was doing lots of things that have got names but I wasn't aware of it. I was just trying to prepare myself for the competition and it can be right the way through the complete build-up for the competition, all through training and to the competition. I do it whenever I think it's necessary. But it's not a deliberate thing'. When asked what she actually did, Sue replied: 'I visualize myself doing whatever move it is easily and with good rhythm and no panic, so it's very slow and rhythmical. I think back to when things have been going really well, like really high moments in my trampolining career, and I think about how I felt then and try and feel like that again so it fills me with confidence and ease and that hopefully relaxes me. Sometimes I just switch off for a couple of minutes and think "OK, I'm just going to sleep for a couple of minutes", or whatever, where the intention is not to think about it because my tendency is to go over and over everything in my mind all the time'. Interestingly, she stated that she does not 'try and get rid of the physical symptoms. I think they take care of themselves if your mind is right'. Sue's strategy just before performing is to 'adjust my adrenaline by walking at different speeds. Walking is very good because if you feel that you're getting a little too anxious you can just walk very slowly'.

Mary Nevill said that she does not use relaxation during the pre-competition period but does during a match. She does this by relaxing her shoulders by 'just dropping them' and taking a deep breath. Mary usually tries to relax before stick-stopping a penalty corner, a time when she feels some pressure on her: 'It would just be a moment to physically relax, and also I think I just need a quiet moment to prepare myself for a very important event. If I miss that stop we could lose a goal because you have quite a fair chance of scoring off a penalty corner'. She occasionally practises this during training and feels it helps: 'If I go into it without any forethought I think there is more chance of me missing (the stop) than there is if I just take a moment or two to relax before the next one'.

Finally, Alan Edge reported three strategies that he used as a means of relaxing prior to big events. As has already been mentioned, during the weeks prior to important competitions, Alan used his teaching job as a way of taking his mind off the event. On the day of competitions, he identified that his pre-competition ritual, and particularly his early morning warm-up at approximately 6.30 am, were the most important factors in establishing the calm and relaxed manner for which he was renowned. With regard to more specific relaxation strategies, Alan stated that 'funnily enough, I knew nothing about any strategies for relaxation really . . . all my awareness about these things came after my best result. I did have my own ways of coping with things that, in a layman's sense, were versions of relaxation, but they were much less than some of the things that I did after, and have subsequently coached'. Later on in the interview, Alan enlarged on this statement by describing several imagery-based dissociation-type strategies that he used as a means of relaxing. He could not recall whether these dissociation strategies that he used had paddling-related images or totally unrelated images, but he was quite definite that they were not about the course or the competition. Some of the strategies that he reported using were very creative, for example imaging what it would feel like to perform a golf swing, or an off-break (in cricket), or some skill really well, even though he was unable to actually perform those skills himself. He added that 'things like that make me feel really good and have a relaxing effect as well'. One final strategy which Alan used to help him relax, both prior to and in between runs, was listening to music.

These responses indicate that all of the athletes interviewed used some form of relaxation technique, although it was also apparent that they had experienced little if any formal training in them. Their use of relaxation seemed to be part of the natural preparation which they had developed, and often appeared to take place in a fairly unstructured manner. The techniques adopted by the athletes varied, as did their reasons for using them; some of them seemed to use relaxation strategies to control cognitive anxiety, while others indicated that they used them to control their physiological arousal. Pre-competition warm-up rituals also seemed to play an important part in anxiety reduction for some of the athletes (see Boutcher, Chapter 9 in this book).

Visualization

Visualization has been shown to be a powerful means of enhancing performance (Feltz and Landers, 1983), particularly among elite performers (see Hemery, 1986). More specifically, the empirical literature suggests that visualization can be used to reduce warm-up decrement (Hardy and Wyatt, 1986), to reduce anxiety (Burton, Chapter 7 in this book; Davidson and Schwartz, 1976; Mace, Chapter 8 in this book) and to increase self-confidence (Bandura, 1977; Burton, Chapter 7 and Mace, Chapter 8 in this book). The series of questions which comprised this section of the interview asked the athletes about their use of visualization in training and during competition. The questions also enquired about the precise form which their visualization took, and their perception of its influence upon self-confidence and anxiety levels.

Steve Backley reported practising visualization 'absolutely all the time—it's almost an obsession'. He visualizes himself performing the perfect throw: 'I sometimes visualize myself throwing 90 metres (the world record is 87.66 metres) (see note 1). I can even visualize what would happen afterwards (it should be noted that this could constitute a subtle form of goal setting). I do it (visualize) without thinking I should do it. I train at it three or four hours a day—it's always on my mind. If I'm lifting in the gym I visualize myself throwing between lifts. I never really snap out of it'. In competition there is usually about 30 minutes between throws: 'I'd sit down for 10 minutes and forget everything, then spend five minutes getting back into it and then another five minutes of really intense visualization. What I tend to do is stand there and watch myself move away, almost step out of myself and then carry on and I can watch myself almost getting smaller and then throwing at the end. I have a tremendous feeling of what the throw is like'. Steve further commented that he uses visualization to enhance his confidence and, through this, is able to handle any stress.

David Hemery also reported using visualization every day. Indeed, it became clear during the interview that, like goal setting, visualization was a major weapon in his psychological armoury. Prior to his major races, David mentally rehearsed every conceivable condition that he could think of in every heat and the final in order to reinforce his attention control plan for the race, and also to enhance his confidence that he could stick to that plan. He also reported rehearsing his training sessions, particularly if they were going to be difficult, and used an imagery-based dissociation strategy to help him control his anxiety if he got distracted from his plan before a race (see previous section). It was clear that David was extremely skilful at imagery, with the ability to create vivid images in a number of different sensory modalities at once.

Mary Nevill said that she used imagery frequently when she had a spare few minutes or was driving the car: 'I'd be thinking about certain skills and things which I wish to improve on the ball all the time'. She practises visualization more frequently as a competition approaches. One skill she often visualizes is the stick stop: 'I imagine the ball coming, moving towards the ball, where I put my feet, where I put the stick, where my head is and so on, going through the whole procedure when it is working well. Another example would be in the open field of play, visualizing myself beating an opponent and making a good pass. A specific example would be picking up the ball and moving down the left wing, pulling it out wide to the side of me and sending it back to a player directly behind me. That can be quite a complex move in hockey because of the obstruction laws'. Mary added that she visualizes skills which she perceives herself to be good at and any new skills that she has not performed in a match before. In the case of a new skill, she might visualize and physically practise it in training for weeks before actually trying it in a game. She also reported using internal as opposed to external visualization every time she images. Mary said that during a match she only visualises the closed skills she performs, such as stick-stops and penalty strokes.

James May reported that he used visualization both prior to competing and in training when he was learning a new move, or when he cut down the number of routines he was doing in each training session during the lead-up to a competition. Like David Hemery, he used visualization as a form of simulation training prior to competitions, and he also reported re-running any rehearsals that went wrong until they went right. Like many gymnasts, James used a multimodal form of visualization with both visual and kinesthetic images: 'The way I go through a routine is by imagining what I will be feeling in terms of my body and what I am actually going to be seeing while I am doing the move. Obviously, when you are doing a move you are not looking at everything. If you do a double back (somersault) your eyes aren't open all the time. So, say you are going around in the first somersault, halfway over you are *feeling* that you are halfway over, and what I do is spot the ground after one somersault. Then I know how much more somersault I have got to do in the second one before I can open out and see the ground. So, if I was rehearsing that, I would be feeling the first part. I would see it halfway through, feel the second half, and then spot the landing.'

Alan Edge used visualization a great deal in slalom canoeing, both to work out how to paddle different sections of the course and to rehearse paddling the whole course prior to performing. After the course is set slalom conoeists get one practice run down it and then two timed runs with the best time counting. Consequently, an ability to accurately predict the best way to paddle the river is clearly an important asset. Alan reported always using internal visual imagery, and occasionally using kinesthetic imagery, when he rehearsed. He also reported that, prior to performance, he always rehearsed the whole course, just once or twice, from starting gate to finish. He never rehearsed individual sections or gates at this stage so as to 'avoid the bogey gate syndrome'. Finally, in spite of the fact that he clearly used visualization techniques a great deal at races, Alan was quite critical of the fact that he did not practise his visualization techniques enough in training: 'In training I was not as thorough and as structured as I would like to have been. The more experience you get, the more you can prescribe what is needed, that is the key to it. If you get it right in practice, you are more likely to get it right under pressure. It's hard to teach (this skill) very quickly. It's a question of going to a lot of different sites and saying "OK, there's that bit of water there, no gate on it. What's that bit of water going to do to your boat? Can you feel what it's going to do to your boat before you even get on the water?" Then when a gate is put on it, you know "well there's a gate just after that bit of water, it's going to whack me sideways and put a wobble on. I must be on the right-hand blade, the gate is there so I need a target there". That kind of preparation definitely went on then (when I was paddling), but we weren't as consistent I don't think because it became something that we used at big competitions. We didn't give ourselves enough time in training. You have got to give yourself enough time with mental rehearsal. It is not compatible with some physiological recovery periods and so there has got to be a time when it is accepted that you will not work at all'.

Sue Challis reported that she used visualization extensively in training and also when she has an injury which prevents physical practice: 'Because I've had an injury I've been going into the gym and standing on the trampoline visualizing my routine. I even put my leotard on one day and did it'. When visualizing she goes through the whole routine: 'And it's funny how things that go wrong when you're actually jumping go wrong in your imagination. I get to a specific move and I always struggle even when I'm mentally rehearsing. In training, I practise (by both visualization and physical practice) the bits that go wrong so that I deliberately drill in the techniques. I might work on a whole routine while just bouncing on the trampoline. I always face the way of the first move and imagine myself doing the first move. Then I do a half twist and imagine myself doing a back somersault, and so on'. Sue does not visualize the perfect routine, only as well as she thinks she can do it. She uses both internal and external visualization but finds internal visualization more powerful. She also reported that it alleviates stress to some extent because 'it reinforces the idea that you have recently practised doing the right things and teaches me to get used to and cope with the feelings of anxiety in the jumps'.

It is clear from the above discussion that all the athletes used visualization extensively as a part of both their routine training and their preparation for competitions. This finding is, of course, reminiscent of Orlick and Partington's (1988) previous finding that successful Olympians reported better imagery skills than less successful Olympians. For the most part, it appeared that the athletes practised visualization every day, so that they were very proficient at it (see Mace, Chapter 8 in this book for a discussion of the amount of practice required to acquire metacognitive skills).

The precise details of application(s) varied between athletes but, in general terms, they used visualization to mentally rehearse new skills; to practise and refine existing skills (cf. Feltz and Landers, 1983); to rehearse successfully coping with the competitive environment (cf. Bandura, 1977; Burton, Chapter 7 and Mace, Chapter 8 in this book); to relax (cf. Davidson and Schwartz,

1976); and to warm up (cf. Ainscoe and Hardy, 1987; Hardy and Wyatt, 1986; Boutcher, Chapter 9 in this book). Several of them also reported using visualization to review their performances. Although there was certainly no universal consensus amongst the athletes regarding the content of their visualization, it was clear that kinesthetic imagery formed a most important component and there was a suggestion that internal visual perspectives were more popular than external visual perspectives (cf. Mahoney and Avener, 1977).

CONCENTRATION AND SIMULATION TRAINING

The competitive environment clearly includes several factors which are not present to the same degree in training, all of which constitute a source of stress. Consequently, recent researchers have proposed that performers should attempt to simulate some of the stresses of competition during training (Jones, Chapter 2 in this book; Jones and Hardy, 1989). The rationale behind this proposal is, first, that it can desensitize the performer to the stress, and secondly, it can enhance the performer's ability to concentrate or control his/her attention. Consequently, it would appear that simulation training which emphasizes concentration training is a valuable part of the preparation process.

Alan Edge reported definitely using simulation training as much as he possibly could; not just simulation of the moves which would probably be encountered on a course but also where on the course they would come. For example, he would simulate a particularly hard move that might come late in a course by paddling very hard for five minutes and then going straight into the move. Conversely, he would practise difficult moves that required him to slow the boat down at the end of very fast stretches of water so that he had to 'take the speed off the boat' when he did not want to. Alan also reported simulating the format of competitions by mentally rehearsing courses from the bank, having only one practice run at courses, and even on occasions doing timed runs without a practice run 'to overload' as he put it. It was clear that mental rehearsal played an important part in these practices. Having said all this, Alan was critical that he did not use either mental rehearsal or simulation training as much as he might have done when he was a performer: 'The majority of the time now we say you never paddle on gates without it, never put yourself in the position of finding out by doing. Another thing we didn't do was to change the course enough in those days either. We tended to do eight reps of a course and, it's ridiculous you know, because if you weren't getting it right on the fourth, fifth or sixth time, then there was something wrong anyway. So now we tend to work in blocks of three and change the course every three runs. You can still do as many as you want but it's a different course after three.' As has already been indicated in the section on goal setting. Alan always prepared a very detailed race plan with clearly defined process-oriented goals about how he wanted to paddle each section of the course. Because this plan included subgoals about what to do if he made any mistakes, it was theoretically possible for him to stick to the plan regardless of anything that happened during a run. It became clear during the interview that Alan attached a great deal of significance to having this sort of plan, and used it to help him focus his attention and feel in control. It also seems highly likely that focusing his attention on this plan helped him to 'block out' any mistakes he made during a run, an attribute which Alan identified as one of his strongest as a performer.

David Hemery reported using a number of different strategies to help him maintain an appropriate attentional focus in stressful situations. These included having an extremely detailed race plan, constant mental rehearsal of this plan in the face of all the different possible situations that could arise, and dissociation strategies for use if the presence of another runner distracted him from his pre-race preparation. David's race plan had as its cornerstone an internal focus of attention upon his body so as to monitor his process-oriented goals for the race: 'It was a feeling; I focused on the feeling that generated the pace. I couldn't tell you what it was . . . a percentage of effort was how it came. And certainly there was a focus on the track. You have got to stay within a few inches of the inside of the lane because every lane is four yards in every bend. You have got to take off a precise distance from each hurdle, so there were adjustments going on there. But far more, it had to do with how much percentage of effort you were going to put into each section of the race . . . going down the back straight at 80 per cent, but then accelerating the legs and running wide because I hadn't learned to hurdle off the other leg sufficiently well, and I had to put in two extra strides so I revved higher around the second bend intentionally . . . and took a foot off every stride'. David's simulation training was similarly detailed. He reported regularly mentally rehearsing 'every lane and condition that I could conceivably think of: drawn in lane one and having people hare off, but maintaining my control; drawn in the outside lane and not being able to see and still having sufficient confidence in my going for world record pace, so if I couldn't see anyone I would still go for it, not letting them determine my aim. It was my aim, and if it was good enough then fine. . . If it wasn't then I had done the best I could'.

Steve Backley said that he did not deliberately practise concentration training despite the fact that he identified this as a potential source of concern after performing a good first throw. However, he did say that he sometimes structured his training in an attempt to put himself under the same sort of pressure as that he experiences on the qualifying day of a major competition: 'I'd have three throws to get over 75 or 76 metres and put the mark out and actually go through the process of trying to simulate the pressure. If I've got a minor club competition, I'll slip in a "qualifying round" the day before to create the physical fatigue the day after and also the mental stress, but it's never to the same degree as in a big competition'. Steve also used visualization to simulate the stress of competition. Specifically, he visualized himself 'in the last round of a major competition losing and with only one throw left. That sort of training through the winter and imagining myself in that position and succeeding made me feel stronger in the (last) summer'.

Mary Nevill stated that she did not practise attention control but perceived herself to have reasonably good concentration anyway. She did state that an attempt to simulate the competitive environment is made during international squad training weekends: 'For example, we would have penalty corner competitions and also very competitive games amongst ourselves. It's linked to the kind of pattern that we would play in an international match. Obviously, a lot of the pressure is missing, but we do try and simulate it as closely as possible'. Mary found this form of practice very useful: 'I think the penalty corner competitions are successful because it's a very close simulation of what happens . . . the actual training games are also a close simulation'.

James May reported that he generally coped quite well with minor distractions during competitions: 'At the World Championships I jumped up on the parallel bars and a balloon burst after I had done the first move. I knew it was a big bang and I registered it, but the thing that immediately sprang to my mind was "undersommy, straddle clip", which was the next move'. With more serious distractions, such as doubts about performing a particular move, James reported using a combination of reviewing previously successful performances of the move to recapture its feeling and the key points, followed by rehearsal of those key points. Although James did not specifically structure training situations to practise coping with such distractions, he reported that he did practise coping with them whenever they occurred naturally during training; 'It's not like a programme, it just happens when people mess about. You try and use it. You try and concentrate when people are trying to put you off. It can be a very useful part of a training programme'. James indicated that he did use simulation training prior to competitions. Features of this simulation training included: declaring to the coach that 'this routine is the one'; performing in front of a judge; and performing a routine without a warm-up 'to handicap himself'. As the interview progressed, it became clear that James identified at least three factors which contribute to his ability to maintain his concentration under high levels of stress: enough repetitions of his routines to be totally certain that nothing could possibly go wrong with them; positive self-talk to remind himself of his ability; a detailed but flexible competition plan which specifies how he wants to warm up, and also includes key points for each piece of apparatus. Like David Hemery, James rehearses his competition plan prior to the event to reassure himself that he knows how to cope with the stress.

Sue Challis said that 'when you are completely prepared and in the right frame of mind you're not aware of anything else'. She does not deliberately practise attention control as such but reported that in 1984, when she won the World Championship, she deliberately thought about and imagined all the distractions that might occur in order to get used to them. Sue regarded herself as being very successful in simulating competitive conditions in training: 'I actually do the routine in training and imagine that I've got one chance. I present to the judges and make it as near to the competition as possible. I often get quite uptight if I don't get it right, but if it's good it really boosts my confidence'.

Simulation training was obviously a high priority for all the athletes. This training was achieved by two means: physical practice in the presence of simulated competition stressors and mental rehearsal of the actual competitive event. An important and consistent feature of this training was the variety of situations that were practised or rehearsed. It seemed clear from the interviews that the athletes intuitively felt that this variety of practice would lead to better transfer to actual competitive environments, an intuition which compares quite favourably with Schmidt's (1975) schema theory for discrete motor actions. Perhaps these performers' skills were so well rehearsed that they were to all intents and purposes discrete.

Perhaps the most fundamental attention control strategies employed by the athletes were their competition plans (cf. Orlick and Partington, 1988; Boutcher, Chapter 9 in this book). These were usually detailed plans which specified how the athletes would achieve the performance goals they had set for themselves. Perhaps inevitably, these competition plans had process-oriented goals as their central feature. Little empirical research has been performed upon process-oriented goals, but several empirical researchers have suggested that such goals should improve attentional focus, at least in complex tasks (cf. Hardy and Fazey, 1990; Hardy and Nelson, 1988; Beggs, Chapter 6 and Boutcher, Chapter 9 in this book).

Another feature of these athletes' preparation which may well have enhanced their concentration was the emphasis which they all placed on overlearning the skills which they were required to reproduce during competition. It seemed clear from the interviews that the athletes were unanimous in their feeling that skills had to be overlearned to the extent that, no matter what situation arose, they would not have the slightest doubt in their ability to produce. While no empirical research has directly addressed the question of how much overlearning is required to achieve such a state, it seems likely to be a very large amount from the anecdotal evidence which was presented. There is, of course, a substantial empirical literature which indicates the value of overlearning in general terms (cf. Eysenck, 1982; Hockey and Hamilton, 1983; Humphreys and Revelle, 1984; Parfitt, Jones and Hardy, Chapter 3 in this book).

SELF-CONFIDENCE

A theme that has repeatedly recurred throughout the earlier sections of this book is the role of self-confidence (or self-efficacy) in performing optimally under stressful conditions (Parfitt, Jones and Hardy, Chapter 3; Hardy, Chapter 4; Beggs, Chapter 6; Burton, Chapter 7; and Mace, Chapter 8). Consequently, this section of the interview comprised questions which examined the athlete's confidence in their ability to perform certain routines, moves, etc., which they had performed successfully many times in training, under the conditions of competitive stress. The athletes were also asked about any strategies which they had for enhancing or maintaining self-confidence.

In the long term, David Hemery identified that his self-confidence was most strongly determined by his long history of achieving performance improvement goals and by the confidence that he gained from beating other competitors. He described his history of goal achievement as being a self-perpetuating spiral, with every step making him feel 'stronger, fitter, faster'. On the confidence he gained from beating other performers, David said: 'I don't know where that comes from. It's a bit of the Dr Jekyll and Mr Hyde, but once the gun went off there was a determination that was matched on the training track, and once I beat them, there was no way that they would beat me again'. In the shorter term, David reported that he gained a lot of confidence from rehearsing his race plan, and also from his warm-up, which was a part of this plan. The warm-up was a chance to 'rev the engine', to check out his stride length and leg speed: 'It wasn't until the warm-up that I could tell whether the legs were springy and resilient . . . I could always run close to my best, but only if that feeling was there'.

Sue Challis said that she builds her confidence by 'training very hard. I like to do what I'm going to do in competition over and over again. Most trampolinists don't do that . . . they do bits and pieces, but I like to have done the whole routine many times so I really know that, whatever happens, I can do it'. Sue stated that she had occasionally doubted her ability to perform moves of a sufficient quality to the extent that she has 'set off to do one and then done another, easier move'. She elaborated on this by saying, 'the routine I am doing is one that has been built up over the years and only small changes happen at once. It is a progression . . . if something goes wrong or if you panic, or if you decide you can't cope, you can go back to what you were doing before. I've got 10 double somersaults in my routine, but I've got lots of alternatives, so if I get to a point where I don't think I can do the next double, I can put in a single that is obviously much easier . . . I can always go back to what I was doing before and play safe'.

Perhaps the most significant influence upon Alan Edge's self-confidence was 'the plan'. An important part of this plan was his early morning warm-up ritual. This was quite a strenuous warm-up which Alan performed at 6.30 a.m. on the morning of a race. He reported that 'the warm-up was important and it became a way of physically giving me confidence that I was on the right countdown'. However, he identified that the people he was with and the music he could listen to were also important influences upon his self-confidence on race days. Finally, Alan reported that playing with 'rodeo' type tricks at the end of a session or paddling an open course 'fast and clean' were both things he liked to do during training sessions to feel good and confident.

Steve Backley reported that practising psychological skills 'over the past few months' had made him psychologically stronger, and had greatly enhanced his self-confidence in particular. 'The difference between being confident and slightly doubting is psychological training'. Visualization clearly played an important part in enhancing and maintaining Steve's self-confidence, as described in earlier sections, plus his ability to dismiss negative thoughts 'and create something positive instead'. Steve Backley cited an instance during the 1988 World Junior Championships when a lack of confidence had negatively affected his performance: 'I was put in the position where I had one last throw. I was leading the whole competition and this guy came through in the fifth round to take the lead. I had one last throw. It was a distance that I was easily capable of, I hadn't thrown it in training because I'm never that aroused in training but I'd thrown it in many competitions. But on this occasion I doubted that I could do it, and didn't'. Steve attributed this to the fact that he lacked the confidence: 'If you're slightly down and doubting yourself then you've lost . . . you've lost that battle with yourself to create a highly skilled performance'.

Mary Nevill said that she gained confidence from being thoroughly prepared, 'by knowing that I've done everything I'm supposed to do . . . I've (physically) practised and mentally rehearsed. I couldn't do any more . . . I am as well prepared as I could possibly be'. She also appeared to be very proficient at getting rid of any negative thoughts and images and replacing them with positive ones; for example, 'if I miss a stick-stop (from a penalty corner) then I can put that behind me until the next one. I might have this negative flash through my mind that I missed the last one, but I would immediately think of an image of positively stopping it'. Mary also reported, however, that she did doubt her ability to perform certain skills 'just occasionally. For example, for a long time in training I've been working on dummies over the ball and also mentally rehearsing it, but I think it's only recently, after about two years of practising, that I've actually begun to try dummies in a match, and it's still infrequently. It takes a long time before you've actually got the confidence to do it'. Mary attributed this to the increased pressure in a match situation, and particularly the time constraints: 'In training I have time to think about doing it (the dummy) . . . in a match situation you are put under so much pressure by the opposition and by the situation that you don't have time to think'.

Self-confidence was clearly a crucial factor in James May's success. Equally clear was that James perceived the primary determinant of his self-confidence to be his previous experiences of success at performing his routines: 'The more times you go through a routine successfully, then you are going to feel more confident about going through the performance on the day. If you've got to cut out things from your routine so that you haven't got the full requirement (of difficult moves), then it must be much better to do that and go through with only that little deduction than to go through with the full routine but lose more by failing on the other things'. Because of this belief, James tried to gear the whole of his competition preparation, from a considerable time before the event until right up to the warm-up, towards ensuring that he experienced success, and had total confidence in his routines. Positive self-talk and the competition plan were important parts of this process.

It seemed clear from these interviews that self-confidence was one of *the* factors which the athletes perceived to be important to their competitive performances. At the end of the discussion, one cannot escape the feeling that in these athletes' minds there was absolutely no room for even the slightest doubts if they were to attain the levels of performance which they sought. With corroborative evidence from more quantitative research, such views would not sit easily alongside pure distraction theories of anxiety and perform- ance (cf. Martens *et al.*, 1990; Wine, 1971, 1980), since these theories predict that small doubts should not have such catastrophic effects upon performance. The interviews also seemed to suggest that the athletes viewed self-confidence as some sort of inoculation against anxiety effects (cf. Hardy, Chapter 4 and Mace, Chapter 8 in this book). However, the athletes also reported that their confidence in their ability to perform moves or skills could be reduced by the stress of competition (see Cale and Jones, 1989; Hardy, Maiden and Sherry, 1986).

The factors which the athletes identified as having a major influence upon their self-confidence generally fitted very neatly into Bandura's (1977) self- efficacy theory. Previous experience of success with its concomitant implica- tions for overlearning was universally accepted as the major determinant of self-confidence, while David Hemery also reported some classic use of struc- tured goal setting (see Beggs, Chapter 6 in this book) to achieve his world record run in 1968. Similarly, visualization was just as extensively used as a means of obtaining vicarious experience of success (see also Burton, Chapter 7 and Mace, Chapter 8 in this book; Orlick and Partington, 1988). Verbal persuasion emerged as another means of enhancing self-confidence in some of the athletes. Interpretation of their physiological arousal was also clearly important to all the athletes. It seems likely that this was one of the reasons why several of the athletes emphasized their warm-up as an opportunity to check that their body was 'feeling good'.

One final factor which seemed to be an important source of self-confidence was the competition plan (cf. Orlick and Partington, 1988). As indicated in the previous section, all the athletes had fairly detailed competition plans, and some had quite explicit alternative plans which they could use to enable them to cope with any conceivable situation that arose. This sort of strategy has, of course, much in common with the philosophy underlying stress inoculation training (Meichenbaum, 1977; Burton, Chapter 7 and Mace, Chapter 8 in this book) and Lazarus and Folkman's (1984) ways of coping.

CONCLUSIONS

The major purpose of this chapter has been to examine the practical applications and implications of many of the theoretical issues addressed in the previous chapters. The interviews which were conducted towards this end provided an opportunity to gain a valuable insight into the experiences of some elite athletes who have competed at the highest level in their sports. Of primary interest were the athletes' experiences of stress, its effects upon performance, and the psychological techniques which the athletes employed to help them cope with the stress of competition.

The responses generally demonstrated that stress was a major factor in sport, at least at the highest level. However, it became increasingly evident during the course of the interviews that stress was not necessarily a negative factor in sport and could be, as Steve Backley stated, 'a huge positive factor'. Another conclusion which could be drawn from the athletes' responses was that they had generally developed very effective psychological skills in the areas of goal setting, relaxation, visualization, attention control and confidence enhancement (cf. Hardy and Nelson, 1988). Visualization, in particular, emerged as a skill which all of them appeared to excel at, and which they perceived to be extremely powerful.

Note: Since this interview was conducted Steve has become the first man to break 90 metres and currently holds the World Record at 90.98 metres.

REFERENCES

Ainscoe, M. W. and Hardy, L. (1987). Cognitive warm up in a cyclical gymnastics skill, *International Journal of Sport Psychology*, **18**, 269–275.

Bandura, A. (1977). Self-efficacy: toward a unifying theory of behavioural change, *Psychological Review*, **84**, 191–215.

Cale, A. and Jones, J. G. (1989). Relationships between expectations of success, multidimensional anxiety and perceptuo-motor performance. Paper presented at the Annual Conference of the North American Society for the Psychology of Sport and Physical Activity, Kent State University, Ohio, USA, September.

Davidson, R. J. and Schwartz G. E. (1976). The psychobiology of relaxation and related states: a multiprocess theory, in D. Mostofsky (ed.). *Behavioural Control and Modification of Physiological Activity*. Englewood Cliffs, New Jersey: Prentice-Hall.

Eysenck, M. W. (1982). *Attention and Arousal: Cognition and Performance*. New York: Springer-Verlag.

Feltz, D. L. and Landers, D. M. (1983). The effects of mental practice on motor skill learning and performance: a meta-analysis, *Journal of Sport Psychology*, **5**, 25-57.

Fenz, W. D. (1975). Coping mechanisms and performance under stress, in D. M. Landers and R. W. Christina (eds). *Psychology of Sport and Motor Behaviour II*. The Pennsylvania State University.

Fisher, S. (1984). *Stress and the Perception of Control*. Hillsdale, New Jersey: Lawrence Erlbaum.

Gould, D. and Krane, V. (in press). The arousal–athletic performance relationship: current status and future directions, in T. Horn (ed.). *Advances in Sport Psychology*. Champaign, Illinois: Human Kinetics.

Hardy, L. and Fazey, J. A. F. (1990). *Mental Training*. Leeds: The National Coaching Foundation.

Hardy, L., Maiden, D. S. and Sherry, K. (1986). Goal setting and performance: the effects of performance anxiety, *Journal of Sports Sciences*, **4**, 233–234.

Hardy, L. and Nelson, D. (1988). Self-regulation training in sport and work, *Ergonomics*, **31**, 1573–1585.

Hardy, L. and Whitehead, R. (1984). Specific modes of anxiety and arousal, *Current Psychological Research and Reviews*, **3**, 14–24.

Hardy, L. and Wyatt, S. (1986). Immediate effects of imagery upon skilful motor performance, in D. G. Russell and D. Marks (eds). *Imagery 2*. New Zealand: Human Performance Associates.

Hemery, D. (1986). *The Pursuit of Sporting Excellence*. London: Collins.

Hockey, G. R. J. and Hamilton, P. (1983). The cognitive patterning of stress states, in G. R. J. Hockey (ed.). *Stress and Fatigue in Human Performance*. Chichester: Wiley.

Humphreys, M. S. and Revelle, E. (1984). Personality, motivation, and performance: a theory of the relationship between individual differences and information processing, *Psychological Review*, **91**, 153–184.

Jones, J. G. (in press). Recent developments and current issues in competitive state anxiety research. *The Psychologist*.

Jones, J. G. and Cale, A. (1989). Relationships between multidimensional competitive state anxiety and cognitive and motor subcomponents of performance, *Journal of Sports Sciences*, **7**, 129–140.

Jones, J. G. and Hardy, L. (1989). Stress and cognitive functioning in sport, *Journal of Sports Sciences*, **7**, 41–63.

Lazarus, R. S. and Folkman, S. (1984). *Stress, Appraisal and Coping*. New York: Springer.

Locke, E. A. and Latham, G. P. (1985). The application of goal setting to sports, *Journal of Sport Psychology*, **7**, 205–222.

Mahoney, M. J. and Avener, M. (1977). Psychology of the elite athlete: an exploratory study, *Cognitive Therapy and Research,* **1**, 135–141.

Martens, R. (1987). Science, knowledge and sport psychology, *The Sport Psychologist,* **1**, 29–55.

Martens, R., Burton, D., Vealey, R. S., Bump, L. A. and Smith, D. E. (1990). Competitive State Anxiety Inventory-2, in R. Martens, R. S. Vealey, and Burton (eds). *Competitive Anxiety in Sport.* Champaign, Illinois: Human Kinetics.

Meichenbaum, D. (1977). *Cognitive Behaviour Modification.* New York: Plenum.

Orlick, T and Partington, J. (1988). Mental links to excellence, *The Sport Psychologist,* **2**, 105–130.

Parfitt, C. G. and Hardy, L. (1987). Further evidence for the differential effects of competitive anxiety upon a number of cognitive and motor sub-systems, *Journal of Sports Sciences,* **5**, 62–63.

Patton, M. Q. (1980). *Qualitative Evaluation Methods.* Beverley Hills, California: Sage.

Scanlan, T. K., Ravizza, K. and Stein, G. L. (1989). An in-depth study of former elite figure skaters. I. Introduction to the project, *Journal of Sport and Exercise Psychology.* **11**, 54–64.

Scanlan, T. K., Stein, G. L. and Ravizza, K. (1989). An in-depth study of former elite figure skaters. II. Sources of enjoyment, *Journal of Sport and Exercise Psychology.* **11**, 65–83.

Schmidt, R. A. (1975). A schema theory of discrete motor skill learning, *Psychological Review.* **82**, 225–260.

Thayer, R. E. (1978). Toward a psychological theory of multidimensional activation (arousal), *Motivation and Emotion,* **2**, 1–34.

Wine, J. D. (1971). Test anxiety and direction of attention, *Psychological Bulletin,* **76**, 92–104.

Wine, J. D. (1980). Cognitive-attentional theory of test anxiety, in I. G. Sarason (ed.). *Test Anxiety: Theory, Research and Applications.* Hillsdale, New Jersey: Lawrence Erlbaum.

3

STRESS IN SPORT:
FUTURE RESEARCH DIRECTIONS

Chapter 11

Future directions for research into stress in sport

Lew Hardy and J. Graham Jones

University of Wales, Bangor and Loughborough University

The primary objective of this book has been to explore the area of stress in sport from three different perspectives. The first section of the book discussed the experimental literature which has addressed the question of how stress affects performance. The majority of the second section examined the experimental literature on stress control interventions and strategies. Finally, Chapter 10 employed more qualitative research methods to investigate the personal strategies and skills which have been employed by elite sports performers to control the effects of stress upon their sports performance.

This chapter attempts to draw together some of the common threads and major proposals of the preceding chapters. It comprises five sections which address the central issues that have been raised in the text. Each section ends with a series of consensus statements regarding the current state of knowledge in that particular area, and a list of research questions which are considered worthy of further investigation. Unfortunately, the distinction between that which is consensus and that which is a question is not always as clear as one might like, so that personal interpretations may have sometimes influenced which side of 'the line' an issue has been placed. However, it is hoped that these 'grey areas' have been clearly indicated in the text.

BASIC CONCEPTS IN STRESS RESEARCH

Perhaps the most obvious starting point for any discussion of consensus is the fact that great care is needed regarding even the definitions of the basic concepts involved in stress research. For example, stress, arousal, activation and anxiety are clearly not synonymous. Stress can be a positive or a negative experience (Kerr, Chapter 5) and can have a positive, a negative, or no observable effect upon performance (see particularly Parfitt, Jones and Hardy,

---

Stress and Performance in Sport. Edited by J. Graham Jones and Lew Hardy.

Chapter 3). Arousal and activation are not easily defined, and consensus regarding their definitions may not yet exist. Perhaps the nearest that one can get to a consensus is Pribram and McGuiness' (1975) definition of a multidimensional system in which activation is a tonic state of readiness to respond (possibly reflecting organized response programming) and arousal is a phasic response to input (see Jones, Chapter 2). Consensus regarding anxiety is a little easier to achieve. Anxiety is generally regarded as a multidimensional construct which can be considered from both state and trait perspectives, each of which comprises at least two components: cognitive anxiety and somatic anxiety (see Jones, Chapter 2; Parfitt, Hardy and Jones, Chapter 3; Burton, Chapter 7; Martens et al., 1990; Smith, Smoll and Schutz in press).

The precise role of self-confidence in stress and anxiety research is not yet entirely clear. Nevertheless, there was a general consensus among all the sport psychologists and performers who contributed to this book that self-confidence was a very important variable in sports performance (cf. Bandura, 1977, 1986). This apparently obvious position contrasts quite markedly with the view held by certain rather more clinically oriented psychologists that self-confidence (or, more precisely, self-efficacy) is simply an epiphenomenon reflecting a lack of anxiety (e.g. Borkovec, 1978; Eysenck, 1982). Furthermore, although it might be somewhat premature to describe it as a consensus, several authors (Parfitt, Jones and Hardy, Chapter 3; Hardy, Chapter 4; Kerr, Chapter 5; Mace, Chapter 8) seemed to suggest that self-confidence might be orthogonal to cognitive anxiety, as opposed to being at the opposite end of the same continuum (see also Hardy and Whitehead, 1984; Thayer, 1978). Such a proposal, if confirmed, could have important consequences for understanding how it is that anxiety can have both debilitative and facilitative effects upon performance (see later section on performance effects, and also Beggs, Chapter 6).

In many of the studies which have been reported throughout this book, competitive state anxiety has been measured using Martens et al.'s (1990) Competitive State Anxiety Inventory-2 (CSAI-2), and there seems little doubt that the vast majority of researchers would regard this as entirely appropriate. However, this approach to the measurement of competitive anxiety is not universally favoured. For example, Kerr (Chapter 5) has based much of his research on the telic state measure of metamotivational states. Similarly, Hardy's (Chapter 4) work suggests the possibility that it is the negative attribution of perceived physiological arousal by cognitively anxious performers that leads to decrements in performance, rather than simply their perception of it. If proven, such a position would imply that the interpretation of somatic symptoms is much more important than somatic anxiety per se (see also Schachter, 1964; Bandura, 1977). Furthermore, advances in psychophysiological measurement may also provide a means of evaluating anxiety levels actually during performance, rather than simply prior to it (see Boutcher,

Chapter 9). Finally, it may prove necessary to radically rethink the measurement of state and trait anxiety if suggestions regarding the importance of considering the frequency, intensity and direction of cognitive intrusions are empirically substantiated (Jones, in press; Parfitt, Jones and Hardy, Chapter 3; Burton, Chapter 7). Mace's (Chapter 8) 'automatic thoughts' may also have some bearing upon this issue.

Using the CSAI-2, several researchers have demonstrated that cognitive and somatic anxiety follow different time courses during the period leading up to an important competition (see Parfitt, Jones and Hardy, Chapter 3; Burton, Chapter 7). Cognitive anxiety is generally elevated and fairly stable for some days prior to the event, while somatic anxiety tends to peak late and fast upon arrival at the site of the competition. However, the majority of research in this area has employed male subjects and recent studies by Jones and Cale (1989) and Jones, Swain and Cale (in press) suggest that this finding may not generalize to female populations.

Most of the authors who contributed to the book considered the possible causes of anxiety, although some did this more explicitly than others (see particularly Parfitt, Jones and Hardy, Chapter 3; Kerr, Chapter 5; Beggs, Chapter 6; Jones and Hardy, Chapter 10). Furthermore, there did seem to be some consensus among them in identifying the importance of the event, the precise nature of the performer's goal and the performer's perceived readiness to perform as important determinants of anxiety. Several authors also suggested that anxiety could occur because of a mismatch between preferred physiological states and actual physiological states, although only Kerr (Chapter 5) offered direct experimental support for this.

Consensus statements

1. Researchers must take great care to explain their use of basic terminology such as stress, arousal, activation and anxiety.
2. Stress can be perceived to be either positive or negative.
3. Self-confidence (self-efficacy) is an important variable in competitive stress research which seems to be at least partially independent of cognitive anxiety.
4. The CSAI-2 is a valid and reliable instrument for the assessment of the intensity of competitive state anxiety.
5. Using the CSAI-2, the cognitive and somatic components of anxiety dissociate under a time-to-event paradigm for male subjects. However, they may not dissociate in the same way for female subjects.
6. The antecedents of anxiety include the importance of the event, the precise nature of the performers' goals, their perceived readiness to perform, and the degree of mismatch between their actual and their preferred physiological state.

Research questions

1. How important are the frequency and direction of cognitive intrusions in the competitive state anxiety response?
2. How reliably does telic state predict positive and negative perceptions of stress? Are these perceptions influenced by other metacognitive variables?
3. How does self-confidence (self-efficacy) interact with cognitive anxiety, physiological arousal and other metacognitive variables (such as the perception of control) to influence performance?
4. Can psychophysiological techniques be devised to predict different metacognitive states during performance?
5. How stable are the gender differences which have been reported in the temporal patterning of the anxiety components? What factors predict these differences?
6. Are the antecedents of the different anxiety components different for different sports? How stable are the gender differences which have been reported in these antecedents? What causes these differences?

THE EFFECTS OF STRESS UPON PERFORMANCE

There was a consensus among almost all the authors who contributed to this book that stress can have either a positive or a negative effect upon performance. The principal aim of this section is to draw together what is known about the precise conditions under which these performance effects occur and how they are caused.

Modelling the effects of stress upon performance

Two models of performance anxiety which have been presented in this book are Hardy and Fazey's (1987) catastrophe model (see Hardy, Chapter 4) and Apter's (1982) reversal theory model (see Kerr, Chapter 5). Both these models represent radically different ways of looking at the problem of performance anxiety—Apter's model perhaps more so than Hardy and Fazey's. Nevertheless, both appear to possess some potential, and interestingly share some common characteristics. For example, both models are based on bistable systems and attempt to describe the interaction between metacognitive and physiological states in terms of affect and performance, respectively. The intriguing possibility exists that the models have other common factors; for example, could the catastrophe model's upper and lower performance surfaces reflect paratelic and telic states in the stressed performer? Accurately modelling the stress–performance relationship is an important precursor to determining the precise mechanisms *via* which (competitive) performance anxiety exerts its influence upon performance. However, one must seriously doubt whether this is possible without also considering at least some other metacognitive variables such as self-confidence and the perception of control. To get a clearer view of the seriousness of this criticism, the reader is invited to consider for a moment how much more complex the anxiety–performance relationship becomes when one includes interactions between cognitive anxiety and physiological arousal, as in Hardy and Fazey's catastrophe model, rather than simply considering their main effects, as in Martens *et al.*'s (1990) multidimensional model (see also Burton, 1988; Gould *et al.*, 1987). The inclusion of further variables, such as self-confidence and the perception of control, in such a catastrophe model leads one into five-dimensional catastrophes at the very least. These are not easy to imagine, let alone draw!

Explaining the effects of anxiety upon performance

There seemed to be consensus among most authors that inverted-U type explanations of stress effects in terms of some sort of generalized arousal construct were not really very appropriate. This is not, of course, to say that physiological arousal does not have any effect upon performance, but only that stress and anxiety effects cannot be satisfactorily explained in terms of any such arousal construct alone (see particularly Jones, Chapter 2). Indeed, both Kerr (Chapter 5) and Hardy (Chapter 4) argued that performers' perceptions and interpretations of their physiological states were principal determinants of stress effects upon performance.

Relatively strong evidence was also put forward for the notion of different anxiety components exerting differential effects upon different subcomponents of performance (see particularly Parfitt, Jones and Hardy, Chapter 3). However, it is clear that much more still needs to be known about the precise patterning of any such effects. One tantalizing possibility is that the subcomponents of performance which are affected by competitive stress are precisely those which are perceived to be important. This notion is suggested by several different lines of reasoning. First, there is Hardy's (Chapter 4) notion of anxious performers trying 'too hard'. Coupled with Burton's (Chapter 7) and Mace's (Chapter 8) description of the inner dialogue of anxious performers, together with Boutcher's (Chapter 9) arguments regarding the inefficiency of conscious control, this suggests that anxious performers may experience a breakdown in precisely those aspects of performance which they perceive to be important.

Secondly, Hardy (Chapter 4), Beggs (Chapter 6) and others before them (cf. Kahneman, 1973; Revelle and Michaels, 1976; Eysenck, 1982) have pointed out that moderate levels of cognitive anxiety can lead to increased on-task effort, provided that the task (goal) is perceived to be achievable. Thus, competitive anxiety may lead to enhanced performance in subcomponents which the performer perceives to be important but not too difficult (see

Parfitt, Jones and Hardy, Chapter 3; Beggs, Chapter 6). However, direct empirical support for these predictions is still awaited.

Other possible mechanisms also exist to explain the differential effects of competitive stress upon performance. The most classical of these is the distraction hypothesis, which states that anxious subjects use up attentional resources by focusing upon task-irrelevant cues such as their own negative cognitions (see Jones, Chapter 2; Parfitt, Hardy and Jones, Chapter 3; Hardy, Chapter 4; Burton, Chapter 7; Mace, Chapter 8; Boutcher, Chapter 9). Alternatively, the physiological arousal which is associated with the anxiety response could also affect different aspects of performance *via* selectivity of attention (Easterbrook, 1959; Boutcher, Chapter 9), changes in the activation set (Parfitt, Jones and Hardy, Chapter 3; Boutcher, Chapter 9) or discrepancies between the preferred and the actual levels of perceived physiological arousal (Kerr, Chapter 5). From these arguments, it is clear that there is a consensus that competitive anxiety may affect performance *via* at least three different mechanisms: motivation, attention and physiological arousal. Interestingly, these three mechanisms coincide precisely with the three factors of competitive trait anxiety which have recently been identified by Smith, Smoll and Schutz (in press).

Consensus statements

1. Stress effects upon performance can be either positive or negative.
2. Inverted-U type explanations of the stress–performance relationship in terms of a generalized arousal response are seriously flawed.
3. Competitive stress can affect performance *via* at least three different mechanisms: motivation, attention and physiological arousal. All three of these paths can produce either positive or negative effects, depending upon certain (unknown?) performer-by-situation characteristics.

Research questions

1. Current models of the stress–performance relationship include cognitive anxiety and performers' perceptions of their physiological arousal. However, accurate modelling may only be possible by including additional meta-cognitive variables such as self-confidence and the perception of control. Knowledge about how such variables interact with cognitive anxiety and (the perception of) physiological arousal is urgently required.
2. There are several possible explanations of the stress–performance relationship which would fit Hardy and Fazey's catastrophe model. However, direct empirical tests of these explanations have not yet been performed.
3. What are the links between Hardy and Fazey's catastrophe model and Apter's reversal theory model?

4. How do other metamotivational pairs such as sympathy–mastery interact with perceived physiological arousal in the reversal theory model of stress and performance?
5. What are the major subcomponents of different sports skills?
6. Different anxiety components seem to have differential effects upon different subcomponents of performance, but we need to know more about the precise patterns of these effects for different sports skills.
7. It seems to be possible to account for the present results on the differential effects of anxiety upon different subcomponents of performance in terms of two arousal systems (Parfitt, Jones and Hardy, Chapter 3). However, researchers in other fields (e.g. Hockey and Hamilton, 1983; Sanders, 1983) argue that more than two are necessary. How many arousal systems are necessary, and how are they related to each other?

STRESS CONTROL IN SPORT

One implicit or explicit thread of optimism which runs throughout this book is that cognitive behavioural interventions do work: that is to say, we can do something about stress in sport. All of the authors in the stress control section of the book presented empirical evidence in support of the use of cognitive behavioural interventions, while the performers who were interviewed spoke of many similar skills or strategies which they had developed to help them control and use stress. What is not quite so clear yet is exactly how all these different strategies work. Not surprisingly, researchers have adopted different theoretical positions from which to present their different cognitive behavioural strategies. For example, Beggs (Chapter 6) and Mace (Chapter 8) both suggested that changes in self-confidence (self-efficacy) may mediate the effects of cognitive behavioural interventions upon performance. However, Burton (Chapter 7) adopted an anxiety reduction model based upon the matching hypothesis for his chapter on stress management, while Boutcher (Chapter 9) identified that there were at least three different possible explanations of the effectiveness of the pre-performance routines. Finally, Beggs (Chapter 6) and others (for example Burton, 1989a) have suggested that the setting of appropriate goals might help performers to experience less stress in the first place, although Beggs also indicated that goal-setting theories about sport are in fairly short supply.

What is really required, of course, is a composite theory that indicates precisely how stress interacts with self-concept and other individual difference variables to influence both affective states and performance, thereby predicting which metacognitive skills are required to maximize the beneficial effects. We are clearly still some distance away from such a model. Nevertheless, it is hoped that this book has advanced us at least a small way towards such a position. For example, several authors (Hardy, Chapter 4; Kerr, Chapter 5; Burton, Chapter 7; Mace, Chapter 8) suggested that reductions in physiological arousal were not the only possible, and might not always be the most effective, intervention with highly anxious performers. Rather, more cognitively based restructuring strategies should enable performers to perceive situations from a more positive perspective (cf. Lazarus and Folkman, 1984). It is perhaps worth noting at this stage that the stress management strategy reported by Burton (Chapter 7), which consisted of physiological arousal reduction followed by cognitive restructuring and then reactivation, is exactly that which is predicted by Hardy's (Chapter 4) catastrophe model.

Several authors have also suggested that different components of anxiety are likely to affect different aspects of performance differently, and that these effects may be mediated by motivational, attentional and physiological arousal processes (see Chapters 2–5 and the previous section of this chapter). Furthermore, these different mediational processes do have some implications for cognitive behavioural intervention. For example, Parfitt, Jones and Hardy (Chapter 3), Beggs (Chapter 6), Burton (Chapter 7) and Mace (Chapter 8) have all reported evidence which suggests that performers' cognitive appraisals of the situation are important determinants of motivational state and attentional strategies; Boutcher (Chapter 9) has suggested that pre-performance routines should contain attention control strategies, physiological arousal-controlling strategies and general task cues to discourage the performer from lapsing into conscious processing of information. This latter suggestion is particularly interesting for two reasons. At a theoretical level, it offers one possible explanation of how performance catastrophes might occur; at a practical level, it may have important implications for when to use imagery and goal-setting strategies, which can perhaps be thought of as encouraging more and less automatic control, respectively (cf. Burton, Chapter 7).

Several of the researchers who have written chapters in this book indicated that in order to evaluate the effectiveness of cognitive behavioural interventions there was an urgent need to develop valid, reliable and objective measures of both metacognitive skills and performance (see particularly Beggs, Chapter 6; Burton, Chapter 7; Mace, Chapter 8; Boutcher, Chapter 9). While the assessment of performance is not particularly problematic in some sports, it is clearly very difficult in others. However, the theoretically based match analysis procedures which have been proposed by Parfitt, Jones and Hardy (Chapter 3) may at least offer a starting point.

The objective evaluation of metacognitive skills presents a rather more serious problem, since most sports performers acquire metacognitive skills in very specific situational contexts. However, at least two self-report questionnaires exist which have been used for the assessment of metacognitive skills. The first is Mahoney, Gabriel and Perkins' (1987) Psychological Skills Inventory for Sports (PSIS). This yields scores on six subscales: anxiety control, concentration, confidence, mental preparation, motivation, and team orientation. However, as the authors emphasized, the psychometric properties of this questionnaire are at present unknown. Furthermore, several problems seem to exist with the method of item selection, the samples used to validate the questionnaire, and the face validity of certain factors. Consequently, its wholesale use for the evaluation of metacognitive skills can hardly be recommended.

Because of these psychometric problems with the PSIS, Nelson and Hardy (1990) developed a new metacognitive skills questionnaire, called the Sport-Related Psychological Skills Questionnaire (SPSQ), which has more desirable psychometric properties. This questionnaire gives scores on seven subscales which were identified by factor analysis: imaginal skills, mental preparation, self-efficacy, cognitive anxiety, concentration skill, relaxation skill, and motivation skill. Each subscale has eight items, and a Cronbach's alpha of 0.78 or greater.

Perhaps at some stage more objective tests of metacognitive skills will be devised along the lines suggested by Boutcher (Chapter 9). Such tests might utilize the analysis of electroencephalograms, cardiac activity, signal detections, overt behaviour and projective techniques. However, it is perhaps worth noting that the construction of objective tests to measure metacognitive skills has proved elusive during the history of psychology, and is unlikely to be straightforward.

Consensus statements

1. Appropriate cognitive behavioural interventions and strategies do seem to have a beneficial effect upon both anxiety and performance. In particular, the following metacognitive skills appear to be beneficial to athletic performance: goal setting, self-talk, imagery, relaxation, activation, attention control, restructuring, and positive self-evaluation skills.
2. Straightforward reductions in physiological arousal may not be the most effective intervention with highly anxious performers.
3. Pre-performance routines may provide an important means of controlling the effects of anxiety upon performance.

Research questions

1. While cognitive behavioural interventions do appear to exert some influence upon performance under stressful conditions, the precise means by which they exert this influence need to be better understood.
2. What is the most appropriate content for pre-performance routines for different sports (and different performers)?

3. How well does the matching hypothesis stand up to direct empirical scrutiny in the context of sport?
4. What are the motivational and stress management effects of goal setting in sport?
5. How can goal setting best be used with complex tasks?
6. Can a metric be developed for measuring goal-setting skill?
7. Can objective measures of attention control be developed?
8. What are the most effective ways of enhancing attention control during performance?
9. Are metacognitive skills best taught in some packaged form or as a set of separate skills from which performers construct their own personal stress management strategies?
10. What are the most effective methods of teaching metacognitive skills? In particular, how well do distance-learning packages of mental training work?

INDIVIDUAL DIFFERENCES

Although individual differences were not explicitly addressed by all of the contributors, there did seem to be a general consensus that individual differences were important in both perceptions of, and responses to, stress in sport. While most of the chapters in the first section of the book focused upon that which is common in performers' experiences of stress, Kerr (Chapter 5) did consider individual differences explicitly. He proposed that individual differences in telic state determine whether performers perceive high levels of stress to be challenging or threatening. Such differences may, therefore, be an important variable in the personalization of goals to optimize performance, referred to by Beggs (Chapter 6). Beggs also considered the roles of self-confidence (self-efficacy) and self-esteem in goal setting, finding that both were important positive influences upon goal difficulty, goal commitment and performance.

As Beggs pointed out, goals are something of a 'double-edged sword' in sport, since they can be thought of as both a source of stress and a means of reducing it (cf. Burton, 1989a). Consequently, self-concept variables such as self-confidence and self-esteem may provide a means of explaining the facilitative and debilitative effects which competitive anxiety can have upon performance (see Parfitt, Jones and Hardy, Chapter 3; Hardy, Chapter 4; Mace, Chapter 8). Of course, the study of such interactions may require fairly complex paradigms and analytical methods (see next section), so that it is perhaps not surprising that these speculations await empirical investigation.

The individualization of mental training programmes to meet performers' needs was clearly an 'ever present' in the second section of the book. Burton

(Chapter 7) and Mace (Chapter 8) discussed the need to consider performers' dominant modes of anxiety response in stress management training, while Burton (Chapter 7), Mace (Chapter 8) and Boutcher (Chapter 9) all suggested that mental training should be fine-tuned to the needs of both the performer and the sport (for example teaching respiration control as a relaxation strategy for divers). However, these authors also acknowledged that, as always, empirical research lagged some way behind clinical and educational practice.

To date, most individual difference research is of a fairly crude nature, examining gender differences (see, for example, Chapter 3) or differences due to trait anxiety (see, for example, Martens, 1977; Smith, Smoll and Schutz, in press). While such differences may be very important at a practical level, they seem unlikely to unravel all the mysteries of what is actually happening when athletes perform under stressful conditions. What is really required is research which examines the details of the interactions which must take place between self-concept, anxiety and other personality variables (for example need for achievement) in such situations.

Consensus statements

1. Individual differences do exist in both perceptions of, and responses to, high levels of stress in sport.
2. There are gender differences in competitive state anxiety, although the precise reason for these are not fully understood.
3. Self-efficacy and self-esteem appear to be important determinants of the relationship between goal difficulty and performance.
4. At a clinical and educational level, it is recognized that stress management programmes should take account of both individual and situational differences.

Research questions

1. What are the major determinants of whether competitive state anxiety has a facilitative or a debilitative effect?
2. Goal difficulty has been identified as an important antecedent of anxiety, and a potential determinant of performance. However, some sort of goal challenge metric is needed to further examine this influence.
3. To what extent does telic state determine the optimal level of goal difficulty?
4. Can theories of stress and performance be developed which include such individual difference variables as self-efficacy and the perception of control, as well as anxiety?

METHODOLOGICAL ISSUES

The importance of situational relevance and ecological validity runs as a theme throughout this book. Indeed, as stated by Beggs in Chapter 6, they are distinguishing features of stress research in sport. However, this does not mean that researchers are automatically committed to the *post hoc* analysis of associations between variables. Many of the empirical findings which have been discussed in the preceding chapters were obtained from quasi-experimental, or even true experimental, paradigms in which at least some control was maintained over the independent variables.

The results which were reported from these studies show some similarities and also some important differences between competitive sports stress and other stressors which have been considered elsewhere (see Eysenck, 1982; Hockey and Hamilton, 1983; Jones, Chapter 2; Parfitt, Jones and Hardy, Chapter 3; Beggs, Chapter 6). For example, although many of the findings which are discussed in Parfitt, Jones and Hardy (Chapter 3) can be accounted for by the models of stress and cognitive performance which have been presented by Eysenck (1982), there is clearly a much greater emphasis placed upon motor memory in the former than there is in the latter. Similarly, while it seems likely that many of the goal-setting findings from organizational psychology will transfer to sport psychology (Barnett and Stanicek, 1979; Burton, 1989b; Hall and Byrne, 1988; Locke and Latham, 1985), there also seem to be some distinctive features of sport which make sports settings very different from organizational settings (cf. Beggs, Chapter 6; Eysenck, 1982).

One of the most striking features of a book like the present one is that it draws attention to different ways of addressing the same problem. Indeed, careful scrutiny of some of the chapters (for example Parfitt, Jones and Hardy, Chapter 3; Burton, Chapter 7) reveals that the use of different paradigms can lead to quite fundamentally different conclusions about the influence of cognitive and somatic anxiety upon motor performance. Rather than viewing such findings as contradictory and attempting to 'brush them under the carpet', it is important that we actively seek out radically new and different ways of examining stress in sport (cf. Martens, 1987). If higher-order interactions between different metacognitive variables produce novel and complex models of performance, then let us produce equally novel paradigms and statistical procedures to handle them. For example, a number of new statistical procedures have been derived during the last decade to handle non-linear multidimensional models (see particularly Cobb, 1981; Guastello, 1987; Oliva *et al.*, 1987).

In the area of interventions and stress management training, all of the authors in the second section of the book identified a need to develop valid and reliable measures of both metacognitive skills and sports performance. While the measurement of sports performance is relatively trivial in some sports, it is clearly a highly complex problem in others. These authors were also unanimous in their call for the need to control for placebo effects in intervention studies. Finally, Mace (Chapter 8) discussed in detail many of the problems which beset stress management research, and proposed the use of multiple baseline single-subject designs as a means of controlling for individual differences in such studies. While empirical research into individual differences in sport is in its infancy, such a suggestion has much to commend it. However, it is to be hoped that one day we will know enough about the complex interactions which determine sports performance to be able to control for individual differences in a slightly more refined way.

Consensus statements

1. Despite many areas of common ground between research on stress in sport and research on other types of stress, there remain several important differences between them.
2. Different paradigms and analyses in stress–performance research yield paradoxical results. However, such findings are not necessarily contradictory and should be explored rather than ignored.
3. The use of multiple baseline single-subject designs is recommended for exploratory research in the areas of intervention and stress management.
4. All intervention-type studies should include some means of controlling for placebo effects.

Research questions

1. Designs and analyses capable of examining the complex interactions which make up sports performance are urgently required.
2. Valid and reliable measures of performance are required in many sports.
3. Length of training has been identified as an important variable in intervention research. However, there have been few (if any) controlled studies of how long is required for different types of subject to learn different interventions.
4. Most intervention studies which have employed group designs have used novice subjects. There is a need to understand more about the effects of stress management interventions upon experienced performers.

EPILOGUE

This chapter has attempted to draw together the common elements which have been presented by the different contributors to this book and identify priority areas for future research. There was almost universal agreement among the contributors that stress could be perceived to be either a positive or a negative phenomenon. Furthermore, positive perceptions should be experienced as excitement, while negative perceptions should be experienced as anxiety. Such anxiety responses have been shown to comprise at least two different components: cognitive anxiety and somatic anxiety.

It has been proposed that these different components of anxiety affect performance in different ways *via* motivational, attentional and physiological mechanisms. These effects are not always negative, and it has been suggested that self-confidence may be an important determinant of whether anxiety effects are positive or negative. Other determinants appear to include the cognitive load of the task; or put another way, the extent of overlearning on the task. None of these hypotheses has as yet been the subject of direct empirical testing.

At the level of interventions, there was general consensus that, because of the complexity of the variables involved, multimodal interventions were much more likely to control anxiety and enhance self-confidence than were unimodal approaches. Several contributors to the book also suggested that the precise nature of the performer's goals may have important consequences for both motivation and stress management. Consequently, teaching performers appropriate goal setting and attributional strategies may prove to be a highly productive and as yet little explored intervention.

To conclude, current models of stress and performance in sport tend to include at most two predictor variables and even then do not usually examine the interactions which must take place between these variables. What is required is a composite theory which indicates precisely how stress interacts with self-concept and other individual difference variables to influence both affective states and performance. The theory should then predict which metacognitive skills are required to maximize performance. Having constructed such a theory in the morning, the researcher concerned might like to celebrate by running a three-minute mile in the afternoon!

REFERENCES

Apter, M. J. (1982). *The Experience of Motivation: The Theory of Psychological Reversals*. London: Academic Press.

Bandura, A. (1977). Self-efficacy: toward a unifying theory of behavioural change, *Psychological Review*, **84**, 191–215.

Bandura, A. (1986). *Social Foundations of Thought and Actions: A Social Cognitive Theory*. Englewood Cliffs, NJ: Prentice-Hall.

Barnett, M. L. and Stanicek, J. A. (1979). Effects of goal-setting on achievement in archery, *Research Quarterly*, **50**, 328–332.

Borkovec, T. D. (1978). Self-efficacy: cause or reflection of behavioural change, in S. Rachman (ed.). *Advances in Behavioural Research and Therapy*, Vol. 1. Oxford: Pergamon.

Burton, D. (1988). Do anxious swimmers swim slower? Re-examining the elusive anxiety performance relationship, *Journal of Sport Psychology*, **10**, 45–61.

Burton, D. (1989a). Winning isn't everything: examining the impact of performance goals on collegiate swimmers' cognitions and performance, *Journal of Sport Psychology*, **3**, 105–132.

Burton, D. (1989b). The impact of goal specificity and task complexity on basketball skill development, *The Sport Psychologist*, **3**, 34–47.

Cobb, L. (1981). Parameter estimation for the cusp catastrophe model, *Behavioural Science*, **26**, 75–78.

Easterbrook, J. A. (1959). The effect of emotion on cue utilization and the organization of behaviour, *Psychological Review*, **66**, 183–201.

Eysenck, M. W. (1982). *Attention and Arousal: Cognition and Performance*. Berlin: Springer-Verlag.

Gould, D., Petlichkoff, L., Simons, J. and Vevera, M. (1987). Relationship between Competitive State Anxiety Inventory-2 subscale scores and pistol shooting performance, *Journal of Sport Psychology*, **9**, 33–42.

Guastello, S. J. (1987). A butterfly catastrophe model of motivation in organizations: academic performance, *Journal of Applied Psychology*, **72**, 161–182.

Hall, H. K. and Byrne, A. T. J. (1988). Goal setting in sport: clarifying recent anomalies, *Journal of Sport and Exercise Psychology*, **10**, 184–198.

Hardy, L. and Fazey, J. (1987). The inverted-U hypothesis: a catastrophe for sport psychology? Paper presented at the Annual Conference of the North American Society for the Psychology of Sport and Physical Activity, Vancouver, June.

Hardy, L. and Whitehead, R. (1984). Specific modes of anxiety and arousal, *Current Psychological Research and Reviews*, **3**, 14–24.

Hockey, G. R. J. and Hamilton P. (1983). The cognitive patterning of stress states, in G. R. J. Hockey (ed.). *Stress and Fatigue in Human Performance*. Chichester: Wiley.

Jones, J.G. (in press). Recent developments and current issues in competitive state anxiety research. *The Psychologist*.

Jones, J. G. and Cale, A. (1989). Precompetition temporal patterning of anxiety and self-confidence in males and females, *Journal of Sport Behaviour*, **12**, 183–195.

Jones, J. G., Swain, A. and Cale, A. (in press). Gender differences in precompetition temporal patterning and antecedents of anxiety and self-confidence. *Journal of Sport and Exercise Psychology*.

Kahneman, D. (1973). *Attention and Effort*. Englewood Cliffs, NJ: Prentice-Hall.

Lazarus, R. S. and Folkman, S. (1984). *Stress, Appraisal and Coping*. New York: Raven.

Locke, E. A. and Latham, G. P. (1985). The application of goal setting to sports, *Journal of Sport Psychology*, **7**, 205–222.

Mahoney, M. J., Gabriel, T. J. and Perkins, T. S. (1987). Psychological skills and exceptional athletic performance, *The Sport Psychologist*, **1**, 181–199.

Martens, R. (1977). *Sport Competition Anxiety Test (SCAT)*. Champaign, Illinois: Human Kinetics.

Martens, R. (1987). Science, knowledge, and sport psychology, *The Sport Psychologist*, **1**, 29–55.

Martens, R., Burton, D., Vealey, R. S., Bump, L. A. and Smith, D. E. (1990). The Competitive State Anxiety Inventory-2, in R. Martens, R. Vealey and D. Burton (eds.). *Competitive Anxiety in Sport*. Champaign, Illinois: Human Kinetics.

Nelson, D. and Hardy, L. (1990). The development of an empirically validated tool for measuring psychological skill in sport. *Journal of Sports Sciences*, **8**, 71.

Oliva, T. A., Descarbo, W. S., Day, D. L. and Jedidi, K. (1987). Gemcat: a general multivariate methodology for estimating catastrophe models, *Behavioural Science*, **32**, 121–137.

Pribram, K. H. and McGuinness, D. (1975). Arousal, activation and effort in the control of attention, *Psychological Review*, **82**, 116–149.

Revelle, W. and Michaels, E. J. (1976). The theory of achievement motivation revisited: the implication of inertial tendencies, *Psychological Review*, **83**, 394–404.

Sanders, A. F. (1983). Towards a model of stress and human performance, *Acta Psychologica*, **53**, 64–97.

Schachter S. (1964). The interaction of cognitive and physiological determinants of emotional state. In L. Berkowitz (ed.), *Advances in Experimental and Social Psychology*. New York: Academic Press.

Smith, R. E., Smoll, F. L. and Schutz, R. W. (in press). Measurement and correlates of sport-specific cognitive and somatic trait anxiety: The Sport Anxiety Scale, *Anxiety Research*.

Swain, A. B. J., Jones, J. G. and Cale, A. (1990). Temporal patterning and antecedents of competitive state anxiety in males and females. *Journal of Sports Sciences*, **8**, 84–85.

Thayer, R. E. (1978). Toward a psychological theory of multidimensional activation (arousal), *Motivation and Emotion*, **2**, 1–34.

Index